Evaluation and Management of Blepharoptosis

Adam J. Cohen • David A. Weinberg
Editors

Evaluation and Management of Blepharoptosis

"Foreword by George Brian Bartley, MD"

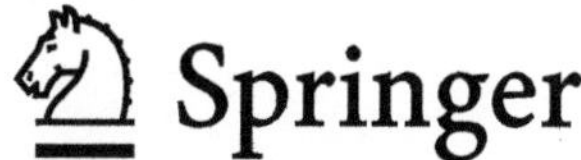

Editors
Adam J. Cohen
Private Practice
The Art of Eyes
Skokie, IL
USA
acohen@theartofeyes.com

David A. Weinberg
Concord Eye Care
Concord, NH
and
Department of Surgery (Ophthalmology)
Dartmouth Medical School
Hanover, NH
USA
daweinberg@hotmail.com

ISBN 978-0-387-92854-8 ISBN 978-0-387-92855-5 (eBook)

DOI 10.1007/978-0-387-92855-5
Springer New York Dordrecht Heidelberg London

Printed on acid-free paper

Springer is part of Springer Science+Business Media (www.springer.com)

Dedicated to the memory of Bartley R. Frueh, MD –

a superb clinician, scientist, and teacher

Foreword

You are reading this book, presumably, because you want to know more about treating patients with ptotic eyelids (or perhaps that one particularly vexing patient whose droopy eyelid refuses to respond to your normally successful surgical expertise). The good news: any eyelid can be lifted. But more about that later.

First, reflect for a moment on the supreme elegance of the eyelid. Less than an organ but far more than mere tissue, the eyelid is both subtle and sublime. Our eyes can detect, with a quick glance, asymmetries of eyelid height and abnormalities of eyelid contour that measure less than a millimeter. Think of how much nonverbal information can be conveyed by a blink, a wink, a squint, or a glare; eyelids are the primary drivers of facial expression. Twinkling eyes, sad eyes, bedroom eyes, pop-eyes – extraordinarily different subjectively, amazingly similar objectively.

We should pause and ponder, however, if we think that a ptotic eyelid is a ptotic eyelid is a ptotic eyelid. Yes, patients with weak levators walk into our clinics every day, but, given enough time in practice, so also will patients with myasthenia gravis, aneurysms, tumors, chronic progressive external ophthalmoplegia, Marcus Gunn jaw winking, Kearns–Sayre syndrome, blepharophimosis, oculopharyngeal dystrophy, and a host of other unusual but important systemic conditions that we had better not miss. Ptosis keeps odd company and late hours.

When we take a patient with ptosis to the operating room, we must be intimately familiar with the eyelid's anatomy. It is not intuitive. For example, why does the levator aponeurosis insert on the inferior portion of the tarsal plate rather than to its superior border, where a committee of anatomists probably would design it to terminate? Why are the aponeurotic attachments to the lateral orbital rim so much more robust than their relatively flimsy medial counterparts? Why is Whitnall's ligament so variable from person to person – and what is it doing there in the first place? Why is our understanding of the relationship between the levator and the superior rectus, and the levator and Müller muscle, so rudimentary? Given that there is so much that we do not know, perhaps we should be surprised by how often we are able to achieve a satisfactory result when we venture forth to treat ptosis.

Unfortunately, surgery for blepharoptosis will likely be one of the last holdouts against the protocolization of medicine. Some practitioners use an anterior approach, levator aponeurotic advancement for virtually every patient – even those with Horner syndrome in which the malfunction is clearly related to Müller muscle. Other operators swear by the posterior approach, Müller muscle – conjunctiva resection, regardless of whether a preoperative phenylephrine test temporarily elevates the eyelid. More subtle technical variations abound. Should one use epinephrine and/or hyaluronidase in the local anesthetic or not? Should one release the septal attachments widely and secure the advanced levator aponeurosis with several sutures or make a small buttonhole in the septum and move the aponeurosis forward with a single stitch? And should those sutures be permanent or absorbable? Should every patient be brought to the upright position intraoperatively to check the eyelid position (such a nuisance…) or can predictable results be achieved by allowing the patient to remain supine throughout the procedure? Should the eyelid crease be purposefully re-created in every case, or will it "find its own level?" Given the overall high rates of success for the various methods of ptosis repair, a randomized clinical trial that was sufficiently powered to demonstrate statistically significant differences when all the above variables are considered would require an untenably large number of enrollees. Surgery for droopy eyelids seems destined to remain as much art as science.

But artists and scientists need humility. As soon as we begin to get confident (or, caveat chirurgeon, begin to get cocky) that ptosis surgery is "routine," a soap-bubble aponeurosis will chasten us. Or a child with severe unilateral congenital ptosis will be brought to our office by parents who refuse to accept that the eyelid cannot be "fixed" to perfection. (As an aside, in 25 years of discussing the option of extirpating the normal levator and placing bilateral frontalis slings – the Beard operation – I have yet to encounter a patient whose parents embraced the idea.)

Ultimately, for better or for worse, any eyelid can be lifted. We are obliged, therefore, to understand why it is ptotic, what therapeutic options are reasonable, and what consequences may ensue. The treatment of blepharoptosis is a study in balance: between the goal of elevating the eyelid and the need for the eye to be protected, between the relative positions of the upper and lower eyelids which yield the palpebral fissure, and between the eyelid retractors and the eyelid protractors and the muscles of the forehead. Sometimes it takes very little to disrupt the balance. I recall a patient with chronic progressive external ophthalmoplegia whose severe blepharoptosis significantly obscured his vision. Raising his eyelids a single millimeter tipped the balance from comfortable eyes to intolerable exposure, from clear corneas to penlight-visible Rose Bengal staining. The patient and I eventually achieved a visually acceptable state of ophthalmic détente, but it was a sobering lesson for both of us.

Useful lessons abound in this book, which will serve as a valued resource for the thoughtful reader. The collected experience of its esteemed authors represents the state of the art of contemporary ptosis surgery. But…we still have much to learn.

Rochester, MN George Brian Bartley, MD

Preface

Blepharoptosis (ptosis) is a widely prevalent disorder that is encountered by virtually every clinician, whether one is working with an adult or pediatric population. Therefore, it behooves the medical practitioner to be familiar with this condition from the diagnostic standpoint, particularly with respect to identifying a serious underlying disorder, such as an aneurysm, tumor, carotid artery dissection, or myasthenia gravis. Any surgeon who manages ptosis should be well-acquainted with the various surgical approaches to repair since different techniques are often particularly applicable to certain scenarios.

Landmark treatises on ptosis, such as *Beard's Ptosis*, are unfortunately out-of-print. Furthermore, while certain aspects of this subject, such as the general technique for external levator resection surgery, may not have changed significantly over the years, there have been major advances in our understanding of the underlying genetics and our ability to identify and classify disorders based on the genetic analysis. This is especially relevant to the various inherited myopathies that are often associated with ptosis, which are reviewed in this book. Admittedly, a comprehensive discussion of myopathic disorders is beyond the scope of this text, and we have condensed that subject to a review of myopathies relevant to the ophthalmologist and ptosis surgeon. As scientific research progresses, we have no doubt that there will be much more to say about pathophysiology and genetics of ptosis in the future.

While many books have been published in the field of oculoplastic surgery, most provide only a limited discussion of blepharoptosis, emphasizing the key points of diagnosis and surgical management. It was our intent to provide a practical reference that offered a 360° view of blepharoptosis – from etiology to management. We begin with a historical perspective, then move on to a review of relevant eyelid anatomy and physiology, how to evaluate the ptosis patient, and then differential diagnosis. Other ocular and periocular disorders may be confused with ptosis, and these are discussed in the chapter on pseudoptosis. After reviewing the various categories of ptosis, classified based on etiology, we cover the management of ptosis, including nonsurgical modalities and the various surgical procedures for ptosis correction, as well as tips regarding anesthesia and analgesia during surgery in order to optimize the surgical experience for both the patient and the surgeon. The significance of patient ethnicity and gender is reviewed. The book would not be complete without a discussion of surgical complications and the basis for surgery failure and its management. The chapter entitled "Perspective of a Risk Manager" provides a thoughtful analysis of the physician–patient relationship, with suggestions regarding how to establish a favorable rapport with the patient and reduce the likelihood of an unhappy patient, regardless of the outcome of surgery.

This is a multiauthored textbook that is written by experts in the fields of oculofacial plastic surgery and neuro-ophthalmology. This subject matter is relevant to physicians and surgeons in all disciplines that deal with eyelid ptosis, from both a diagnostic and therapeutic perspective. It is our hope that this reference text will be helpful to clinicians in a wide range of specialties and ptosis surgeons, from the novice to the expert.

Skokie,IL — Adam J. Cohen,M D
Concord, NH — David A. Weinberg,M D

Acknowledgments

I would like to acknowledge, with gratitude, my parents, family, friends, teachers, and patients.

—Adam J. Cohen

To my wife, Rebecca, whose editorial support was immeasurably helpful, and my three wonderful children, Elena, Sara, and Jonathan.

—David A. Weinberg

Contents

Part V Other Considerations

Contributors

Heather Baldwin
Department of Ophthalmology, Rayne Institute, St. Thomas' Hospital, London, England, UK

George Brian Bartley
DepartmentofO phthalmology, MayoC linic, Rochester, MN, USA

C. RobertB ernardino
Department of Ophthalmology, Yale Eye Center and YaleN ewH avenH ospital, NewH aven, CT, USA

Jurij R. Bilyk
Department of Ophthalmology, Jefferson University Hospitals and ThomasJ effersonU niversityM edicalC ollege, Philadelphia, PA, USA

Nariman S. Boyle
Assistant Professor of Ophthalmology, Ophthalmic Plastic, Orbital and Reconstructive Surgery, Department of Ophthalmology, State University ofN ewY orka tSton yB rook, StonyB rook, NY, USA

Adam G. Buchanan
WashingtonU niversityEye C enter, St.Louis , MO, USA

Eli L. Chang
Department of Ophthalmology, Doheny Eye Institute, Los Angeles, CA, USA

Shu-Hong Chang
Division of Oculoplastic Surgery, Jules Stein Eye Institute, UCLASc hoolofM edicine, LosA ngeles, CA, USA

Adam J.C ohen
PrivatePra ctice, Skokie, IL, USA

Vikram D. Durairaj
Associate Professor of Ophthalmology and Otolaryngology, Head and Neck Surgery, Oculoplastic and Orbital Surgery; Fellowship Director, Associate Residency Program Director, Department of Ophthalmology, UniversityofC oloradoD enverSc hoolo fM edicine, Denver, CO, USA

Jonathan J. Dutton
Department of Ophthalmology, University of North Carolina – Chapel Hill, ChapelH ill, NC, USA

Ian C. Francis
The Ocular Plastics Unit, Prince of Wales Hospital and Sydney Children's Hospital, TheU niversityofN ewSouthW ales, Sydney, Australia

Bartley R. Frueh
Department of Ophthalmology, Kellogg Eye Center, Universityo fM ichigan, AnnA rbor, MI, USA

Mithra O. Gonzalez
Flaum Eye Institute and Department of Ophthalmology, University of RochesterSc hoolofM edicinea ndD entistry, Rochester, NY, USA

Milad Hakimbashi
Department of Clinical Ophthalmology, Shiley Eye Center, UniversityofC alifornia–Sa nD iego, LaJ olla, CA, USA

Andrew R. Harrison
Department of Ophthalmology and Otolaryngology, University of Minnesota, Minneapolis, MN, USA

Morris Hartstein
Department of Ophthalmology, St. Louis University School of Medicine, St.Louis , MO, USA

John T. Harvey
Department of Ophthalmology, McMaster University Medical Centre, Hamilton, ON, Canada

John B. Holds
Departments of Ophthalmology and Otolaryngology/Head and NeckSur gery, St.Louis U niversity, St.Louis , MO, USA

Kim Jebodhsingh
Department of Ophthalmology and Vision Sciences, University of Toronto, Toronto, ON, Canada

Natan D. Kahn
MaineEye C enter, Portland, ME, USA

Robert Kersten
Department of Ophthalmology, University of California-San Francisco, SanFra ncisco, CA, USA

Don O. Kikkawa
Department of Clinical Ophthalmology, Division of Ophthalmic Plastic and Reconstructive Surgery, Shiley Eye Center, University of California – SanD iego, LaJ olla, CA, USA

Jonathan W. Kim
Department of Ophthalmology, Stanford Medical Center, Stanford, CA, USA

Bobby S. Korn
Department of Clinical Ophthalmology, Shiley Eye Center, UniversityofC alifornia–Sa nD iego, LaJ olla, CA, USA

Michael S.L ee
Department of Ophthalmology, Neurology and Neurosurgery, UniversityofM innesota, Minneapolis, MN, USA

Ippolit C.A. Matjucha
Neuro-opthalmologist, Comprehensive Surgical Opthalmologist, PrivatePra ctice, Sudbury, MA, USA

Jill Melicher
Fellow Physician, Department of Ophthalmic Plastic and ReconstructiveSur gery, CincinnatiEye Institute, Cincinnati, OH, USA

Dale R. Meyer
Lions Eye Institute and Department of Ophthalmology, AlbanyM edicalC enter, Albany, NY, USA

Eve E. Moscato
Department of Ophthalmology, University of California-San Francisco SchoolofM edicine, SanF rancisco, CA, USA

Ann P. Murchison
Department of Ophthalmology, Jefferson University Hospitals and ThomasJ effersonU niversityM edicalC ollege, Philadelphia, PA, USA

Jefferey A. Nerad
Ophthalmic Plastic and Reconstructive Surgery, Cincinnati Eye Institute; Professor of Ophthalmology, University of Cincinnati, Cincinnati, OH, USA

James Oestreicher
Department of Ophthalmology and Vision Sciences, University of Toronto, Toronto, Ontario, Canada

Jed Poll
MountO gdenEye C enter, Ogden, UT, USA

Stuart R. Seiff
Department of Ophthalmology, University of California-San Francisco SchoolofM edicine, SanFra ncisco, CA, USA

John Shore
TexasO culoplasticC onsultants, Austin, TX, USA

Norm Shorr
Division of Oculoplastic Surgery, Jules Stein Eye Institute, UCLASc hoolofM edicine, LosA ngeles, CA, USA

David I. Silbert
ArmestoEye A ssociates, Mechanicsburg, PA, USA

Guy JonathanB en Simon
Department of Orbital, Ophthalmic Plastic and Lacrimal Surgery, The Goldschleger Eye Institute, Sheba Medical Center, Tel Hashomer, Israel

Alon Skaat
Department of Ophthalmology, The Goldschleger Eye Institute, ShebaM edicalC enter, TelH ashomer, Israel

Chris Thiagarajah
Oculofacial Surgeon, Neuro-ophthalmologist, The Eye Care and Surgery Center of New Jersey, Westfield, NJ, USA

JoseL uis Tovilla
DepartmentofO phthalmology, ClínicaFlorida Sa telite, Naucalpán, Mexico

David A. Weinberg
Concord Eye Care, Concord, NH and Department of Surgery (Ophthalmology), DartmouthM edicalSc hool, Hanover, NH, USA

Geoff Wilcsek
The Ocular Plastics Unit, Prince of Wales Hospital and Sydney Children's Hospital, TheU niversityofN ewSouthW ales, Sydney, Australia

EdwardJ . Wladis
DepartmentofO phthalmology, AlbanyM edicalC enter, Albany, NY, USA

Edward J. Yen
Department of Ophthalmology, Baylor College of Medicine, Houston, TX, USA

Renzo A. Zaldivar
AestheticF aciala ndO cularPla sticSur geryC enter, ChapelH ill, NC, USA

PartI
Introduction

Chapter 1
Introduction

Adam J. Cohen and David A. Weinberg

Abstract Blepharoptosis, or drooping of the upper eyelid, is one of the most common surgical eyelid disorders. The word "ptosis", which derives from the Greek πτῶσις ("fall" or "falling"), refers to "abnormal lowering or prolapse of an organ or body part".[1] While one may apply the term "ptosis" to describe any anatomical structure, such as breast or chin ptosis, "ptosis" will be used interchangeably with "blepharoptosis" in this book, strictly referring to the eyelid disorder.

There may be some debate as to what constitutes a ptotic eyelid. One could try to define it quantitatively, based on the margin reflex distance (MRD1), which is the distance from the corneal light reflex to the central upper eyelid margin. Yet, there is a relatively wide variation in eyelid position in the general population, and ethnic and racial differences have been described.[2,3] When comparing whites, African Americans, Latinos, and Asians in a similar age bracket, whites displayed the highest mean MRD1 (5.1 mm), while Asians had the lowest (3.8 mm).[2] The normal upper eyelid margin rests somewhere between the superior edge of the pupil and the superior limbus, typically around a MRD1 of 4, give or take a millimeter. There would be little argument that a MRD1 of 0 represents a ptotic eyelid, and a MRD1 of 7 indicates lid retraction. However, where does one draw the line between a "normal" eyelid and a ptotic eyelid? Should ptosis be defined as a MRD1 below 3 mm? 2.5 mm? 2 mm? It is more difficult to define mild ptosis precisely in individuals with symmetric upper eyelids, as opposed to those with asymmetric upper eyelids, i.e., unilateral ptosis. Another way to define ptosis is from a functional standpoint, or qualitatively. Perhaps an eyelid should be considered ptotic if it is low enough to obstruct the visual axis, i.e., below the superior edge of the pupil, since that is the primary functional consequence of ptosis. How low an upper eyelid needs to be in order to obstruct vision depends on the pupil size, and that is affected by ambient lighting conditions, degree of arousal, and systemic or topical drugs, among other factors. By this definition, an upper eyelid would not be functionally ptotic in a patient with a MRD1 of 1.5–2 mm and a pupil size of 3 mm, since the upper edge of the pupil is 1.5 mm above the corneal light reflex.

There is also patient perception. Some individuals may desire wider palpebral fissures that make them appear more alert, even if their vision is not obstructed by the upper eyelid position, while others may wish for the ptotic "bedroom eyes" look of Marilyn Monroe or Marlene Dietrich. Thus, what is "normal" or "abnormal", and what is desirable vs. undesirable, is in the eyes of the beholder, and so treatment needs to be individualized.

Management of the ptosis patient poses challenges with respect to both diagnosis and

A.J.C ohen(✉)
PrivatePra ctice, TheA rtof Eye s,Sk okie IL, USA
e-mail:a cohen@theartofeyes.com

A.J. Cohen and D.A. Weinberg (eds.), *Evaluation and Management of Blepharoptosis*,
DOI 10.1007/978-0-387-92855-5_1,

treatment. From a diagnostic standpoint, ptosis can be the hallmark of numerous diverse and potentially serious disorders, underscoring the importance of identifying the etiology of the ptosis. This will set the framework for ptosis management and helps establish whether a patient needs surgery and what type of surgery.

There are many considerations involved in the evaluation and management of the patient with blepharoptosis. In the chapters that follow, we examine this subject from a wide range of perspectives, with the hope of providing a broad overview of this common yet complex eyelid disorder.

References

1. The American Heritage Dictionary of the English Language. 4th ed. Boston:Houghton Mifflin;2000.
2. Murchison AP, Sires BA, Amadi AJ. Margin reflex distance in different ethnic groups. Arch Facial Plast Surg.2009; 11:303–5.
3. Price KM, Gupta PK, Woodward JA, Stinnett SS, Murchison AP. Eyebrow and eyelid dimensions: an anthropometric analysis of African Americans and Caucasians.P lastR econstrS urg.2009; 124:615–23.

Chapter2
TheHi storyo fPt osisSur gery

Mithra O. Gonzalez and Vikram D. Durairaj

Abstract From an inexact origin of trial and error, blepharoptosis surgery has become a scientific art. The arc of its technical development parallels that of anatomical discoveries and surgical materials. Approaches have varied, as have the tissues of interest, and with increasingly reliable results in the reconstructive domain came greater expectations and the development of its cosmetic counterpart. That said, for some diseases associated with blepharoptosis, an ideal surgery remains elusive. This chapter provides a chronological account of the treatment of blepharoptosis with attention paid to the tissues involved. The rich history of blepharoptosis surgery provides a fertile matrix for the field of oculofacial plastic surgery, and in return, the field continues to evolve blepharoptosis' surgical treatment.

The history and evolution of eyelid ptosis surgery can be analyzed in terms of chronology and tissue. A discussion of its chronology is inviting because this method allows for an understanding of the field's consecutive advances. One is able to appreciate the "who, what, when," and in some cases, the more complex questions of "why" and "how" of a particular technique and understand its ultimate favor or disfavor. In a chronological discussion, one may see the subject matter's natural arch, which unfortunately, can be confusing at times. On the other hand, a discussion of the tissues involved in eyelid ptosis surgery allows for an artificially coherent history by abstracting the salient subject matter from its historical context and ignoring the tempo of evolution. Such abstraction dispossess the matter of elements potentially useful to those responsible for the next generation of surgical innovations.

Authors on the history of ptosis surgery tend to use one approach or the other. Beard used the tissue approach in his writing on the history of ptosis surgery [1, 2]. Servat and Mantilla and Thaller and Collin, as well as Julius Hirschberg, chose the chronological approach [3–5]. In this chapter, the latter approach is utilized with sensitivity paid to the tissues involved and the intention of providing the best attributes of both methods.

According to Rycroft and commonly cited in historical accounts of ptosis surgery, "ancient Arabian ophthalmologists" provide the first reference of eyelid surgery for the treatment of ptosis [1–3, 6]. In what amounted to a blepharoplasty, the " ancient Arabian" procedure involved resecting from the medial part of the upper lid an ellipse of skin that varied in size as a function of the amount of ptosis present. Others claim that about 100 ad, the encyclopedist of Greek and Roman surgery, Aulus Cornelius Celsus first documented the resection of eyelid skin for the treatment of ptosis in De Re Medica [7].

On the contrary, Hirschberg argues that neither did Celsus invent a blepharoplasty nor is

V.D.D urairaj (✉)
DepartmentofO phthalmology,
University of Colorado Denver School of Medicine,
7651E.8thA venue, Denver, CO 80230, USA
e-mail:vikra m.durairaj@uchsc.edu
e-mail:vikra m.durairaj@ucdenver.edu

A.J. Cohen and D.A. Weinberg (eds.), *Evaluation and Management of Blepharoptosis*,
DOI 10.1007/978-0-387-92855-5_2, © Springer Science+Business Media, LLC 2011

there any mention of such a procedure in the Greek and Roman repertoire of surgery [5]. Instead Hirschberg credits C.F. von Graefe and Dzondi with performing eyelid reconstruction in 1818 and Johann Karl Georg with the first monograph on blepharoplasty published in 1829 [5].

Regardless of its ancient origins, the history of ptosis surgery seems to unify with the 1806 publication of *Practical Observations on the Principle and Disease of the Eye* by the Italian anatomist and surgeon Antonio Scarpa. In this work, he describes a resection of "integuments at the upper part of the relaxed eyelid in the vicinity and direction of the superior arch of the orbit" thatis inte ndedtoe levatethe lid [1, 2, 6].

Henceforth, the wealth of publications allows for a logical narration with few opportunities for conflicting opinions. After 1806, ptosis surgery undergoes many revolutions as knowledge of anatomy and physiology progresses and as types of materials expand. At its core, however, Beard keenly notes that ptosis surgery essentially falls into one of six categories: skin resection, frontalis suspension, tarsus resection, levator resection, superior rectus muscle suspension, or a combination of the aforementioned categories [1]. With these facts in mind, the tour of the history of ptosis surgery continues.

In 1831, Hunt realizes that Scarpa's procedure is in fact a frontalis suspension by virtue of its ability to tether eyelid to frontalis muscle by way of skin shortening [8]. The lifting effect is short-lived and the ptosis recurs, so alternative procedures are sought. A few years later, in 1855, though some sources suggest that it was not until 1882, A. von Graefe devises a technique in which a transcutaneous approach is used to excise approximately 10 mm of skin and orbicularis [3, 9]. The procedure seeks to weaken the protractors and consequently enhance the effective power of the retractors. Interest in this approach waxes and wanes with published reports until as recently as 2006 [10]. Two years after von Graefe's report, and for the first time, Bowman targets the retractors [11]. Using an internal and external approach, he resects both levator palpebrae superioris and tarsus.

Interest in the frontalis suspension technique is renewed with Dransart in 1880 as he uses buried catgut sutures to suspend the lid to the brow [12]. Dransart believes a scar serves as the true suspender once the suture is absorbed through inflammation. A year later, Pagenstecher places a temporary silk suture between the lid and the brow [13]. Hess also uses silk sutures, suspending the lid to the brow and removing them 3 weeks later [14]. Stepping away from the use of pure exogenous materials, De Wecker in the year 1882, uses a combination of skin, orbicularis and silk suture as a suspender, thus employing the first partial autogenous sling [4]. Pannus improves on the use of the skin sling and addresses the early and late infections associated with the procedure [2, 15]. Tansley in 1895 uses more differently shaped skin than that used by his predecessors, and Darier in 1897 uses orbicularis muscle as the brow suspension [4, 16].

A novel approach to ptosis surgery is devised in 1897 when Motais and Parinaud use the superior rectus muscle to provide lid elevation [17, 18]. Motais' technique uses part of the actual muscle, while Parinaud uses part of the tendon, with both operations resulting in attachment of muscle or tendon to tarsus. Forty years later, Wheeler uses strips of orbicularis to attach the lidtothe s uperiorre ctusmus cle [19].

Although a new source of lid-lifting power, namely, the superior rectus muscle, had been identified, the lion's share of attention, as evidenced by the number of publications, remains with the frontalis suspension. Koster used buried nonabsorbable sutures in 1899, Mules, a subcutaneous central gold wire in 1907, and Angelucci, levator to suspend the lid to the brow [4, 20, 21]. Payr's implementation of thigh fascia in 1909 marks a significant advance in autologous slings [22]. Over the next 20 years, several variations of the above procedures are devised. Be it differently fashioned strips of skin or fascia, all techniques are dependent on the frontalis muscle for power [23–28].

The levator again becomes the tissue of interest as Everbusch describes a levator tuck operation performed via an external approach in 1883 [29]. In the same year, Snellen reports on having successfully treated ptosis with a levator tendon or aponeurosis resection [30]. Wolff in 1896 recommends isolating, mobilizing, and advancing the levator palpebrae superioris [31]. Blaskovics devises an internal approach with excision of the tarsal plate and levator in 1909, which he further develops with increasing attention to the lid creasein1929 [32, 33].

The year prior to Blaskovics' lid crease technique, Kirby returns interest to the superior rectus muscle as a source of lid-lifting power and sparks a fury of publications [27]. Calling the procedure a "modified Motais operation," Kirby sutures the superior rectus tendon to the tarsus and combines it with a temporary frontalis sling. Seven years later, Trainor resects the superior edge of tarsus and, by the strip of resected tarsus' length, attaches the residual tarsus of the lid to the superior rectus tendon [34]. A year later, in 1936, Dickey uses fascia lata to link tarsus to the superior rectus tendon [35]. 1949 sees Berke reporting on a successful technique wherein he resects superior rectus muscle and, using the excised tendon, links the resected superior rectus musclea nde yelid [36].

Attention returns to the levator as Agaston reports on a refinement of the internal levator resection procedure in 1942 [37]. Ten years later, Berke modifies Blaskovics' original internal approach [38]. In the same year, Fox brings enthusiasm for the external approach to levator resection, an enthusiasm that is continued by Leahey in 1953, Johnson in 1954, and Berke in 1959 [39–42]. Around the same time, Iliff publishes on the virtues of the internal approach to levator resection [43]. Schimek reports that once the levator is resected it may be used as an autologous suspender in the same operation, thus providing both levator resection and frontalis sling [44].

In 1961, the conjunctival-tarsal-Müllerectomy, otherwise known as the Fasanella–Servat procedure, is published [46]. The simplicity and predictability of the procedure makes it attractive and, according to some, helps bring ptosis surgery to a greater number of ophthalmologists and thus patients. Initially, it is thought of as a type of levator resection but is later understood to work in part, because of its resection of Müller's muscle. 1964 is remarkable in the history of ptosis surgery as an anatomist Jones suggests that the sympathetically innervated Müller's muscle could be employed in the treatment of mild ptosis [45]. He devises a surgery that advances the levator aponeurosis, but preserves Müller's muscle [45]. The technique is modified by Collins and Beard but does not gain popularity [1].

Rycroft continues to evolve the frontalis slings and recommends the use of extensor longus from the small toe as the suspender in 1962 [47]. In the subsequent 2 years, Yasuna describes a successful frontalis sling using cadaveric fascia lata as Iliff uses reconstituted collagen [6, 48]. Of note, Tillet and Tillet recommend the use of Number 40 silicone strips in lid-brow suspensions, and, near the same time, Bodian uses scleraa sthe s uspender [49, 50].

Much development occurs during the 1960s and 1970s with new methods of lid elevation, and newer technologies. Although reported in the French and Argentinean literature, Guy and Ransohoff report on the use of a palpebral spring in the treatment of severe paralytic ptosis [51]. In 1967, Jones and Wilson report on the use of the corrugator supercilii muscle as a power source in the treatment of ptosis [52]. Mustarde describes a technically challenging surgery that tucks the levator to the roof of the orbit [53]. Singh and Singh utilize the power of the superior rectus by attaching it to the lid [54]. Conway describes a procedure in which magnets are implanted in the eyelid and applied to the rims of glasses as a means of elevation [55]. Sometime later, eyelid crutchesa rede scribed [56].

1969 marks the next chapter in the history of ptosis surgery and is remarkable for the founding of the American Society of Ophthalmic Plastic and Reconstructive Surgery (ASOPRS). With its establishment, research in and publications on ptosis surgery flourish. Older procedures are rediscovered; modifications are made, while materials are varied as anatomical knowledge increases.

In 1972, Putterman devises a clamp for a modified Fasanella–Servat procedure [57]. Putterman continues to improve his technique that resects Müller's muscle and conjunctiva while sparing the tarsus [58]. Carbajal resects levator and Müller's muscle through a combined internal and external approach [59]. In 1975, Lauring reports on the success of a sutureless Fasanella–Servat operation, and Bodian uses 5-0 nylon suture that is secured externally to avoid corneal irritation [60–62]. Weinstein uses a marking suture to more easily isolate Müller's muscle and place the Putterman clamp [63]. Iliff uses a Fasanella-like approach but incorporates levator aponeurosis into the operative site [64]. Dortzbach recognizes the utility of phenylephrine as a means of preoperatively determining postoperative lid position of a Müller's muscle resection [65]. Most recently, in 2008, Khooshabeh and associates describe an "open sky" surgery that isolates and resects Müller's muscle while leaving conjunctiva largely intact, exceptingthe inc ision [66, 67].

The frontalis sling continues in popularity. During the 1970s, fascia lata slings undergo extensive investigation. Incisions are varied, postoperative adjustments made, and long-term results reported on their outcomes [68–70]. The frontalis silicone sling receives further attention, and its use continues to this day [71, 72]. In 1986, Anderson describes a procedure in which the needle is passed through the brow and then behind the septum on its course to the eyelid margin [73]. This results in a more natural-appearing lid crease and thus a more cosmetically acceptable appearance [73]. Goldberger in 1991 reports on the use of a double rhomboid silicone rod frontalis sling [74]. Downes uses a Mersilene mesh sling in ptosis repair [75]. Again varying the suspensory material, Sternberg successfully uses preserved placental umbilical vein as a sling [76]. Han transposes a frontalis muscle flap and attaches it to tarsus as a treatment of the ptotic lid [77]. Leibsohn rotates a periosteal flap, and Ibrahim uses the levator muscle as the suspensorye lement [78, 79].

The anatomical studies of Jones, Quickert, Anderson, and the like, during the 1970s, usher in the age of levator palpebrae superioris aponeurosis surgery [45, 80, 81]. Although aponeurosis surgery has had been previously conceived, performed, and described at the end of the nineteenth century, unreliable results and more reliable alternatives diminished its popularity [29, 31]. With improved understanding of eyelid anatomy and physiology, interest in aponeurosis repair returns. In 1975, Jones et al. and Older report on aponeurosis repair, while Harris and Dortzbach report on levator muscle and aponeurosis tucking [80, 82, 83]. Fox notes that levator function and not the degree of ptosis should dictate the amount of repair [84]. Anderson, a great champion of aponeurosis repair surgery for the treatment of ptosis, reports extensively on its anatomy, its use in neuromyopathic, involutional, and milder cases of congenital ptosis, and deems the 1980s the Age of Aponeurotic Awareness [81, 85–88]. Variations are carried out during this period of enthusiasm that include the manner of aponeurotic repair, i.e., an A-frame repair versus a single suture or the size or location of the incision made by a variety of instruments – CO_2 laser versus surgical steel [89–92]. In 2001, Meltzer describes an external aponeurotic repair using a single 5-0 silk that may be adjusted by postoperative day 4 [93]. To this day, aponeurosis repair remains a popular approach to ptosis surgery.

All told, the history of ptosis surgery is a story of success and failure, of procedures invented, rejected, and forgotten, only to be rediscovered as surgical material, knowledge, and technique improve, making yesterday's imdpossible today's standard of care. As the understanding of eyelid anatomy and physiology increases and technologies employed in surgical repair advance, greater satisfaction by both the surgeon and patient may be achieved. One may be certain that though much progress has been made in the treatment of eyelid ptosis, much remains undiscovered and consequently,a ne nticingpur suit.

References

1. Beard C. Ptosis. St. Louis: Mosby Company; 1976.
2. Beard C. History of ptosis surgery. Adv Ophthalmic Plast Reconstr Surg. 1986;5:125–31.
3. Servat J, Mantilla M. The history of ptosis surgery. Adv Ophthalmic Plast Reconstr Surg. 1986;5:133–7.
4. Thaller VT, Collin JR. History of ophthalmic plastic surgery in Europe. Adv Ophthalmic Plast Reconstr Surg.1986;5:223– 31.
5. Hirschberg J. The history of ophthalmology, vol. 5: the renaissance of ophthalmology in the eighteenth century (Part 3)/the first half of the nineteenth century (Part 1) as translated by Frederick C. Blodi. Bonn: Wayenborgh;1985.
6. Rycroft BW. The transconjunctival and transcutaneous approach to levator resection in the treatment of ptosis. In: Troutman R, Converse J, Smith B, editors. Plastics and reconstructive surgery of the eye and adenexa. London: Butter-worth; 1962.
7. AulusC orneliusC elsus,D eR eM edica.
8. Hunt RT, cited by Fox SA. Surgery of ptosis. 1980.
9. Beard C. Ophthalmic surgery. 2nd ed. Philadelphia: P. Blakiston's Son & Company; 1914. p. 231, 241, 370.
10. Singh D. Orbicularis plication for ptosis: a third alternative. Ann Ophthalmol. 2006;38(3):185–93.
11. Bowman WP, cited by Bader D. Report of the chief operations performed at the Royal Ophthalmic Hospital for the quarter ending September 1857. Ophthal Hosp Rep. 1857;1:1857–1859, 34.
12. Dransart HN. Un cas de blepharoptose opere par un procede special a l' auteur. Ann Ocul. 1880;84:88.
13. Pagenstecher A, cited by Fuchs E. Textbook of ophthalmology. 1977. p. 964.
14. Graefe AV. Operation du ptosis. Albrecht von Graefes Arch Klin Exp Ophthalmol. 1863;91:57.
15. Hess C. Operation methode gegen ptosis. Arch Augenheilkd.1893; 28:22.
16. Panas P. D'un noveau procede operatoire applicable au ptosis congenital et au ptosis paralitique. 1886.
17. Tansley JO. A congenital ptosis case and operation. Trans Am Ophthalmol Soc. 1895;7:427.
18. Motais M. Operation du ptosis par la graffe tarsienne d/une languette du tendon du muscle droit superieur. Ann Ocul. 1897;118:5.
19. Parinaud H. Nouveau procede operatorie du ptosis. Ann Ocul. 1897;118:13.
20. Wheeler JM. Correction of ptosis by attachment of strips of orbicularis muscle to the superior rectus muscle. Arch Ophthalmol. 1939;21:1.
21. Koster W. De verbouding van den musculus tarsalis superior mulleri bij ptosis congenital. Ned Tijdschr Geneeskd.1899;35 :417.
22. Mules PH, cited by Grismdale H, Brewerton, E. A textbook of ophthalmic operations. 1907. p. 63.
23. Payr E. Plastik mittels freier faszien transplantation bei ptosis. Dtsch Med Wochenschr. 1909;35:822.
24. Machek P. An operation for ptosis with the formation of a fold in the upper lid. Arch Ophthalmol. 1915; 44:539.
25. Wright WW. The use of living sutures in the treatment of ptosis. Arch Ophthalmol. 1922;51:99.
26. Reese RG. An operation for blepharoptosis with formation of a fold in the lid. Arch Ophthalmol. 1924;53:26.
27. Hunt HL. Plastic surgery of the head, face, and neck. Philadelphia: Lea and Febiger; 1926.
28. Kirby DB. A modified Motais operation for blepharoptosis. Arch Ophthalmol. 1928;57:327.
29. Friedenwald JS, Guyton JS. A simple ptosis operation: utilization of the frontalis by means of a rhomboid-shaped suture. Am J Ophthalmol. 1948;31:411.
30. Everbusch O. Zur operationen der congenitalen blepharoptosis. Klin Monatsbl Augenheilkd. 1883;21:100.
31. Snellen H. Levator tendon shortening for ptosis. Heidelberg: Report of the German Ophthalmology Society;1883.
32. Tessier P, Rougier J, Hervouet F, Woillez M, Lekieffre M, Derome P. Plastic surgery of the orbit and eyelids. New York: Masson; 1981. p. 272.
33. Wolff H. Der verlagerung des musculus levator palpebrae superioris mit durchtrennung der insertion: Zwei neue methoden gegen ptosis congenital. Arch Augenheilkd.1896; 33:125.
34. Blaskovics L. A new operation for ptosis with shortening of the levator and tarsus. Arch Ophthalmol. 1923;52:563.
35. Blaskovics L. Treatment for ptosis: formation of a fold in the eyelid and resection of the levator and tarsus. Arch Ophthalmol. 1929;57:315.
36. Trainor ME. Operation for lid ptosis. Trans Sect Ophthalmol.1935: 93.
37. Dickey CA. Superior rectus fascia lata sling in the correction of ptosis. Am J Ophthalmol. 1935;19: 660.
38. Berke RN. An operation for ptosis utilizing the superior rectus muscle. Trans Am Acad Ophthalmol Otolaryngol.1949; 53:499.
39. Agaston SA. Resection of levator palpebrae muscle by the conjunctival route for ptosis. Arch Ophthalmol. 1942;27:994.
40. Berke RN. A simplified Blaskovics operation for blepharoptosis. Arch Ophthalmol. 1952;48:460.
41. Fox SA. Ophthalmic plastic surgery. Orlando, FL: Grune & Stratton; 1952.
42. Leahey BD. Simplified ptosis surgery: resection of the levator palpebrae by the external route. Arch Ophthalmol.1953; 50:588.
43. Johnson C. Blepharoptosis: a general consideration of surgical methods with results in 162 operations. Am J Ophthalmol. 1954;38:129.
44. Berke R. Results of resection of the levator muscle through a skin incision in congenital ptosis. Arch Ophthalmol.1959; 61:177.
45. Iliff C. A simplified ptosis operation. Am J Ophthalmol. 1954;37:529.

46. Schimek RA. A new ptosis operation utilizing both levator and frontalis. Arch Ophthalmol. 1955; 54:92.
47. Jones LT. The anatomy of the upper eyelid and its relation to ptosis surgery. Am J Ophthalmol. 1960; 57:943.
48. Fasanella R, Servat J. Levator resection for minimal ptosis. Another simplified operation. Arch Ophthalmol. 1961;65:493.
49. Yasuna E. Use of prepared fascia in correction of ptosis. Am J Ophthalmol. 1962;54:1097.
50. Iliff CE. Surgical management of ptosis. Sommerville, NY: Ethicon; 1962.
51. Tilllet CW, Tillett GM. Silicone sling in the correction of ptosis. Am J Ophthalmol. 1966;62:521.
52. Bodian M. Repair of ptosis using human sclera. Am J Ophthalmol.1968 ;65:352.
53. Guy CL, Ransohoff J. The palpebral spring for paralysis of the upper eyelid in facila never paralysis: technical note. J Neurosurg. 1968;29(4):431–3.
54. Jones LT, Wilson WA. Transplantation of the corrugator supercilii muscle for the cure of ptosis. Trans Am Acad Ophthalmol Otolaryngol. 1967;71:889.
55. Mustarde JC. Experiences in ptosis correction. Trans Am Acad Ophthalmol Otolaryngol. 1968;72:173.
56. Singh D, Singh M. Total transplantation of the superior rectus muscle for ptosis. Trans Ophthalmol Soc UK.1978;98:71.
57. Conway JS. Alleviation of myogenic ptosis by magnetic force. Br J Ophthalmol. 1973;57:315.
58. Lapid O, Lapid-Gortzak R, Barr J, Rosenberg L. Eyelid crutches for ptosis: a forgotten solution. Plast Reconstr Surg. 2000;106(5):1213–4.
59. Putterman AM. A clamp for strengthening Müller's muscle in the treatment of ptosis. Modification, theory and clamp for the Fasanella-Servat ptosis operation. Arch Ophthalmol. 1972;87(6):665–7.
60. Putterman AM, Urist MJ. Müller's muscle-conjunctival resection in the treatment of blepharoptosis. Arch Ophthalmol.1975; 93:619.
61. Carbajal UM. Levator-Müller's muscle resection through combined internal and external approach. Eye Ear Nose Throat Mon. 1972;51(9):348–54.
62. Lauring L. Letter: sutureless Fasanella-Servat belpharoptosis correction. Am J Ophthalmol. 1975;80(4): 778.
63. Lauring L. Blepharoptosis correction with the sutureless Fasanella-Servat operation. Arch Ophthalmol. 1977;95(4):671–4.
64. Bodian M. A revised Fasanella-Servat ptosis operation. Ann Ophthalmol. 1975;7(4):603–5.
65. Weinstein GS, Bueurger GF. Modification of the Müller's muscle-conjunctival resection operation for blepharoptosis. Am J Ophthalmol. 1982;93(5):647–51.
66. Ilif CE. In Duane TD, editor. Clinical ophthalmology. Hagerstown, MD. 1976.
67. Dortzbach RK. Superior tarsal muscle resection to correct belpharoptosis. Ophthalmology. 1979;86(10): 1883–91.
68. Khooshabeh R, Baldwin HC. Isolated Müller's muscle resection for the correction of blepharoptosis. Eye.2009; 23(5):1236.
69. Lake S, Mohammad-Ali FH, Khooshabeh R. Open sky Müller's muscle-conjunctiva resection for ptosis surgery. Eye. 2003;17(9):1008–12.
70. Argamaso RV. An adjustable fascia lata sling for the correction of blepharoptosis. Br J Plast Surg. 1974; 27(3):274–5.
71. Argamaso RV, Lewin ML. Fascia lata sling in blepharoptosis: enhancement of result by postoperative adjustment. J Pediatr Ophthalmol. 1976;13(1):51–5.
72. Crawford JS. Repair of ptosis using frontalis muscle and fascia lata: a 20-year review. Ophthalmic Surg. 1977;8(4):31–40.
73. Rowan PJ, Hayes GS. Silicone sling for ptosis. South Med J. 1977;70(1):68–9.
74. Leone Jr CR, Rylander G. A modified silicone frontalis sling for the correction of blepharoptosis. Am J Ophthalmol.1978; 85(6):802–5.
75. Patrinely JR, Anderson RL. The septal pulley in frontalis suspension. Arch Ophthalmol. 1986;104(11): 1707–10.
76. Goldberger S, Conn H, Lemor M. Double rhomboid silicone rod frontalis suspension. Ophthalmic Plast Reconstr Surg. 1991;7(1):48–53.
77. Downes RN, Collin JR. The mersilene mesh ptosis sling. Eye. 1990;4(3):456–63.
78. Sternberg I, Seelenfreund MH, Sternberg N. A new sling material for ptosis patients. Ophthalmic Surg. 1988;19(1):64–6.
79. Han K, Kang J. Tripartite frontalis muscle flap transposition for blepharoptosis. Ann Plast Surg. 1993; 30(3):224–32.
80. Leibsohn JM. Blepharoptosis repair by supraorbital rim periosteal rotation flaps. Ophthalmic Plast Reconstr Surg. 1995;11(1):16–21.
81. Ibrahim HA. Use of levator muscle as a frontalis sling. Ophthalmic Plast Reconstr Surg. 2007;23(5): 376–80.
82. Jones LT, Quickert MH, Wobig JL. The cure of ptosis by aponeurosis repair. Arch Ophthalmol. 1975;93: 629–34.
83. Anderson RL, Beard C. The levator aponeurosis. Attachments and their clinical significance. Arch Ophthalmol.1977; 95:1437–41.
84. Harris WA, Dortzbach RK. Levator tuck: a simplified blepharoptosis procedure. Ann Ophthalmol. 1975;7(6): 873–88.
85. Older JJ. Levator aponeurosis tuck: a treatment for ptosis. Ophthalmic Surg. 1978;9(4):102–10.
86. Fox SA. A simple levator resection operation. Ann Ophthalmol.1975; 7(2):315–8.
87. Anderson RL, Dixon RS. Neuromyopathic ptosis: a new surgical approach. Arch Ophthalmol. 1979;97(6):1129–31.
88. Anderson RL, Dixon RS. The roll of Whitnall's ligament in ptosis surgery. Arch Ophthalmol. 1979;97: 705–7.

89. Anderson RL, Dixon RS. Aponeurotic ptosis surgery. Arch Ophthalmol. 1979;13:1123–8.
90. Anderson RL. Age of aponeurotic awareness. Plast Reconstr Surg. 1985;1:77–9.
91. Small RG. The A-frame operation for acquired blepharoptosis. Arch Ophthalmol. 1980;98(3):516–9.
92. Baker SS, Muenzler WS, Small RG, Leonard JE. Carbon dioxide laser blepharoplasty. Ophthalmology. 1984;91(3):238–44.
93. Meltzer MA, Elahi E, Taupeka P, Flores E. A simplified technique of ptosis repair using a single adjustables uture.O phthalmology.2001; 108(10):1889–92.

Chapter3
Eyelid Anatomy and Physiology with Reference toB lepharoptosis

Jonathan J. Dutton and Bartley R. Frueh

Abstract The eyelids provide mechanical protection to the globe, produce chemical elements to the precorneal tear film, and help distribute these layers evenly over the surface of the eye. Eyelid motility requires a sophisticated interplay of muscles and suspensory systems that are intimately related to ocular movements, coordinated by fine sensory and motor control mechanisms. This chapter reviews anatomy and physiology of the eyelids and its suspensory system as a foundation for later chapters on evaluation and surgery for blepharoptosis repair. We also discuss the forces that determine eyelid position and complex blinking movements. These include those forces exerted by the levator and supratarsal muscles and the nature of their attachments, the anterior/posterior position of the eye, and the forces of gravity. Specific fiber types and their metabolic differences are important factors in understanding the function of the levator muscle, Müller's sympathetic muscle, and their relationship to extraocular and other skeletal muscles.

Introduction

The eyelids serve several valuable functions. Most importantly, they provide mechanical protection to the globe. They also provide vital chemical elements to the precorneal tear film, and help distribute these layers evenly over the surface of the eye. During the blink phase, the eyelids propel tears to the medial canthus where they enter the puncta of the lacrimal drainage system. The eyelashes along the lid margins sweep air-borne particles from in front of the eye, and the constant voluntary and reflex movements of the eyelids protect the cornea from injury and glare. The ability of the eyelids to cover the eye and rapidly retract requires a sophisticated interplay of muscles and suspensory systems that are intimately related to ocular movements, coordinated by fine sensory and motor control mechanisms.

EyelidA natomy

In the young adult, the interpalpebral fissure measures 10–11 mm in vertical height. In middle age, this is reduced to only about 8–10 mm [1], and in old age the fissure may be only 6–8 mm. In the primary position of gaze, the upper eyelid margin usually lies at the superior corneal limbus in children and 1.5–2.0 mm below it in the adult. In the presence of ptosis, the margin of the upper eyelid will typically overhang the superior corneal limbus by at least 1 mm beyond these limits, although there is no specific definition in terms of palpebral fissure measurement.

The margin of each eyelid is about 2-mm thick. Posteriorly, the marginal tarsal surface is covered with conjunctival epithelium, interrupted

J.J.D utton (✉)
DepartmentofO phthalmology,
University of North Carolina – Chapel Hill,
ChapelH ill, NC USA
e-mail:jona than_dutton@med.unc.edu

A.J. Cohen and D.A. Weinberg (eds.), *Evaluation and Management of Blepharoptosis*,
DOI 10.1007/978-0-387-92855-5_3, © Springer Science+Business Media, LLC 2011

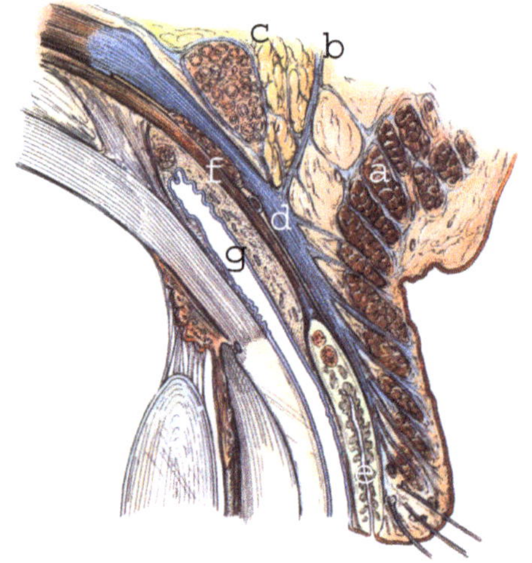

Fig. 3.1 Sagittal cross-section of the upper eyelid. (**a**) Orbicularis muscle; (**b**) orbital septum; (**c**) preaponeurotic fat pad; (**d**) levator aponeurosis; (**e**) tarsal plate; (**f**) Müller's supratarsal muscle; (**g**)c onjunctiva

by the meibomian gland orifices (Fig. 3.1). Anteriorly, the margin is covered with cutaneous epidermis from which emerge the eyelashes. The gray line is a faint linear zone separating these two regions. Between the skin and conjunctiva are layered from front to back the orbicularis muscle, the orbital septum, the preaponeurotic fat pockets, the levator aponeurosis, and Müller's supratarsalmus cle.

Eyelid Skin

The skin covers the external surface of the body and provides significant protection against trauma, solar radiation, temperature extremes, and desiccation. It also allows for major interaction with the environment. It plays a significant role in eyelid function and must be able to flex and stretch without impeding eyelid movement.

The skin of the eyelid is the thinnest in the body owing to only a scant development of the dermis and subcutaneous fat. The epidermis is the outer layer of the skin, averaging about 0.05 mm in thickness, compared to the palms and soles where it can attain a thickness of 1.5 mm. It contains no blood vessels and is dependent upon the underlying dermis for its nutrients. The epidermis also contains several specialized types of cells. Melanocytes of neural crest origin are scattered among the keratinocytes in the deeper layers of the epidermis. They produce melanin that protects the skin from UV radiation. Langerhans cells, or epidermal dendritic cells, serve as antigen-presenting cells that ingest and process foreign antigens.

Beneath the epidermis is the basement membrane and below that the dermis. On the eyelids, the dermis is about 0.3 mm in thickness, and it contains collagen, elastic tissue, and reticular fibers as well as fibroblasts, mast cells, nerve endings, lymphatics, and epidermal appendages surrounded by a ground substance of mucopolysaccharides, chondroitin sulfates, and glycoproteins.

A number of epidermal appendages lined with epithelium lie within the dermis. These include hair follicles associated with an arrectopili muscle attached to the dermal–epidermal junction. Apocrine sweat glands of Moll are coiled glands in the deep dermis that empty into the uppermost portion of the hair follicle. Apocrine glands produce a more viscous secretion with cellular debris and are concentrated along the eyelid margins.

Sebaceous glands contain epithelium that is an outgrowth of the external root sheath of the hair follicle. These produce products of complex oils, fatty acids, wax, and cholesterol esters called sebum. A large sebaceous gland is associated with each hair follicle and empties its secretions directly into the follicle. Additional small sebaceous glands, called glands of Zeis, are present between hair follicles and discharge their contents directly onto the skin surface. Eccrine sweat glands are also present in the dermis and open directly onto the epidermal surface. Eccrine glands secrete a clear fluid composed of water, salts, glycogen, and sialomucin.

Blood vessels and nerve endings course throughout the dermis where they derive from similar structures in the subdermis and deep fascia. Specialized sensory structures called Meissner's and Vater–Pacini corpuscles within the dermis transmit sensations for touch and pressure.

Beneath the dermis is a subcutaneous layer of fat and connective tissue. Subcutaneous fat is very sparse beneath the preseptal portion of the eyelid skin, and absent from the more distal pretarsal portions. Beneath the skin, within the eyelid are also found other structures that can be the focus for disease processes. On the subconjunctival side of the eyelid structures include the accessory lacrimal glands of Krause and Wolfring that are concentrated on the lateral side of the eyelid; the meibomian glands, which are modified sebaceous glands are found diffusely within the tarsal plates.

The Orbicularis Muscle

The orbicularis oculi is a complex striated muscle that lies just below the skin. Its main function is, as a protractor of the eyelid, allowing not only forced closure but also delicate coordinated adjustments in position, working with the levator–Müller's muscle complex and the extraocular muscles. Abnormalities in these coordinated actions can result in eyelid disorders, such as inability to open the eye in apraxia of eyelid opening.

The orbicularis muscle is divided anatomically into three contiguous parts – the orbital, preseptal, and pretarsal portions (Fig. 3.2). The orbital portion overlies the bony orbital rims. It arises from insertions on the frontal process of the maxillary bone, the orbital process of the frontal bone, and from the common medial canthal tendon. Its fibers pass around the orbital rim to form a continuous ellipse without interruption at the lateral palpebral commissure, and insert just below their points of origin.

The palpebral portion of the orbicularis muscle overlies the mobile eyelid from the orbital rims to the eyelid margins. The muscle fibers sweep circumferentially around each lid as a half ellipse, fixed medially and laterally at the canthal tendons. Although this portion forms a single anatomic unit in each eyelid, it is customarily further divided topographically into two parts: the preseptal and pretarsal orbicularis.

The preseptal portion of the muscle is positioned over the orbital septum in both upper and lower eyelids, and its fibers originate perpendicularly along the upper and lower borders of the medial canthal tendon. Fibers arc around the eyelids and insert along the lateral horizontal raphé. The pretarsal portion of the muscle overlies the tarsal plates. Its fibers originate from the

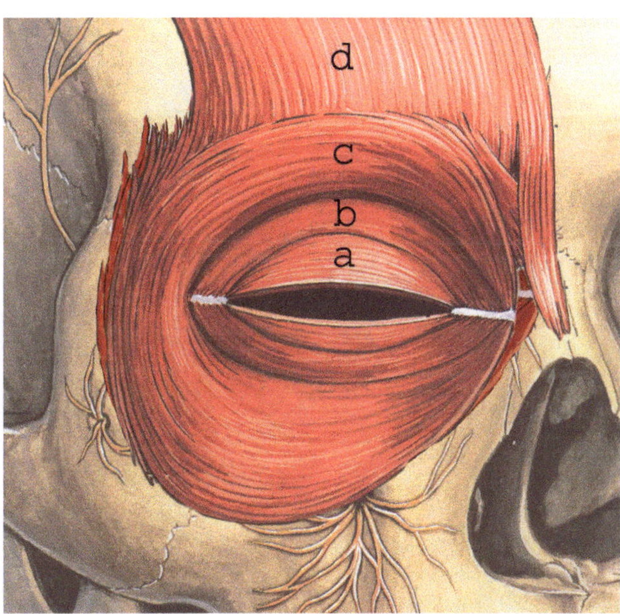

Fig.3.2 Orbicularis and frontalis muscles. (**a**) Pretarsal portion; (**b**) preseptal portion; (**c**) orbital portion; (**d**)f rontalis muscle

medial canthal tendon via separate superficial and deep heads, arch around the lids and insert onto the lateral canthal tendon and raphé. Contraction of these fibers aids in the lacrimal pump mechanism [2]. Medially, the deep heads of the pretarsal fibers fuse to form a prominent bundle of fibers, Horner's muscle, which runs just behind the posterior limb of the canthal tendon. It inserts onto the posterior lacrimal crest. Horner's muscle helps maintain the posterior position of the canthal angle, tightens the eyelids against the globe during eyelid closure, and may aid in the lacrimal pump mechanism [3].

The Orbital Septum

The orbital septum is a thin fibrous multilayered membrane anatomically fused to bone at the arcus marginalis along the orbital rim, and it represents an anterior continuation of the orbital fascial system. Distal fibers of the orbital septum merge into the anterior surface of the levator aponeurosis (Fig. 3.3) [4, 5]. In Caucasians, the point of insertion is usually about 3–5 mm above the tarsal plate, but may be as high as 10–15 mm [6]. In the Asian eyelid, the septum inserts into the aponeurosis closer to the eyelid margin. A loose fascial layer that may sometimes contain significant adipose tissue binds the septal layers to the overlying orbicularis muscle. This fascial layer extends from the septum–levator junction inferiorly along the levator aponeurosis to within a few millimeters of the eyelid margin and serves to weld together the anterior and posterior lamellae below the eyelid crease. This has been referred to as the septal extension [7]. It is important to identify the orbital septum during ptosis surgery. In the lower eyelid, the septum fuses with the capsulopalpebral fascia several millimeters below tarsus, and the common fascial sheet inserts into the inferior tarsal edge [8, 9].

The septum can always be identified at surgery by pulling it distally and noting firm resistance against its bony attachments. Inadvertent shortening of the septum instead of the levator during ptosis surgery can result in significant postoperative lagophthalmos. Immediately behind the septum are yellow fat pockets that lie immediately anterior to the levator aponeurosis in the upper lid and the capsulopalpebral fascia in the lower lid. This anatomical relationship is important to note since identification of the levator aponeurosis is critical in many eyelid surgical procedures. Sometimes, the sub-brow fat pad will extend

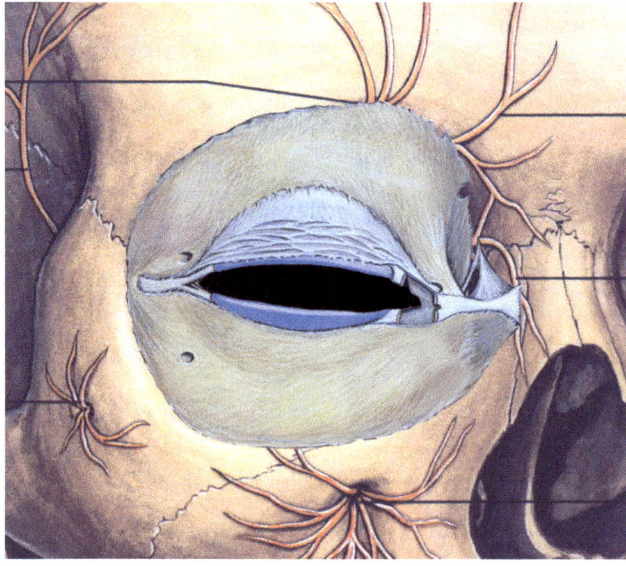

Fig.3.3 Theorbita ls eptum originating from the arcus marginalisof t heor bitalr im

into the eyelid anterior to the septum. In such cases, the septum can be misidentified as the levator aponeurosis.

Any restriction in the movement of the septum with the levator and orbicularis muscles, as with scarring from trauma or previous surgery, can result in a mechanical ptosis, retraction, or lagophthalmos.

The Preaponeurotic Fat Pockets

The preaponeurotic fat pockets in the upper eyelid and the precapsulopalpebral fat pockets in the lower eyelid are anterior extensions of extraconal orbital fat. These eyelid fat pockets are surgically important landmarks and help identify a plane immediately anterior to the major eyelid retractor, which is the levator aponeurosis. In the upper eyelid, there are typically two fat pockets: a medial pocket and a central one. Laterally, the lacrimal gland may be mistaken for a third fat pocket, although the color and texture are different, i.e., the lacrimal gland is more tan or pink in hue and firmer than the preaponeurotic fat. In the lower eyelid, there are three pockets: medial, central, and lateral. Occasionally, there is extensive fatty infiltration of Müller's muscle. During ptosis surgery, it is important to recognize this since in these cases the aponeurosis lies anterior to this fatty layer and the next posterior layer is conjunctiva.

The Major Eyelid Retractors

The retractors of the upper eyelid consist of the striated levator palpebrae muscle and the smooth Müller's sympathetic muscle. They function together to elevate the eyelid in a complex interplay relying on involuntary proprioceptive receptors mainly in Müller's muscle, voluntary contractions of the levator coordinated with the vertical extraocular muscles, and voluntary and reflex arc movements of the orbicularis muscle.

TheL evatorMus cle and Aponeurosis

In congenital ptosis, the levator muscle has been thought to be dystrophic. However, Edmonds et al. failed to find any histochemical differences between levator muscle fibers in normal individuals and those with congenital ptosis [10]. On the other hand, Iljin et al. [11] found that in congenital ptosis the levator muscle shows varying amounts of hypoplasia, decreased number and varying diameter of muscle fibers, collagen proliferation, mitochondrial loss, and hypoplasia in the endomysium and perimysium. They reported that the clinical severity of ptosis correlated with the degree of histopathologic changes.

In involutional ptosis, the pathology is generally thought to result from aponeurotic linkage failure, either disinsertion or more commonly redundancy. However, it has been shown that there is a correlation between degree of ptosis and reduced levator muscle function, suggesting levator muscle dysfunction as a possible additionalc ontributingf actor [12].

The levator muscle arises from the lesser sphenoid wing just above the annulus of Zinn. The muscle runs forward in the superior orbit just above the superior rectus muscle. Near the superior orbital rim, a condensation is seen in the muscle sheath [9], which forms the superior suspensory fascia of the levator system. This suspensory fascia is also referred to as Whitnall's ligament. Its anterior component is formed by a thickening of the levator sheath, and its thicker posterior component represents a thickening of the common sheath separating the levator muscle from the underlying superior rectus muscle [13]. This posterior component has been referred to as the intermuscular transverse ligament by Lukas et al. [14] and appears to be the same structure referred to as the conjoint fascial sheath by Hwang et al. [15]. These fascial bands surrounding the levator muscle attach medially and laterally to the orbital walls and soft tissues, and fibers also blend with Tenon's capsule below. These are important suspensory structures for the levator muscle/aponeurosis complex and

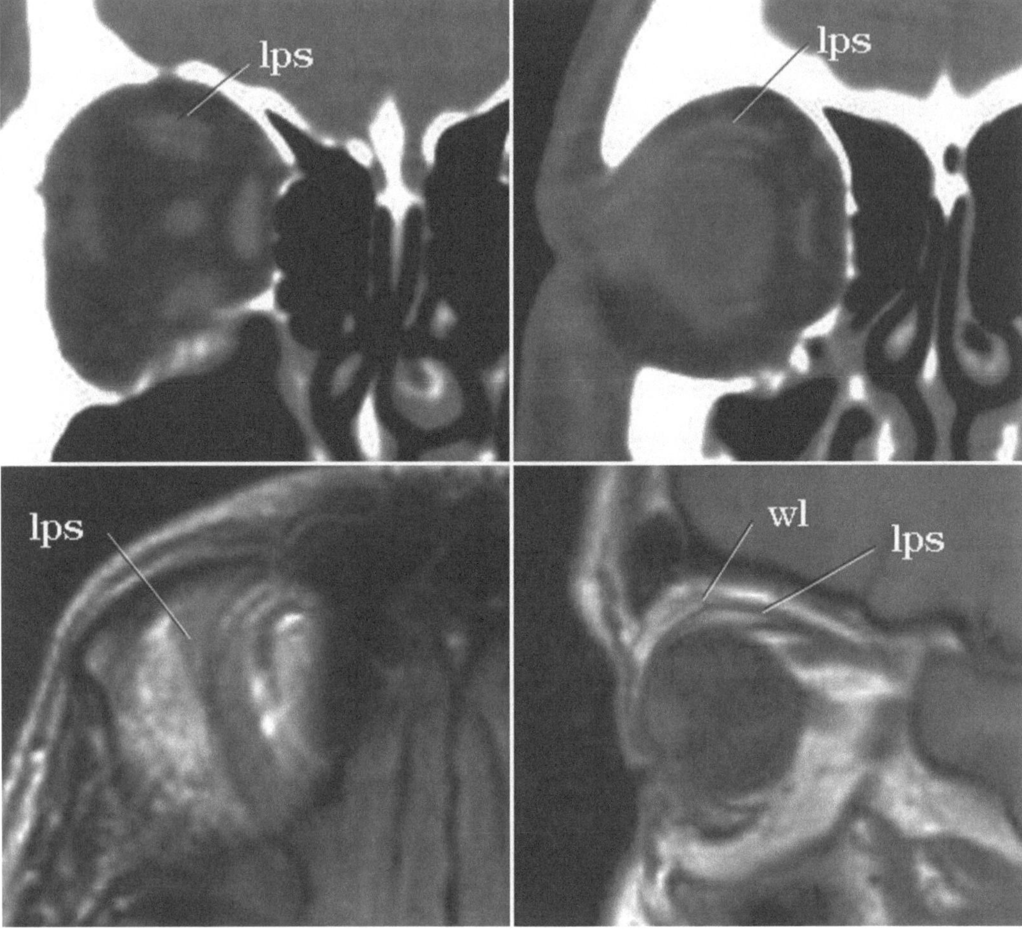

Fig.3.4 Radiologic imaging of the levator muscle. *lps* levator palpebrae superioris muscle, *wl*W hitnall'sl igament

therefore should not be cut during ptosis surgery. A framework of fine fascial strands loosely suspends this fascial structure to the orbital roof. While the exact role of Whitnall's ligament has been a matter of controversy, it appears to provide some support for the orbital fascial systems that maintain spatial relationships between a variety of anatomic structures in the superior orbit. However, the ligament does not correspond to the highest point of levator vector change, and MRI studies have shown that the ligament moves significantly with eyelid elevation, so that it clearly does not act as a fulcrum for the levator as the latter changes its vector from horizontal in the orbit to vertical in the eyelid (Fig. 3.4).

From Whitnall's ligament, the muscle passes into its aponeurosis (Fig. 3.5). This structure has been shown to be made up of several layers. A thicker anterior layer terminates near the junction of the aponeurosis with the orbital septum. In the Caucasian double eyelid, this layer sends numerous delicate interconnecting slips forward and downward through the postorbicular fascial tissue to insert into the interfascicular septa of the pretarsal orbicularis muscle and subcutaneous tissue of the skin. These multilayered slips maintain the close approximation of the skin, muscle, aponeurosis, and tarsal lamellae, thus integrating the distal eyelid as a single functional unit. This relationship defines the upper eyelid crease of the western eyelid [16]. In the single

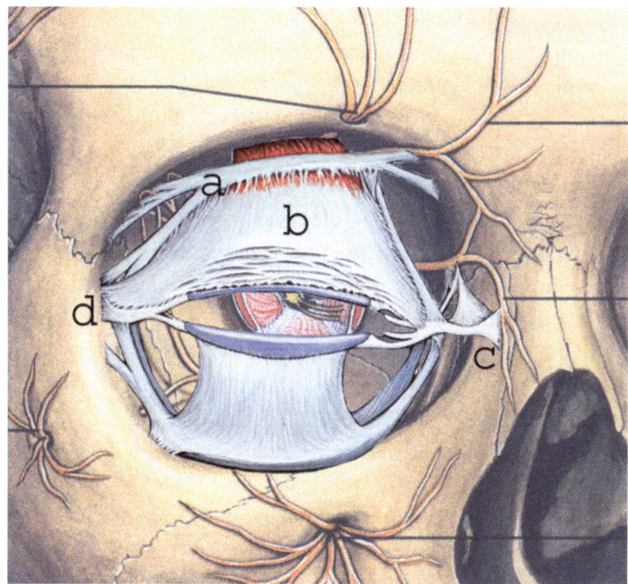

Fig.3.5 Anteriororb italf ascial system. (**a**) Whitnall's ligament; (**b**) levator aponeurosis; (**c**) medial canthal tendon; (**d**)la teralc anthalte ndon

Asian eyelid, these anterior fibrous slips are less well developed or absent [17]. A thinner posterior layer of the aponeurosis is in contact with Müller's supratarsal muscle and fuses with the anterior surface of the tarsus. Reid et al. [7] stressed that failure to recognize this layer could result in failure of ptosis surgery and postoperativela gophthalmos.

Both layers of the aponeurosis contain scattered smooth muscle fibers, more heavily concentratedinthe pos teriorla yer [18].

The levator aponeurosis is most firmly attached at about 3–4 mm above the eyelid margin [19, 20]. While the aponeurosis partially inserts onto the anterior surface of tarsus, most of its fibers insert onto the overlying orbicularis muscle interfascicular sheaths. As the aponeurosis passes into the eyelid from Whitnall's ligament, it broadens to form the medial and lateral "horns." The lateral horn forms a prominent fibrous sheet that indents the posterior aspect of the lacrimal gland, defining its orbital and palpebral lobes. It inserts through numerous slips onto the lateral orbital tubercle of the zygomatic bone, at the lateral retinaculum. The medial horn is less well developed. It blends with the intermediate layer of the orbital septum and inserts onto the posterior crus of the medial canthal tendon and the posterior lacrimal crest. Together, the two horns serve to distribute the forces of the levator muscle along the aponeurosis and the tarsal plate.

In the lower eyelid, the capsulopalpebral fascia is a fibrous sheet arising from Lockwood's ligament and the sheaths around the inferior rectus and inferior oblique muscles. It passes upward and generally fuses with fibers of the orbital septum about 4–5 mm below the tarsal plate. From this junction, a common fascial sheet continues upward and inserts into the lower border of tarsus. Fine fibrous slips pass forward from this fascial sheet to the orbicularis intermuscular septae and subcutaneous tissue, forming the lower eyelid crease and uniting the anterior and posterior lamellae into a single functionalunit.

The Sympathetic Eyelid Retractors

Smooth muscles innervated by the sympathetic nervous system are present in both upper and lower eyelid and serve as accessory retractors [21]. In the upper eyelid, the supratarsal muscle of Müller originates abruptly from the under surface of the levator muscle just anterior to Whitnall's ligament [22]. It runs downward, posterior to the levator aponeurosis, to which it is adherent, and inserts onto the anterior edge of the superior tarsal border. Muscle fibers are intermixed with connective tissue, fat and blood vessels. Laterally, Müller's muscle extends along with the levator aponeurosis between the orbital and palpebral lobes of the lacrimal gland, where it interdigitates with the ductules passing between the two lobes. These lateral fibers may contribute to the lateral flare commonly seen in patients witht hyroide yed isease [23].

In the lower eyelid, the sympathetically innervated inferior tarsal muscle is less well defined. Fibers run behind the capsulopalpebral fascia to insert onto the lower border of tarsus, although they may end 2–5 mm below tarsus [24]. As noted above, the levator aponeurosis does not have any major attachment to the tarsus, and it is likely that Müller's muscle helps transmit the levator force to the tarsal plate and conjunctiva [25]. In fact, it is theorized that the Müller's muscle-conjunctival resection procedure for ptosis correction works by plicating levator and enhancing its effect.

Disruption of sympathetic innervation to these muscles results in Horner's syndrome. This is characterized by the classic triad of ptosis, miosis, and ipsilateral anhidrosis of the face. Specific clinical findings vary according to the location of the lesion along the polysynaptic pathway. The upper eyelid ptosis and elevation ("reverse ptosis") of the lower eyelid result from loss of sympathetic smooth muscle tone and therefore reduction in its action as an accessory eyelidre tractor.

The Tarsal Plates

The tarsal plates consist of dense fibrous tissue, approximately 1–1.5 mm thick, that give structural integrity to the eyelids. Each measures about 25 mm in horizontal length and is gently curved to conform to the contour of the anterior globe. The central vertical height of the tarsal plate is 8–12 mm in the upper eyelid and 3.5–4.0 mm in the lower. Medially and laterally, they taper to 2 mm in height as they pass into the canthal tendons. As these tarsal plates approach the canthal tendons, they widen toward the eyelid margin, thus assuming a more triangular cross-section. Within each tarsus are the Meibomian glands, approximately 25 in the upper lid and 20 in the lower lid. These are holocrine-secreting sebaceous glands not associated with lash follicles. Each gland is multilobulated and empties into a central ductule that opens onto the posterior eyelid margin behind the gray line. They produce the lipid layer of the precorneal tear film.

The Canthal Tendons

Medially, the tarsal plates pass into fibrous bands that form the crura of the medial canthal tendon. These lie between the orbicularis muscle anteriorly and the conjunctiva posteriorly. The superior and inferior crura fuse to form a stout common tendon that inserts via three limbs (Fig. 3.5) [2]. The anterior limb inserts onto the orbital process of the maxillary bone in front of and above the anterior lacrimal crest. It provides the major support for the medial canthal angle. The posterior limb arises from the common tendon near the junction of the superior and inferior crura and passes between the canaliculi. It inserts onto the posterior lacrimal crest just in front of Horner's muscle. The posterior limb (Horner's muscle) directs the vector forces of the canthal angle backward to maintain close approximation with the globe. The superior limb of the medial canthal tendon arises as a broad arc of fibers from both the anterior and posterior limbs. It passes upward to insert onto the orbital process of the frontal bone. The posterior head of the preseptal orbicularis muscle inserts onto this limb, and the unit forms the soft-tissue roof of the lacrimal sac fossa. This tendinous extension may function to provide vertical support to the canthal angle [26], but also appears to play a significant role in the lacrimal pump mechanism.

Laterally, the tarsal plates pass into fibrous strands that interdigitate and blend into the orbital septum. The lateral canthal tendon is a distinct entity, separate from the orbicularis muscle. It measure about 1 mm in thickness, 3 mm in width, and approximately 5–7 mm in length [27]. The insertion of these fibers extends posteriorly along the lateral orbital wall, where it blends with strands of the lateral check ligament from the sheath of the lateral rectus muscle. With age the tendon becomes lax, allowing the canthal angle to move several millimeters with up and downg aze [27].

The Conjunctiva

The conjunctiva is a mucous membrane that covers the posterior surface of the eyelids and the anterior surface of the globe, except for the cornea. The palpebral portion is closely applied to the posterior surface of the tarsal plate and the sympathetic tarsal muscle of Müller. It is continuous around the fornices above and below where it joins the bulbar conjunctiva. Small accessory lacrimal glands are located within the submucosal connective tissue.

At the medial canthal angle is a small mound of tissue called the caruncle. This consists of modified skin containing hairs, sebaceous glands, and sweat glands. Just lateral to the caruncle, there is a vertical fold of conjunctiva, the plica semilunaris. The submucosa of this tissue contains adipose cells and smooth muscle fibers, resembling the nictitating membrane of lower vertebrates. This likely represents a vestigial structure that has been modified to allow enough horizontal slack at the shallow medial fornix for rotation of the globe.

Nerves to the Eyelids

The motor nerves to the orbicularis muscle derive from the facial nerve (N. VII) through its temporal and zygomatic branches (Fig. 3.6). The facial nerve divides into two divisions: an upper temporofacial division and a lower cervicofacial division [28]. The upper division further subdivides into the temporal and zygomatic branches that innervate the frontalis and orbicularis muscles. The lower cervicofacial division gives rise to the buccal, mandibular, and cervical branches, innervating muscles of the lower face and neck. There can be considerable variation in the branching pattern of these nerves, and in some individuals extensive anastomoses interconnect all of these peripheral branches.

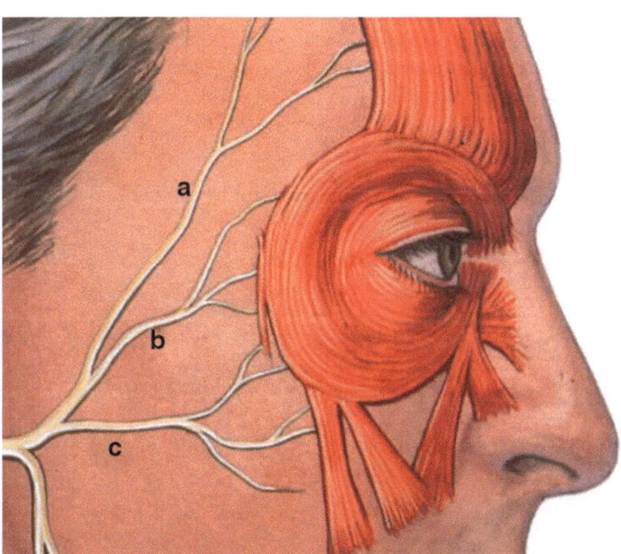

Fig. 3.6 Motor branches of the seventh cranial nerve to the eyelid and brow muscles. (**a**) Frontal branch; (**b**) zygomatic branch; (**c**) buccal branch

The sensory nerves to the eyelids derive from the ophthalmic and maxillary divisions of the trigeminal nerve. Sensory input from the upper lid passes to the ophthalmic division through its main terminal branches, the supraorbital, supratrochlear, and lacrimal nerves. The infratrochlear nerve receives sensory information from the extreme medial portion of both the upper and lower eyelids. The zygomaticotemporal branch of the lacrimal nerve innervates the lateral portion of the upper eyelid and temple. These branches also innervate portions of the adjacent brow, forehead, and nasal bridge. The lower eyelid sends sensory impulses to the maxillary division via the infraorbital nerve. The zygomaticofacial branch from the lacrimal nerve innervates the lateral portion of the lower lid and part of the infratrochlear branch receives input from the medial lower lid.

Vascular Supply to the Eyelids

Vascular supply to the eyelids is extensive. The posterior eyelid lamellae receive blood through the palpebral arterial arcades (Fig. 3.7). In the upper eyelid, a marginal arcade runs about 2 mm above the eyelid margin and a peripheral arcade extends along the upper border of tarsus between the levator aponeurosis and Müller's muscle. These vessels are supplied medially by the superior medial palpebral vessels from the terminal ophthalmic artery and laterally by the superior lateral palpebral vessel from the lacrimal artery. The lower lid arcade receives blood from the medial and lateral inferior palpebral vessels.

The venous drainage system is somewhat less well defined than the arterial system. Drainage is primarily into several large vessels of the facial system (Fig. 3.8). Lymphatic drainage from the

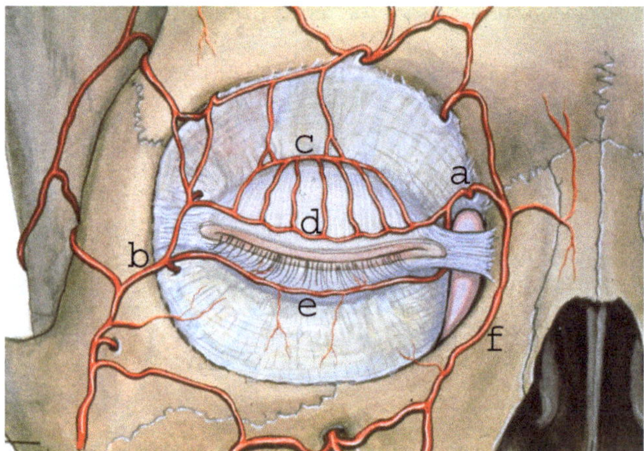

Fig.3.7 Arterial supply to the eyelids. (**a**) Medial palpebral artery; (**b**) lateral palpebral artery; (**c**) superior peripheral arcade; (**d**) superior marginal arcade; (**e**) inferior marginal arcade; (**f**)a ngulara rtery

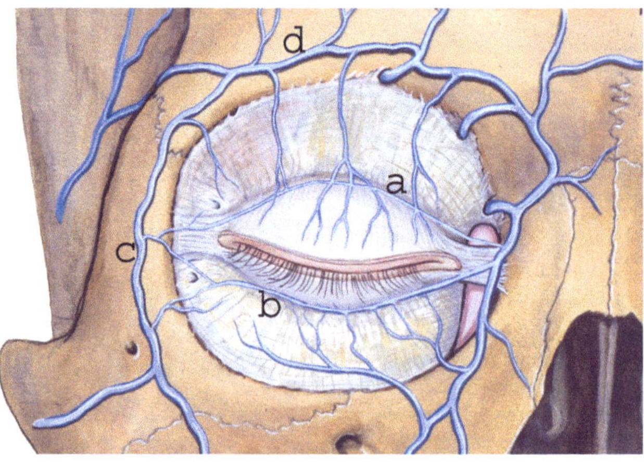

Fig.3.8 Venouss upplyf rom the eyelids. (**a**) Superior venous arcade; (**b**) inferior venous arcade; (**c**) angular vein; (**d**)s uperiorpa lpebral vein

eyelids is restricted to the region anterior to the orbital septum. Drainage from the lateral two-thirds of the upper eyelid and the lateral one-third of the lower eyelid is inferior and lateral into the deep and superficial parotid and sub-mandibular lymph nodes. Drainage from the medial one-third of the upper eyelid and the medial two-thirds of the lower eyelid is medially and inferiorly into the anterior cervical lymph nodes. Extensive excision of subcutaneous eyelid tissues or deep incisions in the inferolateral eyelid or in the deep conjunctival fornix can result in protracted lymphedema due to disruptionofthe sev essels.

UpperEyel idP hysiology

To understand the position of the upper eyelid, we must first understand the forces that determine the position. These will include those forces exerted by the levator muscle and the nature of its attachments, the superior tarsal muscle and the nature of its attachments, the orbicularis oculi muscles, the anterior/posterior position of the eye, and gravity. In this section, we will look at the nature of the three muscles that move the eyelid and their interactions. We will answer the questions (1) What are the elements of the muscle we are assessing when we measure "levator function?" (2) What determines the force a muscle can generate? (3) What is the role of Müller's muscle in eyelid position?

It is appropriate to begin with a quick review of the basic elements of a muscle and then see how they apply to the muscles in question. Striated muscle is made up of bundles of muscle fibers, with each fiber containing multiple, linked sarcomeres, the basic muscle unit, each containing multiple myofibrils. The synaptic terminal of a motor neuron releases acetylcholine. This depolarizes the muscle cell, and an action potential is propagated into the transverse tubules at the ends of the sarcomeres and triggers calcium release from the sarcoplasmic reticulum. In the center of each myofibril sarcomere is the thick filament, which has multiple myosin heads coming off it. These heads contain ATP (adenosine triphosphate) binding sites into which fit ATP, the potential energy for muscle contraction. They also contain actin binding sites, into which fit molecules of actin on the thin filament. The head has a "hinge" at the point where it leaves the core of the thick myofilament, which allows the head to swivel back and forth, and the "swiveling" is what actually causes muscle contraction, as it works its way down the actin molecules on the thin, peripheral filament. There are three proteins on the thin filaments (1) Tropomysin – in a relaxed muscle, the myosin heads of the thick myofilament lie against tropomysin molecules of the thin myofilament. As long as the myosin heads remain in contact with tropomysin nothing happens (i.e., a muscle remains relaxed). (2) Troponin – troponin molecules have binding sites for calcium ions. When a calcium ion fills this site, it causes a change in the shape and position of troponin. And, when troponin shifts, it pulls the tropomysin to which it is attached. When tropomysin is moved, the myosin head that was touching the tropomyosin now comes into contact with an underlying actin molecule. When actin combines with the myosin head, the ATP associated with the head breaks down into ADP (adenosine diphosphate). This reaction releases energy that causes the myosin head to swivel. The maximum a sarcomere can theoretically shorten is the difference between the length of the thick filament within the sarcomere and the length of the sarcomere when there is minimal overlap of the thick and thin filaments. The maximum a muscle can shorten is the amount each sarcomere can shorten multiplied by the number of sarcomeres in series in the muscle. It has been shown that putting a skeletal muscle on stretch causes it to lengthen by adding sarcomeres [29]. This phenomenon in the levator is suggested by the finding that the upper eyelid excursion has a positive correlation with the exophthalmometer reading in normal subjects ands ubjectsw itht hyroide yed isease [30].

The force a muscle can generate is unrelated to length, but rather is proportional to the cross-sectional area of functioning muscle fibers. To normalize this, the force a studied muscle generates is specified as per cross-sectional area (specific force) and is about the same for all skeletal muscles of all species.

The traditional approach to muscle physiology is to divide skeletal muscles into fast and slow muscles, which can be defined with histologic stains of the muscle cross-section and by single skinned fiber testing. It is the percentage of each type of fiber in the muscle that makes a muscle fast or slow. These findings are reasonably consistent across species. The twitch characteristic of a fast muscle is to reach the peak tension more quickly. Fast muscles also relax more quickly. Slow fibers have a moderate velocity of shortening, and so they consume ATP at a moderate rate. These "red" fibers are well supplied with capillaries have lots of mitochondria, and are moderately sized, thus enabling faster rates of oxygen diffusion. Oxidative phosphorylation in the mitochondria, which produces 36 mol ATP/mole of glucose, is more efficient than glycolysis and slow muscles and therefore are more fatigue resistant than fast fibers. Fast fibers have a high velocity of shortening, which requires a high rate of ATP consumption. These paler ("white") fibers tend to have fewer capillaries and a more extensive sarcoplasmic reticulum to facilitate calcium transients. They need higher stimulation frequency to function best. Fast muscles rely on glycolysis (2–3 mol ATP/mole glucose), and therefore fatigue more easily. The myosin heavy chain or myosin isoforms, demonstrated with electrophoresis, are different for different types of muscles.

Extraocular muscles have fairly unique myosin isoforms and are among the fastest muscles in the body, but are intermediate in fatigue resistance between classical fast and slow muscles. As Table 3.1 shows, in a study done in 1994 [31], the levator, which has 89% intermediate or fast fibers, has a mean time to peak tension of 44 ms, similar to that of the completely fast muscle, extensor digitorum longus (EDL) (33 ms), yet with the same fatigue protocol it retained 55% of its initial force, compared with 20% for the EDL. The soleus, which has predominantly slow fibers, had 82% of its initial force with the same fatigue protocol. All skeletal muscles generate the same specific force (force per cross-sectional area), and it is the same in vitro and in vivo. A peculiarity of extraocular muscles is that they exhibit only about 10% of the specific force in vitro that skeletal muscles exhibit, and yet in vivo generate force equal to that of skeletal muscle [32]. The reason for this is not understood. Using skeletal muscle fiber typing for extraocular muscles is a poor method of comparison because they are so different, but it is the language of classical muscle physiology, and what has been analyzed. Skinned fiber evaluation, looking at Ca^{2+}- and Sr^{2+}-activated isometric contractile properties of single fibers, reveals some curious and very different fibers in extraocular muscles that express both fast- and slow-twitch contractile

Table 3.1 Fiber-type percentage, contractile characteristics, and fatiguability of the extensor digitorum longus muscle, a prototypical fast muscle, the soleus muscle, a prototypical slow muscle, the levator muscle, and the superior rectusmus cle

	TypeI (%, based on mATPase activity)	TypeI I (%, based on mATPase activity)	TPT (ms)	1/2R elaxation time[a](ms)	Fatigability[b] (% of initial force)
EDL	4[c]	96[c]	33[c]	28[c]	20[d]
Soleus	95[c]	5[c]	80[c]	142[c]	82[d]
Levator	11[d]	89[d]	44[d]	53[d]	55[d]
Superiorre ctus	13[d]	87[d]	28[d]	57[d]	35[d]

TPT time to peak tension

[a] 1/2 Relaxation time is the time to relax to one-half the peak tension. The faster the muscle, usually the faster it relaxes

[b] Fatigability: the mean force response was measured before and after a repetitive tetanic stimulation protocol, done over a 5-min interval. The same protocol was used for all muscles

[c] Ryalle ta l. [37]

[d] Fruehe ta l. [31]

characteristics [33]. This suggests the coexistence of fast and slow myosins along the length of some of their muscle fibers. These unusual fibers make up about 36% of all fibers in the levator and superior rectus muscles, contributing to their unique, if incompletely understood, behavior.

There are two clinical tests that can be done to measure the levator integrity. Berke and Johnson [34] introduced us to measuring the eyelid excursion shortly after World War II, to give us a clue about the integrity of the levator muscle and termed this "levator function," a title that has stuck. From the preceding discussion, it can be seen that this measurement reflects the number of functioning sarcomeres strung together in the levator. It is probably comparable only in patients with the same exophthalmometer reading. It is only indirectly related to the strength of the muscle, in that a weak muscle cannot shorten against a load (the eyelid) as much. The other measurement of levator integrity, levator force generation, which is a function of the cross-sectional area of functioning muscle fibers, has been shown to be a more sensitive test of the levator muscle integrity [35]. Unfortunately, a commercial device to measure levator force has not yet been marketed.

The contribution of Müller's, or the superior sympathetic, muscle to eyelid position is tonic, not volitional. It is a curious anomaly in anatomy that it runs in series with the levator muscle and in parallel with the levator aponeurosis. It does not affect either the eyelid excursion or the levator force generation since it is tonic. Its effect is best understood by measuring the changes that occur with stimulating and with paralyzing it. Maximally stimulating it with 10% phenylephrine causes a mean elevation of the eyelid of 1.5 mm (SD 0.6 mm, range 0.5–2.4 mm) [36]. Maximally chemically denervating Müller's muscle with guanethidine 5% and thymoxamine hydrochloride 0.5% causes an eyelid to drop a mean of 1.5 mm (SD 0.4 mm, range 0.9–2.2 mm) [36]. Hence, the tonic stimulation of Müller's muscle is in the middle of the possible range. These data are confirmed by the amount of ptosis usuallys eenw ithH orner'ss yndrome.

References

1. Hrecko T, Farkas LG, Katic M. Clinical significance of age-related changes in the palpebral fissure between ages 2 and18 in healthy Caucasians. Acta Chir Plast. 1968;32:194–204.
2. Dutton JJ. Atlas of clinical and surgical orbital anatomy. Philadelphia: W.B. Saunders; 1994.
3. Ahl NC, Hill JC. Horner's muscle and the lacrimal system. Arch Ophthalmol. 1982;100:488–93.
4. Barker DE. Dye injection studies of orbital fat compartments. Plast Reconstr Surg. 1977;59:82–5.
5. Putterman AM, Urist MJ. Surgical anatomy of the orbital septum. Ann Ophthalmol. 1974;6:290–4.
6. Anderson RL, Dixon RS. The role of Whitnall's ligament in ptosis surgery. Arch Ophthalmol. 1979;97: 705–10.
7. Reid RR, Said HK, Yu M, Haines III GK, Few JW. Revisiting upper eyelid anatomy: introduction of the septal extension. Plast Reconstr Surg. 2006;117: 65–6.
8. Harvey JT, Anderson RL. The aponeurotic approach to eyelid retraction. Ophthalmology. 1981;88: 513–24.
9. Meyer DR, Linberg JV, Wobig JL, McCormick SA. Anatomy of the orbital septum and associated eyelid connective tissue. Ophthal Plast Reconstr Surg. 1991;7:104–13.
10. Edmonds B, Manners RM, Weller RO, Steart P, Collin JR. Levator palpebrae superioris fiber size in normals and patients with congenital ptosis. Eye. 1998;12:47–50.
11. Iljin A, Zielinska A, Karasek M, Zielinski A, Omulecka A. Structural abnormalities in the levator palpebral superioris muscle in patients with congenital blepharoptosis. Ophthalmic Surg Lasers Imaging. 2007;38:283–9.
12. Pereira LS, Hwang TN, Kersten RC, Ray K, McCulley TJ. Levator superior muscle function in involutional blepharoptosis. Am J Ophthalmol. 2008;145: 1095–8.
13. Ettle A, Priglinger S, Kramer J, Koornneef L. Functional anatomy of the levator palpebrae superioris muscle and its connective tissue system. Br J Ophthalmol.1996; 80:702–7.
14. Lukas JR, Priglinger S, Denk M, Mayr R. Two fibromuscular transverse ligaments related to the levator palpebrae superioris: Whitnall's ligament and an intermuscular transverse ligament. Anat Rec. 1996; 246:415–22.
15. Hwang K, Shin YH, Kim DJ. Conjoint fascial sheath of the levator and superior rectus attached to the conjunctival fornix. J Craniofac Surg. 2008;19:241–5.
16. Galatoire O, Touitou V, Heran F, Amar N, Jacomet PV, Gheck L, et al. High resolution magnetic resonance imaging of the upper eyelid: correlation with the position of the skin crease in the upper eyelid. Orbit.2007; 26:165–71.

17. Morikawa K, Yamamoto H, Uchinuma E, Yamashina S. Scanning electron microscopic study on double and single eyelids in Orientals. Aesthetic Plast Surg. 2001;25:20–4.
18. Kakizaki H, Zako M, Nakano T, Asamoto K, Miyaishi O, Iwaki M. The levator aponeurosis consists of two layers that include smooth muscle. Ophthal Plast Reconstr Surg. 2005;21:379–82.
19. Anderson RL, Beard C. The levator aponeurosis. Attachments and their clinical significance. Arch Ophthalmol.1977 ;95:1437–41.
20. Collin JRO, Beard C, Wood I. Experimental and clinical data on the insertion of the levator palpebrae superioris muscle. Am J Ophthalmol. 1987;85:792–801.
21. Manson PN, Lazarus RB, Magar R, Iliff N. Pathways of sympathetic innervation to the superior and inferior (Müllers) tarsal muscles. Plast Reconstr Surg. 1986;78:33–40.
22. Kuwabara T, Cogan DG, Johnson CC. Structure of the muscles of the upper eyelid. Arch Ophthalmol. 1975;93:1189–97.
23. Morton AD, Elner VM, White VA. Lateral extensions of the Müller muscle. Arch Ophthalmol. 1996;114: 1496–8.
24. Hawes MJ, Dortzbach RK. The microscopic anatomy of the lower eyelid retractors. Arch Ophthalmol. 1982;100:1313–8.
25. Bang YH, Park SH, Kim JH, Cho JH, Lee CJ, Roh TS. The role of Müller's muscle reconsidered. Plast Reconstr Surg. 1998;101:1200–4.
26. Anderson RL. The medial canthal tendon branches out. Arch Ophthalmol. 1977;95:2951–61.
27. Cruz AA, Távora DB, Martin LF. Effect of eyelid saccades on the position of lateral canthus in young and older subjects. Orbit. 2008;27:1–4.
28. Malone B, Maisel RH. Anatomy of the facial nerve. Am J Otolaryngol. 1988;9:494–504.
29. Maxwell LC, Carlson DS, McNamara JA, Faulkner JA. Adaptation of the masseter and temporalis muscles following alteration in length, with or without surgical detachment. Anat Rec. 1981;200: 127–37.
30. Frueh BR, Garber FW, Musch DC. The effects of Graves' eye disease on levator muscle function. Ophthalmic Surg. 1986;17:142–5.
31. Frueh BR, Hayes A, Lynch GS, Williams DA. Contractile properties and temperature sensitivity of the extraocular muscles, levator and superior rectus of the rabbit. J Physiol. 1994;475(2):327–36.
32. Frueh BR, Gregorevic P, Williams DA, Lynch GS. Specific force of the rat extraocular muscles, levator and superior rectus, measured in situ. J Neurophysiol. 2001;85(3):1027–32.
33. Lynch GS, Frueh BR, Williams DA. Contractile properties of single skinned fibres from the extraocular muscles, levator and superior rectus, of the rabbit. J Physiol. 1994;475(2):337–46.
34. Berke R. Personal communication with Carl C. Johnson.1991.
35. Frueh BR, Musch DC. Evaluation of levator muscle integrity in ptosis with levator force measurements. Ophthalmology.19 96;103:244–50.
36. Felt DP, Frueh BR. A pharmacologic study of the sympathetic eyelid tarsal muscles. Ophthal Plast Reconstr Surg. 1988;4:15–24.
37. Ryall JG, Schertzer JD, Lynch GS. Attenuation of age-related muscle wasting and weakness in rats after formoterol treatment: therapeutic implications for sarcopenia. J Gerontol A Biol Sci Med Sci. 2007;62A:813–23.

PartI I
Approach to the Ptosis Patient

Chapter4
RiskFac torA ssessmentPr iort oPt osisSur gery

David I. Silbert

Abstract Careful documentation of history and physical findings are important in guiding the ptosis surgeon to carefully select the specific procedure most appropriate for any given patient. It will also help establish which patients are at greater risk for complications with surgical intervention. This chapter will detail the thought processes behind testing and history taking as well as discuss documentation necessary prior to scheduling a patient for ptosis repair. It will review a number of medical issues that may impact the surgical outcome and should be considered prior to surgery. Careful attention to the many issues discussed in this chapter will allow the surgeon to realistically present the patient with the risks inherent in their procedure, and keep patient expectations in line with reality.

Introduction

Prior to performing ptosis repair, it is critically important to obtain a good history and perform a thorough physical examination. The history and physical findings will allow the selection of the appropriate ptosis procedure, establish whether additional diagnostic testing is needed, and identify risk factors for ptosis surgery. Early recognition of risk factors will help in avoiding an unhappy patient. One of the most important issues to address prior to undertaking ptosis surgery is the determination of whether a patient can tolerate the procedure.

OcularSur faceDi sease

Dry eye syndrome and other ocular surface problems are best identified and treated preoperatively, as they are likely to become more symptomatic following surgery. Patients may have dry eye symptoms without significant physical findings. Therefore, it is important to question patients concerning ocular discomfort, tearing that worsens outdoors in windy or cold conditions (reflex tearing), or episodic blurring of vision that improves with blinking. Querying patients about the use of prescription or over-the-counter drops, gels or ointments for dry eyes is helpful. Dry eye syndrome may be associated with systemic autoimmune disease or the use of certain oral medication classes. Many eye medications, such as glaucoma drops, over-the-counter topical vasoconstrictors, or any preservative-containing topical drug, may cause ocular surface irritation and inflammation.

It is important to instruct the patient that treatment for dry eye syndrome and exposure keratopathy may need to be initiated or increased after surgery and that the treatment could be required either temporarily or long term. This should be documented in the informed consent. Some surgeons perform tear production testing

D.I.Silbe rt (✉)
FAAP – Family Eye Group, Lancaster PA,
Mechanicsburg, PA USA
e-mail:s ilbert@supernet.com

A.J. Cohen and D.A. Weinberg (eds.), *Evaluation and Management of Blepharoptosis*,
DOI 10.1007/978-0-387-92855-5_4, © Springer Science+Business Media, LLC 2011

prior to ptosis repair, but this is not a universal practice. It is the author's practice to perform Schirmer II testing with topical anesthesia after drying the palpebral conjunctiva with a cotton tip applicator. This is felt to be a better indication of basal tear production compared with Schirmer I testing without anesthesia. The use of proparacaine is preferred over manufactured fluorescein solutions that contain preservatives that may alter Schirmer test results [1]. The amount of wetting is measured at 5 min. Readings under 10 mm are indicative of dry eyes, and under 5 mm, extremely dry. Caution should be exercised when approaching ptosis repair in patients with extremely dry eyes. Starting an aggressive regimen of ocular surface lubrication preoperatively and performing less aggressive lid elevation, in order to reduce the risk of postoperative lagophthalmos, is recommended in such patients.

Assessment of preoperative corneal staining patterns can be a valuable predictor of ocular surface problems postoperatively. Staining can be evaluated with flourescein or rose Bengal. When using fluorescein, it is best to wait a few minutes before checking the cornea since fluorescein staining increases with time. A useful tool to identify staining is the use of a yellow (Tiffen) filter between the ocular of the slit lamp and the patient. Diffuse punctate keratopathy is often indicative of tear film inadequacy, especially when accompanied by a rapid tear film break-up time, although such a pattern of staining is by no means specific. Inferior corneal staining may be more consistent with meibomian gland dysfunction or lagophthalmos. Many other etiologies of corneal staining should be considered, including incomplete or infrequent blink, anterior basement membrane dystrophy, an embedded foreign body beneath the upper eyelid, and medicamentosa, to name a few. Lissamine green staining can be useful in identifying bulbar conjunctival staining in the absence of corneal staining. Rose Bengal staining may be a more sensitive indicator of dry eye than fluorescein staining, but rose Bengal causes more ocular discomfort. Dry eye symptoms can be quite symptomatic in some patients without significant corneal findings. It is prudent to treat any ocular surface disease and other causes of eye discomfort before proceeding with surgery.

Anterior blepharitis, meibomian gland dysfunction (posterior blepharitis), rosacea, and periocular dermatitis can all lead to ocular surface inflammation. Patients with normal Schirmer testing, but with inferior punctate staining, may have one of these conditions. Performing ptosis surgery on an individual without identifying and treating these conditions preoperatively may worsen their ocular symptoms. Appropriate therapy may include warm compresses, eyelid hygiene, bacitracin or erythromycin ointment applied to the eyelid margins, oral flax seed and omega-3 fish oil supplements, artificial tears, azithromycin eye drops, and oral drugs of the tetracycline family.

It is important to identify both ocular and systemic allergy prior to ptosis repair. In addition to allergic eye symptoms that may be exacerbated by eye rubbing, antihistamines and decongestants, both topical and systemic, can worsen dry eye symptoms. In patients with severe seasonal allergy, it is preferable to operate during times of the year when the patient is less symptomatic with respect to their environmental allergies. It is important to be aware of allergies to latex, iodine, or tape, as well as cold-induced urticaria, among other hypersensitivities. Cold urticaria, whether primary or secondary, is rare and can present with angioedema and anaphylactic shock. Obviously, cold compresses should be avoided in these patients [2]. Typically, patients are aware of these issues and will offer the information spontaneously to the surgeon.

Medications

Anticoagulants, such as warfarin, heparin and enoxaparin, and platelet inhibitors, including aspirin, nonsteroidal anti-inflammatory drugs (NSAIDs), clopidogrel, ticlopidine, and dipyridamole increase the risk of excessive bleeding during and after surgery, which may potentially interfere with an optimal surgical outcome. Even more concerning, postoperative hemorrhage can result in devastating visual consequences, such as blindness due to orbital compartment syndrome. Therefore, one should consider stopping any blood thinners before any surgical procedure, but only after a risk–benefit analysis with the input of the patient's other physicians. That being said, certain procedures carry a greater risk of bleeding, such as lacrimal surgery, or more dire consequences, if there is significant bleeding, such as orbital surgery. Eyelid surgery, such as ptosis repair, is typically not high risk for major bleeding or visual loss, although orbital hemorrhage could occur if the orbital septum is opened during the procedure.

A comprehensive list of many drugs and supplements that have the potential to increase bleeding risk may be found elsewhere. Aspirin use is usually halted 7–14 days preoperatively. The half-life varies among different NSAIDs and that will dictate when the medication should be stopped. Cilostazol may be discontinued 2 days, sulfinpyrazone 1 day, and ticlopidine 7–10 days before surgery. Certain herbal and homeopathic medicines (such as garlic, ginseng, gingko, and ginger) have anticoagulative properties and may promote bleeding during surgery. These "alternative" medications should be stopped 1–2 weeks prior to surgery.

Warfarin is often discontinued 4–5 days preoperatively to bring the INR down to a "safer" range (below 1.5–2.0). However, certain patients with hepatic dysfunction may have altered warfarin metabolism, and it might be prudent to check their INR the day before or the day of surgery. Five milligrams of intramuscular vitamin K can always be used to help reverse the effects of warfarin, if necessary. Warfarin may be resumed on the day of or the day following surgery, since it takes a few days for the drug to reach a therapeutic level. Patients considered to be at high risk for a thrombotic event can be started on an IV heparin drip when coumadin is discontinued, although this requires hospital admission. Because of heparin's short half-life, it can be discontinued the night before surgery or even 4–6 h prior to surgery. It is advisable to check the PTT immediately before surgery. Instead of heparin, a patient can be started on enoxaparin, low molecular weight heparin, when the warfarin is discontinued. The half-life of enoxaparin is 4.5 h and is typically stopped the night before surgery. As opposed to IV heparin, the advantages of enoxaparin as bridge therapy are that it is administered subcutaneously and only given 1–2 times daily.

Clopidogrel carries a significant risk of perioperative bleeding, and this medication should be held 7 days before surgery. However, one must be cautious regarding discontinuation of clopidogrel within the first 6–12 months after cardiac stent placement. Recommended guidelines for discontinuing clopidogrel vary with different types of cardiac stents, e.g. drug-eluting versus bare-metal stents. No decisions should be made with regard to stopping any prescribed anticoagulants or platelet inhibitors without the direct input of the patient's primary care provider, cardiologist, and hematologist. This will help to ensure the patient's safety and provide the necessary documentation for medicolegal purposes.

Prostaglandin analogs latanoprost, travoprost, and bimatoprost often cause abnormal eyelash development (hypertrichosis), as well as occasional eyelash ptosis [3]. Even if the eyelid margin is elevated to a satisfactory position, eyelash ptosis may be a source of postoperative patient dissatisfaction. This could theoretically become more of an issue with the use of the product bimatoprost cosmetic (Latisse, Allergan, Irvine, CA, USA) for lash growth.

Prior Ocular and Periocular Surgery

A history of eyelid speculum use may provide an explanation for a patient's ptosis. Eyelid edema, anesthetic toxicity to the levator muscle, and mechanical stretching of attachments between the levator aponeurosis and tarsal plate are thought to be causes of ocular surgery-related blepharoptosis. Speculum-related ptosis may be reversible, as with other forms of traumatic ptosis, and hence it is worthwhile to allow at least a few months for spontaneous improvement.

In patients with a history of previous cataract surgery, it is important to look for pupillary irregularity, e.g., a sector iridectomy, or eccentricity of the intraocular lens implant. Either of these can cause monocular diplopia once the eyelid is elevated. Usage of a retrobulbar block may occasionally produce restrictive strabismus due to myotoxicity to the inferior rectus muscle and/or inferior oblique muscle from the local anesthetic injection. The strabismus may remain asymptomatic until the eyelid is surgically elevated, since the ptotic eyelid may occlude the patient's symptomatic field of gaze, usually upgaze. It is always best to identify and document this prior to surgery so that the ptosis repair will not be blamed as the etiology of any postoperative diplopia.

Glaucoma patients are worthy of a few comments. There is up to a 10% risk of developing ptosis following trabeculectomy [4]. When considering ptosis surgery in patients who have undergone glaucoma filtering surgery, the bleb should be carefully examined. It is important to note the configuration of the bleb (diffuse or cystic) and the thickness of the bleb wall. Patients with elevated, thin, cystic blebs may be at particular risk for bleb injury or infection, if the eyelid is positioned too high. Such patients may benefit from conservative eyelid elevation and avoidance of overcorrection. The surgeon should be especially cautious during surgery not to damage the bleb. Although it may seem safer to perform ptosis surgery via an anterior approach in patients with filtering blebs, Müllerectomy has been demonstrated to be a viable and safe surgicaloptioninthe sepa tients [5, 6].

Patients with a peripheral iridectomy can occasionally develop monocular diplopia following ptosis repair, if the iridectomy is exposed when the upper eyelid is lifted. It is best to ask the patient preoperatively to elevate the eyelid and verify that he or she can tolerate eyelid elevation without diplopia prior to proceeding with ptosis repair.

Previous eyelid surgery can make ptosis surgery more challenging due to scarred tissue planes, adhesions, deficient tarsal tissue, and generally altered anatomy. In such cases, the likelihood of an optimal surgical outcome is somewhat lower than with a nonoperated eyelid, and patients should be made aware of this. Patients who underwent prior lower eyelid surgery, such as transcutaneous lower blepharoplasty or a subciliary approach to the orbital floor, may have cicatricial lower eyelid retraction, placing them at higher risk for postoperative lagophthalmos and exposure keratopathy. The same is true for patients with lower eyelid retraction and inferior scleral show due to any number of causes. In such cases, it may be prudent to correct the lower eyelid malposition prior to ptosis repair, or at least aim for a less aggressive upper eyelid lift. Lagophthalmos and exposure keratopathy are also important to note prior to ptosis repair, since lifting the upper eyelid will only exacerbate the corneal exposure. Patients should be asked about nighttime lagophthalmos and previous episodes of seventh nerve palsy that can impair eyelid closure and blink due to orbicularis oculi muscle weakness. Previous episodes of apparently resolved Bell's palsy can result in subtle impairment of eyelid closure, aberrant regeneration with orbicularis spasm associated with oromotor movements, and a poor or incomplete blink reflex despite the absence of any frank lagophthalmos. In cases with more obvious residual facial motor deficits and resultant unilateral eyebrow ptosis, eyelid symmetry can be difficult to achieve without browlift surgery to raise the lower brow or botulinum toxin to the frontalis muscle to drop the height of the higher brow.

In cases of a nonseeing eye, deformed eye, or an ocular prosthesis, ptosis repair may present additional challenges. Anophthalmic sockets may have soft tissue volume loss, with resultant enophthalmos, or cicatricial entropion of the eyelids with the eyelashes matted to the front of the prosthesis. Exophthalmometry will establish whether the prosthetic eye is enophthalmic or not. It is important to document whether the patient has an orbital implant and, if present, its size, position, and type. If no implant is present or there is simply deficient orbital soft tissue volume due to any number of factors (such as too small of an implant, fat atrophy, expanded orbital volume due to an old orbital floor, or medial wall fracture), it may be difficult to achieve the optimal esthetic result without addressing the volume deficiency by placing a larger intraconal implant, adding one or more additional implants beneath and behind the globe, typically subperiosteally, or transplanting a dermis-fat graft to the socket. Some colleagues have reported inserting expandable hydrogel implants or injecting a filler (such as hydroxyapatite) into the socket as a simpler, less invasive solution. There is a limit to which enophthalmos can be corrected by augmenting the size of the prosthesis, since this will create a heavier prosthesis that will often be poorly supported by the lower eyelid over the long run. Once the orbital volume deficiency and any other socket issues, such as contracted conjunctival fornices, have been corrected, and a satisfactory prosthesis has been fabricated, ptosis repair may be undertaken, with the patient wearing the prosthesis during surgery. Communication with the ocularist is very important, since the prosthesis may be modified to alleviate the ptosis by building up the prosthesis superiorly or adding a ptosis ledge, instead of ptosis surgery.

Patients who have had previous laser vision corrective surgery present special challenges. There is commonly decreased corneal sensation due to transected corneal nerves and greater risk of dry eye issues for up to 6–12 months following the refractive procedure. This transient, iatrogenic, neurotrophic keratopathy increases the likelihood that postoperative lagophthalmos will be symptomatic after ptosis surgery. Therefore, waiting at least 6–12 months after LASIK before performing ptosis surgery is prudent.

Frequently, small amounts of residual refractive error or astigmatism may be masked by ptosis via a slit or pinhole effect. This should be noted preoperatively, when possible, so that the ptosis surgeon will not be blamed for postoperative blurry vision due to preexisting refractive error. There are conflicting data as to whether refraction changes following ptosis repair. While some studies do suggest that corneal topography may be impacted by ptosis repair [7, 8], others have indicated that refractive error changes minimally and often transiently after such surgery. Refractive surgery patients should be forewarned that they might need glasses following ptosis repair, and this should be documented in the informed consent process.

Contact Lens Use

Contact lens use has been reported to cause ptosis from a variety of mechanisms [9]. Contact lens-induced ptosis is found more commonly in patients who use rigid gas permeable (RGP) contact lenses, and this may relate to stretching of the eyelids with insertion and removal of the lenses, causing levator dehiscence [10]. Ptosis may also be caused by giant papillary conjunctivitis (GPC), so it is helpful to evert the upper eyelid and examine the superior tarsal conjunctiva in contact lens wearers. GPC should be treated medically, and there may be improvement or resolution of the associated ptosis, without requiring surgical repair. Ptosis may result from a retained contact lens in the superior fornix that is usually accompanied by conjunctival injection and discharge, or rarely migration of a RGP lens into the tissues of the upper eyelid. Questioning patients as to whether they have lost a contact lens in the eye is important, as well as palpating the eyelid for a mass [11].

Contact lenses, especially RGP lenses, may not fit properly following ptosis surgery due to changes in corneal shape and positioning of the upper eyelid. In patients with ptosis, contact lens fit is often an "under the eyelid" fit. Following ptosis surgery, the RGP lenses may need to be refitted for an interpalpebral fit, requiring a contact lens evaluation by a specialist and potentially investment in a new lens. Contact lens wearers must be informed that they will need to stay out of their lenses for a period of time following the surgery (we recommend at least 1 week) and will need to have a satisfactory pair of glasses available for use. This is important to address before surgery since many contact lens wearers only have an old pair of glasses on hand. Patients should not stretch the upper eyelid to remove RGP lenses as this may compromise the results of the ptosis repair; suction cups may be used to remove the lenses in the postoperative period. Finally, patients can develop lagophthalmos, a deficient blink, increased exposure and drier eyes following ptosis repair. Dry eye tends to be a greater issue with hydrophilic soft contact lenses. This may cause permanent intolerance of contact lens wear in some patients with very dry eyes. It is important to inform patients preoperatively of these issues and document such discussion.

MiscellaneousC onditions

The patient should be questioned about diplopia or strabismus. The presence of diplopia may herald the presence of a serious underlying disorder, such as third nerve palsy, myasthenia gravis (MG) or other neuromuscular disorders, or an orbital process. Appropriate diagnostic testing should be pursued before proceeding with surgery. Strabismus, acute or chronic, and binocular diplopia may be masked by ptosis by occluding the vision in one eye. Therefore, a patient may not report or even notice strabismus that is present preoperatively. During the preoperative exam, one should lift the ptotic eyelid and give the patient the opportunity to see with both eyes and report whether any diplopia is noted. In rare instances, diplopia can be caused by eyelid surgery, but that would be very unusual with ptosis repair. That would most likely be due to damage to the superior rectus or oblique muscle. In light of this, it is important to document preoperative monocular or binocular diplopia so surgery is not blamed as the cause for an existing but previously asymptomatic strabismus, which may need to be addressed following ptosis repair. The author finds it easier to measure and repair the strabismus following ptosis repair. However, some practitioners prefer to correct the strabismus before ptosis surgery in order to avoid diplopia when the upper eyelid is lifted, as well as the risk of compromising a favorable upper eyelid position with another surgical procedure (eye muscle surgery using an eyelid speculum) after the ptosis repair.

Blepharospasm can masquerade as ptosis, especially if there is tonic spasm of the orbicularis muscle, and it can even reportedly produce ptosis by causing levator dehiscence [12]. If blepharospasm is suspected, a trial of botulinum toxin prior to ptosis repair is warranted since the ptosis may resolve following botulinum treatment, obviating the need for surgery. If ptosis repair is performed on patients with blepharospasm, the ptosis often will not fully respond to surgery without continued chemodenervation. Furthermore, if the patient is experiencing reflex blepharospasm due to ocular surface irritation, ptosis surgery can actually worsen the blepharospasm. Patients undergoing scheduled botulinum toxin injections for blepharospasm will have impaired eyelid closure and possibly lagophthalmos. These untoward side effects can worsen dry eyes following ptosis repair.

The patient presenting with ptosis should be asked about previous botulinum toxin use for blepharospasm, hemifacial spasm, or periocular rhytids. In some cases, ptosis may be caused by weakening of the levator muscle by botulinum toxin. This effect will be transient, and the ptosis will resolve as the effect of botulinum toxin wanes [13]. Apraclonidine eye drops may alleviate the ptosis until levator function recovers.

Patients with sleep apnea, especially those using continuous positive airway pressure (CPAP) can be expected to have more edema postoperatively. These patients often have floppy eyelids with associated lash ptosis or frank upper eyelid entropion with trichiasis. In cases of symptomatic floppy eyelid syndrome, it may be necessary to surgically tighten the eyelids, usually via full-thickness wedge resection, if medical therapy is unsuccessful. Both the eyelid ptosis and the lash ptosis may actually improve following horizontal tightening of the upper eyelid. If it does not, then staged ptosis repair may be performed. Lower eyelid laxity is commonly found in these patients, and it may be necessary to tighten and resuspend the lower eyelid to prevent postoperative lagophthalmos and symptomatic corneal exposure following ptosis correction.

Smoking may affect surgery by impairing wound healing and recovery, as can diabetes and various systemic immunomodulatory drugs. Diabetics also have an increased risk for infection. Asthma, COPD, and CPAP usage can lead to increased edema postoperatively and to prolonged recovery. Patients should be asked about episodic swelling of the eyelids, which can be a sign of blepharochalasis syndrome. Patients with this rare hereditary disorder can be expected to have greater than average edema postoperatively, as in patients with renal insufficiency and thyroid disease.

Assessment of hygiene is important. Poor hygiene can predispose to infection. In patients with hygiene concerns, prophylactic systemic antibiotics may be prudent, including an IV antibiotic shortly before making the incision. Past history of MRSA should be documented.

Individuals should be asked about any history of unusual or prominent scarring. Although keloids generally do not affect the thin eyelid skin, there may be an increased risk of hypertrophic scarring especially as the incision approaches the eyebrow, cheek, or temple. Medial canthal webbing may result from hypertrophic scarring or excessive medial upper eyelid skin excision in the concave medial canthal region. For dark-skinned individuals, there is a risk of postoperative wound dyspigmentation, usually hyperpigmentation can be managed with a topical steroid and bleaching agent if persistent.

CongenitalP tosis

In congenital ptosis, gestational history, birth history, and family history may be helpful. The differential diagnosis of ptosis in children and adults is somewhat different. In children, unilateral or asymmetric ptosis may lead to amblyopia due to an obstructed visual axis, which is an indication for prompt surgical repair. A chin-up head position is another reason to operate, as well as the psychosocial impact of ptosis on school-age children. As in adults, measurements of the eyelid-margin distance and upper eyelid excursion are the major determinants of which type of ptosis procedure to perform in children. The difference between adults and children is that this surgery will virtually always be done under general anesthesia in young children, limiting intraoperative titration of the procedure. The gapping method has been shown by McCord [14] to be useful for lid height predictions under general anesthesia and does not require patient cooperation. The usual choice of procedures is between external levator resection and frontalis suspension for congenital ptosis. With unilateral or bilateral asymmetric ptosis, there is always the decision as to whether the surgery should be performed on one or both eyelids. Changes in eyelid position with oromotor movements may be indicative of Marcus Gunn jaw winking. Some patients with congenital ptosis may have dry eyes (familial dysautonomia or Riley-Day syndrome) or lagophthalmos, and caution should be exercised in such patients to avoid corneal complications after ptosis repair.

Conclusion

In conclusion, a thorough assessment of every patient prior to ptosis repair will help identify all risk factors. This will assist the surgeon in selecting the most appropriate ptosis procedure for each patient and identifying those patients who are suboptimal surgical candidates. When indicated, additional testing may be needed to rule out associated systemic disorders. Thorough clinical documentation on the medical record will provide the best chances of satisfying the insurance company and protecting yourself from medicolegall iability.

References

1. Hodkin MJ, Cartwright MJ, Kurumety UR. In vitro alteration of Schirmer's tear strip wetting by commonly instilled anesthetic agents. Cornea. 1995; 14(1):106.
2. Burroughs JR, Patrinely JR, Nugent JS, Soparkar CN, Anderson RL, Pennington JH. Cold urticaria: an under-recognized cause of postsurgical periorbital swelling. Ophthal Plast Reconstr Surg. 2005;21(5): 327–30.
3. Casson RJ, Selva D. Lash ptosis caused by latanoprost. Am J Ophthalmol. 2005;139(5):932–3.
4. Song MS, Shin DH, Spoor TC. Incidence of ptosis following trabeculectomy: a comparative study. Korean J Ophthalmol. 1996;10(2):97–103.
5. Michels KS, Vagefi MR, Steele E, Zwick OM, Torres JJ, Seiff SR, et al. Müller muscle-conjunctiva resection to correct ptosis in high-risk patients. Ophthal Plast Reconstr Surg. 2007;23(5):363–6.
6. Georgescu D, Cole E, Epstein G, Fountain T, Migliori M, Nguyen Q, et al. Müller muscle-conjunctiva resection for blepharoptosis in patients with glaucoma filtering blebs. Ophthal Plast Reconstr Surg. 2007; 23(4):285–7.
7. Gingold MP, Ehlers WH, Rodgers IR, Hornblass A. Changes in refraction and keratometry after surgery for acquired ptosis. Ophthal Plast Reconstr Surg. 1994;10(4):241–6.
8. Griffin RY, Sarici A, Unal M. Acquired ptosis secondary to vernal conjunctivitis in young adults. Ophthal Plast Reconstr Surg. 2006;22(6):438–40.
9. Epstein G, Putterman AM. Acquired blepharoptosis secondary to contact-lens wear. Am J Ophthalmol. 1981;91(5):634–9.
10. Thean JH, McNab AA. Blepharoptosis in RGP and PMMA hard contact lens wearers. Clin Exp Optom. 2004;87(1):11–4.
11. Tossounis CM, Saleh GM, McLean CJ. The long and winding road: contact lens-induced ptosis. Ophthal Plast Reconstr Surg. 2007;23(4):324–5.
12. Bodker FS, Olson JJ, Putterman AM. Acquired blepharoptosis secondary to essential blepharospasm. Ophthalmic Surg. 1993;24(8):546–50.
13. Zagui RM, Matayoshi S, Moura FC. Adverse effects associated with facial application of botulinum toxin: a systematic review with meta-analysis. Arq Bras Oftalmol.2008; 71(6):894–901.
14. McCordCD,SeifyH,CodnerMA.Transblepharoplasty ptosis repair: three-step technique. Plast Reconstr Surg.2007; 120:1037–44.

Chapter5
Ptosis: Nailing the Diagnosis and Considering theDi fferentialDi agnosis

Geoff Wilcsek and Ian C. Francis

Abstract It is essential that the clinician correctly identifies the aetiology of the ptosis, which will allow one to forge ahead with confidence and carry out surgical repair of the ptosis. It is important to remember that ptosis may represent the first manifestation of a systemic and possible neurological illness that could be life-threatening, or at least life-changing.

Recogniset hePt osis!

When a patient enters the doctor's consulting room, it is incumbent upon that doctor to determine whether the patient does or does not have ptosis. In other words, the ptosis must first be recognised.

Moreover, each Ocular Plastic surgeon, comprehensive Ophthalmologist or ophthalmological trainee must recognise the patient's ptosis at the *outset* of the consultation. This is because the patient is often first seen by an ophthalmic technician or, as in Australia, by an orthoptist. The patient's visual acuity and intraocular pressures are often routinely measured, and the patient's pupils dilated with standard cycloplegics and mydriatics. Generally, therefore, because of the sympathomimetic effect of mydriatics, such as phenylephrine, there may no longer be an opportunity to assess true upper or lower lid position by the time the clinician sees the patient, as the ptosis may by then have been "corrected" or abolished pharmacologically. Likewise, abnormalities of the pupil may be obscured, or be impossible to diagnose, after dilation. Moreover, the cornea may have been rendered anaesthetic by the assessment of intraocular pressure, which requires topical anaesthesia when applanation tonometry or a Tono-pen is used. This abolishes any possibility of assessing the relative corneal sensitivity between the two eyes. Thus, by the conclusion of the preliminary examination by the ophthalmic assistant, it may be impossible to evaluate these parameters, and important clinical signs may be unobtainable.

An analogous event, although seemingly somewhat removed, was reported in the LASIK literature, where a moderate myope underwent "uneventful" LASIK [1, 2]. The initial LASIK physicians had neglected to evaluate the patient's pupils and confrontation visual fields preoperatively, an exercise usually requiring about 20 s of the doctor's time. Despite emmetropia, a poor visual outcome was the result of a large perichiasmal craniopharyngioma that may have been detected earlier, if the pupils and fields had been assessed before surgery. This case highlights the importance of doing a complete ophthalmologicale xamination.

I.C.Fra ncis(✉)
Department of Ophthalmology, The Ocular Plastics Unit, Prince of Wales Hospital and Sydney Children's Hospital, The University of New South Wales, HighStre et, Randwick, NSW 2031, Australia
e-mail:ia ncfrancis@gmail.com

A.J. Cohen and D.A. Weinberg (eds.), *Evaluation and Management of Blepharoptosis*,
DOI 10.1007/978-0-387-92855-5_5, © Springer Science+Business Media, LLC 2011

Diagnoset heA etiology of the Ptosis!

Unsafe Ptosis

It is essential that the clinician correctly identifies the aetiology of the ptosis, which will allow one to forge ahead with confidence and carry out surgical repair of the ptosis. It is important to remember that ptosis may represent the first manifestation of a systemic and possible neurological illness that could be life-threatening, or at least life-changing.
Thus, the ophthalmological clinician may be the first medical practitioner to be given the opportunity to identify a serious underlying medical disorder. Illustrating this notion, a modest, although not all-inclusive, series of case scenarios follows:

1. Ptosis can herald a third nerve palsy, and pupil involvement is particularly concerning. In an otherwise perfectly well 35-year-old man or woman with ptosis, in about 11% of cases [3, 4], third nerve palsy results from an expanding arterial aneurysm at the junction of the ipsilateral posterior communicating artery and the internal carotid artery at the circle of Willis. These *"pcomm" aneurysms* may not always be on the verge of rupturing, and so may not always be associated with headache. Therefore, early diagnosis in a patient with isolated ptosis associated with a painless third nerve palsy may save the patient's life, or at least prevent major neurological disability. Modern CT and MR angiography offer sufficient resolution to reveal most of these aneurysms that were previously only detectable with catheter angiography, an invasive procedure that carries significantris k.
2. If, in the setting of a third nerve palsy, the pupil turns out *not* to be involved (a *pupil-sparing third nerve palsy*), especially in a more mature member of the population, this could represent the first manifestation of *diabetes mellitus*. Nevertheless, in a recent Japanese study of 56 patients with *proven pcomm aneurysms*, only six (11%) had a third nerve palsy, but a surprisingly high proportion (indeed 50%) of those six had pupil-sparing palsies [4].
3. The patient presenting with ptosis due to a third nerve palsy may be a middle-aged dermatopath with severely sun-damaged skin. If there has been a history of frontal, malar, or upper or lower lid squamous cell carcinoma in particular, this could represent a definitive manifestation of *perineural spread of the skin cancer* with orbital involvement [5, 6]. Unfortunately, this scenario is relatively common in Australia. The prognosis is generally poor, but fortunately, perhaps, not precipitous until the patient's almost certain demise from theillne ss.
4. If the pupil is not involved, and there is ptosis with an *apparent third nerve palsy*, saccades must be tested both horizontally and vertically. Typical slow saccades in adduction, depression, and elevation will help to confirm a third nerve palsy, but "intrasaccadic fatigue" [7] may direct the clinician towards a diagnosis of *myasthenia gravis*. In this situation, the saccade commences with normal velocity, but slows towards the end of the excursion. Further, if the lid protractor muscles (mainly orbicularis oculi) are also weak, myasthenia is even more likely. We generally use the House–Brackmann scale [8] to assess the severityoff acialw eakness.

   The potentially associated features of myasthenia gravis will definitely assist in the diagnostic process. These include "afternoon" ptosis, diplopia, ectropion, and tearing, all of which are generally worse later in the day. The Ice test can be positive, with lid fatigue on sustained upgaze and the peek sign [9]. Cogan's lid twitch test is generally performed from downgaze to primary position, but may be performed from upgaze to primary [10]. Three or more twitches are diagnostic of myasthenicptos is [10].

   Enhanced ptosis [11] can be useful and is more often seen in myasthenic ptosis than in aponeurotic ptosis. In this situation, the clinician lifts the more ptotic lid, and the opposite upper lid drops. This test depends basically on Hering's law and can be so impressive that it has been named "lid hopping" by Professors

Helen Danesh-Meyer and Peter Savino (personal communication, 2009), as it can be quite rhythmical.

Ultimately, a neurologist will need to assist in the management of the myasthenic patient, because 50–70% of patients with pure ocular myasthenia will develop generalised disease [12], and the associated respiratory failure may be life-threatening.

5. Ptosis may also indicate an ipsilateral *Horner's syndrome*. Dissection of the ipsilateral internal carotid artery can occur following a minor, let alone a major, skiing "headplant"-type injury. Dissection may also occur in a variety of other scenarios, including a spontaneous dissection, i.e., without evident traumatic provocation. These patients may demonstrate little other than mild neck pain and the ptosis of their Horner's syndrome. Dissections can also occur following vigorous neck-stretching at an exercise class in an individual not accustomed to such exercise. In a more sinister fashion, dissection can occur in uncontrolled, high-velocityne ckma nipulation.

We saw a 52-year-old male smoker who presented with 3 months of hoarseness and dysphagia. He had initially been seen at a peripheral hospital. Following an endoscopic laryngeal assessment in that hospital's Outpatient department, he was reassured by the ENT consultant that he simply had vocal cord polyps due to his smoking. Shortly thereafter, he saw us and was noted to have a right Horner's syndrome (Fig. 5.1a). Right supraclavicular lymphadenopathy was

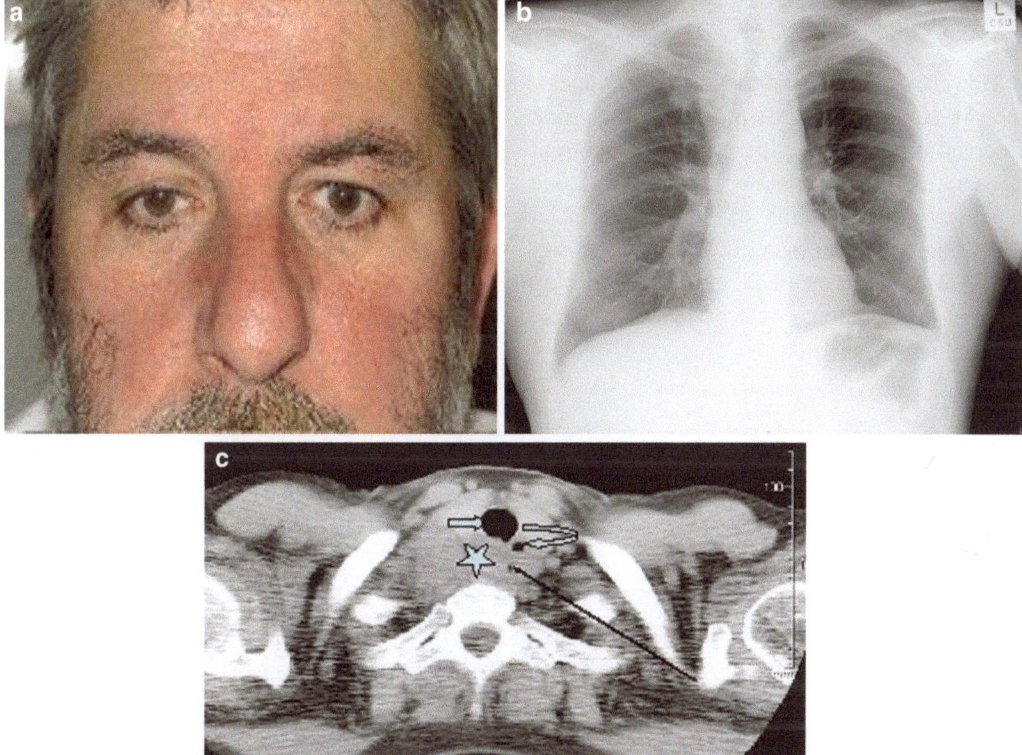

Fig. 5.1 (**a**) Patient with right Horner's syndrome. (**b**) Chest X-ray (PA) of above patient with Horner's syndrome shows subtle narrowing of right aspect of trachea at the level of sternoclavicular joint (*thin arrow*). (**c**) Bony windows axial CT of neck and upper chest demonstrates the trachea surrounded 360° by oesophageal carcinoma (*blue star*), undoubtedly affecting the cervical sympathetics. *Horizontal blue arrow* indicates trachea; *thin black arrow* indicates the narrowed oesophagus; *recurved blue arrow* demonstrates an air-filled oesophageal diverticulum arising anteriorly from necrotic oesophagus

also present. Chest X-ray demonstrated only subtle tracheal narrowing (Fig. 5.1b). CT scanning demonstrated significant compromise of his trachea and oesophagus (Fig. 5.1c). Three days later, after an upper GI biopsy, he was confirmed to have inoperable oesophageal squamous cell carcinoma and was commenced on systemic chemotherapy.

His hoarseness and dysphagia may have been caused by direct invasion of the recurrent laryngeal nerve, along with direct compression of the upper aerodigestive tract.

6. *Ptosis in facial nerve palsy (FNP).* The usual scenario in patients with FNP is ipsilateral lid retraction. However, with the weight of a heavy brow on the upper lid, patients may develop a secondary mechanical or aponeurotic ptosis, especially if the facial nerve palsy does not recover reasonably rapidly. This is seenw ellinFig . 5.2a.

However, this second-most classic appearance is somewhat more interesting than first observed because this patient also had aberrant regeneration of the facial nerve (Fig. 5.2b), due to ephaptic transmission of recovering facial nerve fibres. Indeed, many if not most patients with lower motor neurone FNP will develop aberrant regeneration.

As all cranial nerves can be competently assessed by a careful clinician in about 2.5 min, an associated disorder such as a right cerebellopontine angle lesion might be suspected, if the patient also had ipsilateral deafness and a hypoaesthetic right cornea, as long as the patient had the superior (not the inferior) corneal surface evaluated. This is because the inferior cornea may be exposed due to the FNP and may therefore have become relatively anaesthetic. Moreover, it has been recognised that 5% of the population has nocturnal lagophthalmos [13], and for this reason also may well have a relatively anaesthetic cornea, though to a lesser extent compared with having an FNP.

Safe Ptosis

The aetiology of the ptosis in the large majority of patients does not usually imply a disorder that is life-threatening or life-changing. The commonest type of ptosis is aponeurotic ptosis, previously labelled "involutional" or "senile" ptosis. The latter is clearly a misnomer, since aponeurotic ptosis may occur at birth. It is actually also frequent in relatively young women who have used mascara for several years ("mascara ptosis"),

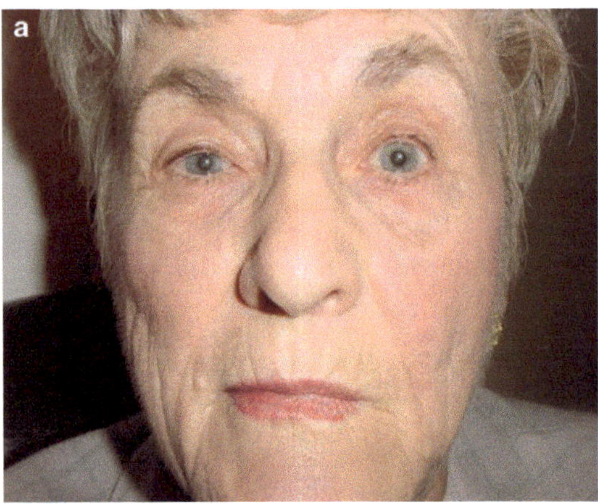

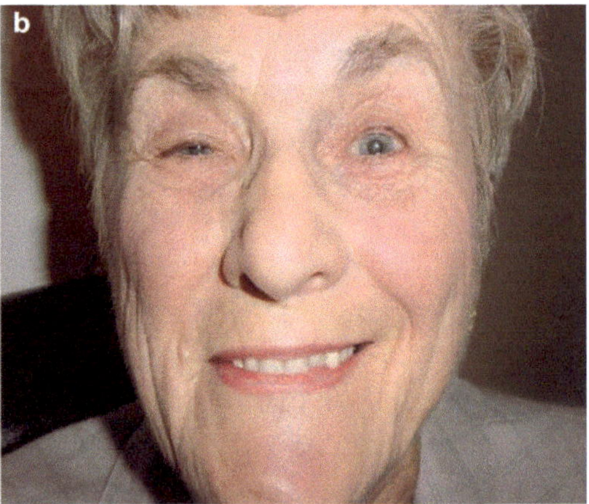

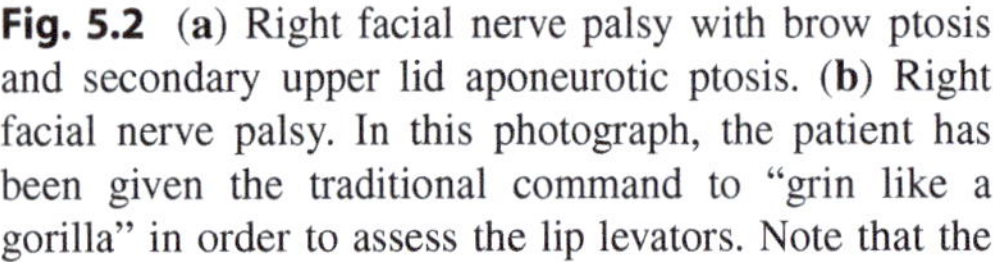

Fig. 5.2 (**a**) Right facial nerve palsy with brow ptosis and secondary upper lid aponeurotic ptosis. (**b**) Right facial nerve palsy. In this photograph, the patient has been given the traditional command to "grin like a gorilla" in order to assess the lip levators. Note that the weak right lip levators do not lift the right angle of the mouth as well as the left. When the lip levators are activated in this patient with aberrant regeneration of the right facial nerve, as she also has, the right upper lid closess ubstantially

but probably most commonly occurs in the mature age group. In the past, it occurred nearly invariably following cataract surgery where a bridle (superior rectus) suture was used to stabilise the eye. It would probably be safe to say that this source of interest for Ocular Plastic surgeons has largely dried up, at least in patients who undergo small incision cataract surgery using phacoemulsification.

Aponeurotic ptosis is dealt with in a subsequent chapter by Dr. Jose Tovilla. Suffice it to say here, apart from moderate ptosis in the more mature age group, or the "mascara" age group, these patients demonstrate not only quite good levator function, but also exhibit thinning of the medial, more than the lateral, horn of the levator. This results in a lateral shift of the levator and tarsal plate. Sometimes the lid is so thin that the patient's iris colour is visible through a gently closed lid. Further, the lid crease elevates, or is completely lost, as the aponeurosis stretches or completelydis inserts.

Distinguishing Safe Ptosis from Unsafe Ptosis

A thorough clinical history of the patient's general health, and also of the ptosis in particular, is essential. It has been said that in Medicine, "More things are missed by not looking than not knowing" [14]. Moreover, Dr. M.B. Kappagoda, probably the foremost clinician in Ophthalmology in Australia until his demise in 2006, stated that the doctor should: "Listen to the patient – the patient is desperately trying to tell you the diagnosis" [14].

All of this must be done in the context of a sound knowledge of general Medicine, but will likely include most branches of Ophthalmology. This will ultimately allow the clinician to recognise and assess ptosis thoroughly and reliably. It may well be true in 2009 that the Ophthalmologist has, or should have, advanced beyond the "battlements of the sclera" [Quote: Dr. Geoff Hipwell (deceased 2009): Sydney, Australia]. One must consider the eye and adnexa in the context of the entire body.

The clinical features of the ptosis both historically and on examination must be carefully ascertained. This has been dealt with in a preceding chapter by Dr. David Silbert on "The history and physical examination." At the risk of possible repetition, we would like to make some salient points.

1. The *duration, timing, and severity of the ptosis* will frequently lend information as to the significance of any underlying diagnosis.
   (a) In relation to the *duration* of the ptosis, congenital ptosis is likely to be benign, but may affect visual development.
   (b) The *timing* of the ptosis can be helpful. Myasthenic ptosis is much more likely to occur later in the day, or after significant exercise. Ptosis after an orbital or eyelid injury is likely to have dated from that time, but old patient photographs such as family snapshots or the patient's driver's licence can be helpful in ascertaining the significance of trauma. Again, ptosis after difficult cataract surgery, glaucoma fistulising or vitreoretinal surgery can help with the aetiology of the diagnosis.
   (c) The *severity* of the ptosis can be helpful. Mild ptosis may simply be aponeurotic in the older age group, but the associated features again are critical to diagnosis. Complete ptosis often indicates a third nerve palsy or may be traumatic.
2. It is essential to identify *any other clinical findings associated with the ptosis*. For instance, new-onset ptosis is likely to be significant in the presence of:
   (a) Diplopia
   (b) A reliable history of worsening of the ptosis later in the day
   (c) Sensorylos sinthe f ace
   (d) Associatedvis uallos s
   (e) Pupil abnormalities which may be noted by the patient
   (f) Bilaterality (midbrain lesions sometimes). That is, the patient should be evaluated appropriately.
3. A competent *cranial nerve examination* should be regarded as a *sine qua non* in the

diagnostic process, since any abnormality of the cranial nerves in the presence of a ptosis needs to be explained. With a little practice, a competent as well as clinically thorough examination of all the cranial nerves should take the ophthalmologist about 2.5 min.

An example of this would include a patient who has nystagmus ipsilateral to the ptosis, the nystagmus beating to the same side as the ptosis, with an associated miosis, ipsilateral loss of pain and temperature sensation on the face and in a crossed fashion on the trunk, nausea and vomiting, and an absent gag reflex. These are all features of the lateral medullary syndrome (Wallenberg's syndrome), which is most often due to an occlusion of one of the branches of the vertebral artery (67%), or the posterior inferior cerebellar artery (10%) [15]. Thus, the cranial nerves should definitely be examined. In this case, surgery on the ptosed lid may not be in the patient's immediate best interests.

4. The *orbit* should be considered. In other words, if there is proptosis or enophthalmos, it is possible that the particular patient's ptosis is not simply an aponeurotic ptosis. Ptosis may be mechanical or neurological due to pathology confined to the orbit. Among many possible orbital aetiologies, ptosis may herald the presence of a malignant orbital process. A recent example seen by us, and indeed one that is well known to Ocular Plastic surgeons, is that of the enophthalmos and mechanical ptosis seen in a woman or man with scirrhous breast carcinomame tastatictothe orbit.

We described a series of patients with enophthalmos due to the silent sinus syndrome who also had diplopia and ptosis. It is encouraging to diagnose this condition, since it is remediable by a combination of functional endoscopic sinuss urgerya ndorbita ls urgery [16].

We have seen a patient whose prosthetic eye could no longer be retained. This was due to a large BCC of the ipsilateral lower lid invading the anophthalmic orbit, resulting in mechanical ptosis of the ipsilateral upper lid, a frozen orbit, and recurrent loss of the prosthesis due to the replacement of the socket with tumour.

If vision is reduced, there may be an involvement of the optic nerve, whether from compression at the orbital apex or more anteriorly. This categorically indicates that more than just an aponeurotic ptosis is present.

We saw an older lady with ptosis secondary to enophthalmos, longstanding phthisis bulbi, and loss of orbital fat. These were all secondary to her original trauma and to multiple surgeries on the eye (Fig. 5.3).

5. The *lid morphology* should be considered. This represents so-called *mechanical ptosis*.

Mechanical causes of ptosis may include eyelid oedema, mass lesions of the eyelid (including benign tumours such as plexiform neurofibroma due to neurofibromatosis type 1, primary and metastatic malignant tumours, or a large chalazion) (Fig. 5.4a, b), eyelid infiltration due to localised skin cancer or amyloid, and other even more rare disorders such as blepharochalasis.

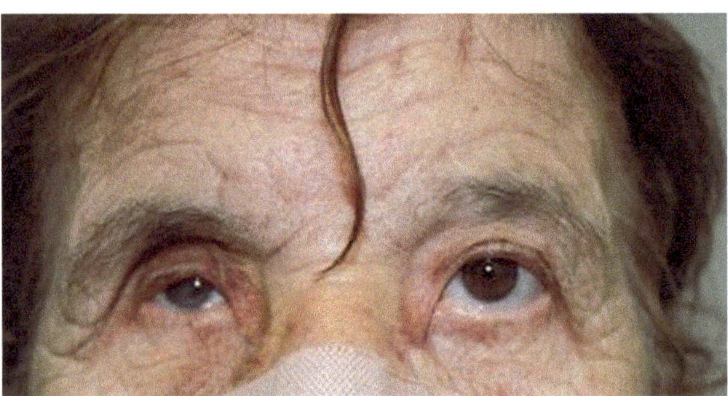

Fig. 5.3 This elderly lady sustained ocular trauma and infection followed by multiple ocular surgeries, with resulting phthisis and loss of orbital fat, all of which contributed to her right ptosis

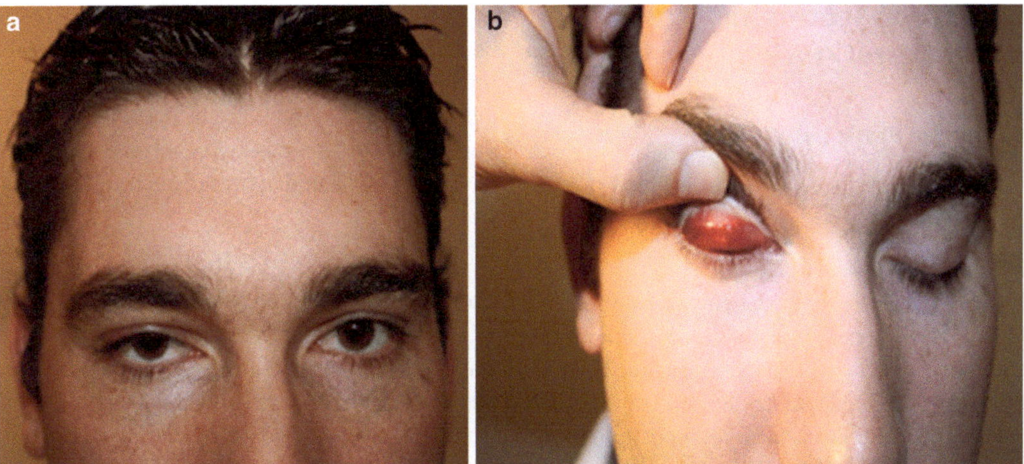

Fig. 5.4 These figures demonstrate a simple right mechanical ptosis (**a**), in this case due to a large chalazion on the affected side (**b**). This diagnosis relies on a thorough clinical examination to exclude other pathology

6. A history regarding any *trauma* should be taken. We were referred a young Sydney surfer with a direct surfboard-nose injury to the upper lid and orbit. Remarkably, his eye was relatively unscathed, but he did demonstrate persistent traumatic mydriasis and marked ipsilateral ptosis. There were no findings that would have suggested any other orbital pathology, and imaging did not suggest a disruption of the levator. Following more than 9 months of watchful expectancy, the patient made a total recovery without surgery.

The secret in making the decision not to operate was based firstly on the fact that the radiology was normal, but secondly, and more importantly, that the velocity of the elevating upper lid saccade was normal, indicating that the ptosis at that stage was likely mechanical and not neurological. Thus, it was anticipated that with the resolution of oedema and local factors, the ptosis might well recover, which indeed it did.

Techniques in Clinical Diagnosis of the Ptosis!

In the practice of Ocular Plastics, a proportion of patients referred for the correction of ptosis does not actually have ptosis. In contrast, some patients referred for conditions such as dermatochalasis and brow ptosis may demonstrate true upper lid ptosis as their main problem.

The following approach may assist the clinician in the diagnosis and therefore the classification of the nature of the patient's ptosis. This may also help to avoid misdiagnosing the aptly named "*ptosis masqueraders*."

Karl Ewald Konstantin Hering (1834–1918) was a German physiologist who worked mostly in Prague. Hering's law of equal innervation [17] is used to explain the conjugacy of saccadic eye movement in stereoptic animals. This law proposes that conjugacy of saccades is due to innate neural connections in which the eye muscles responsible for each eye's movements are innervated equally. We now know that this depends largely on the connections in the pons and midbrain, reliant on the medial longitudinal bundle, and regulated by the neural integrator. This concept is paramount in diagnosing and managing ptosis.

Whenever the clinician examines a patient with an apparent unilateral ptosis, consideration must be given as to whether the ptosis is a true ptosis or is secondary to contralateral upper lid retraction.

Unmasking Subclinical Contralateral Ptosis

Lifting the Ptotic Lid

The simplest way to determine this is for the clinician to lift the ptosed lid with the patient's gaze in primary position.

If the contralateral (higher/more normal) lid falls, then its apparent or relative retraction was due to the effects of an excess of innervation to the ptosed eyelid. Thus, because of Hering's law as it affects the levator, the higher position of the nonptosed upper lid has allowed that lid to appear either slightly retracted, that is, perhaps somewhat more normal, or indeed less ptosed.

In Fig. 5.5a, b, a child with aponeurotic ptosis has a moderately severe right congenital aponeurotic ptosis. When the clinician passively (digitally) elevates the ptotic right upper lid, the left upper lid drops significantly, confirming the nature of this boy's bilateral upper lid aponeurotic ptosis.

ContralateralL idR etraction

The clinician then uses his/her finger to infraduct the higher lid, i.e., gently push the eyelid downward. If the fellow ptosed lid elevates, the clinician is generally bound to suspect lid retraction as the cause of the contralateral ptosis. This is well seen in Fig. 5.6a, b.

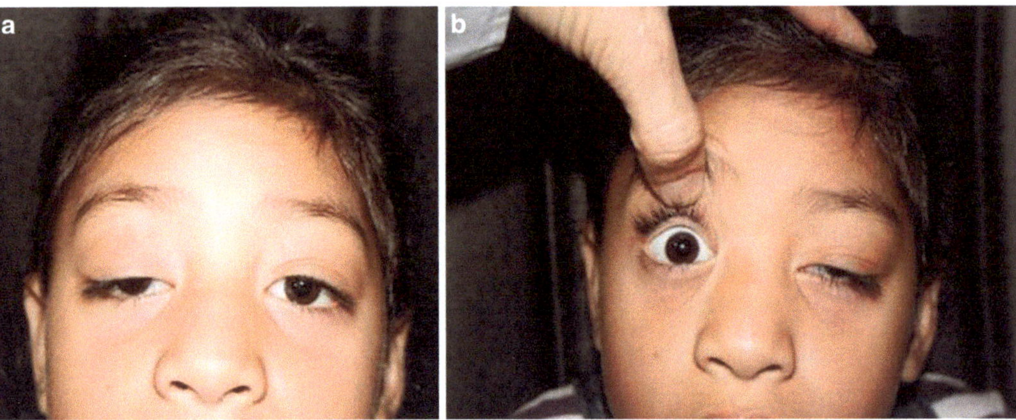

Fig. 5.5 (**a**) Bilateral upper lid aponeurotic ptosis. (**b**) Passive elevation of this boy's right upper lid with subsequent ptosis of this boy's left upper lid confirms that this is a bilateral congenital aponeurotic ptosis

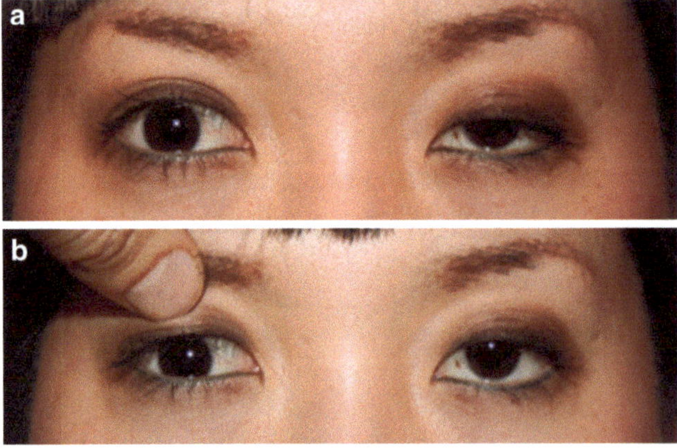

Fig. 5.6 (**a**) Right upper lid retraction in thyroid orbitopathy. (**b**) Infraducting the higher "retracted" lid: the ptotic left lid elevates

The most common cause of lid retraction is thyroid orbitopathy (TO) [18]. This most commonly results from either increased sympathetic tone affecting Müller's muscle and/or mechanical retraction of the levator/Müller's complex by fibrosis.

However, it can also occur if there is fibrotic tightening of the ipsilateral inferior rectus and oblique. In order to maintain orthophoria, the patient attempts to hold the eyes straight by innervating the ipsilateral antagonist superior rectus. Because of Hering's law, there is upper lid retraction. This lid retraction is dealt with by graded muscle recession surgery on the ipsilateral inferior rectus, not the lid.

If each step in the examination described above suggests *retraction of the upper lid*, then the clinician must go on to look for corroborating evidence such as lid hang-up in downgaze (Fig. 5.7a, b) and other features of TO.

1. Lid hang-up or "lag" in downgaze (Fig. 5.7a, b).
2. Other features of TO such as temporal flare, proptosis, limited ocular rotations, resolution of lid retraction in downgaze (due to relaxation of a tight ipsilateral inferior rectus), superior limbic keratoconjunctivitis, significantly raised intraocular pressure in upgaze [19], exposure keratoconjunctivitis, and clinically visible prominence and vascularity of the insertions of the recti muscles.

One summary article reports at least 63 other documented causes of unilateral or bilateral upper lid retraction [20]. Thus, this quite successful clinical approach to assessing the presence of lid retraction may have applications in many disorders other than TO.

ProptosisandEno phthalmos

Enophthalmos can mechanically disadvantage the fulcrum of the levator as it passes over Whitnall's ligament, resulting in either an apparent ptosis or a true ptosis. Similarly, relative proptosis can cause the lid to ride up over the globe.

Nevertheless, in the patient in Fig. 5.8a, b, with left proptosis due to Wegener's disease involving the orbital contents, there was ptosis in theproptos ede ye.

FrontalisOver action

By measuring the upper lid margin to central corneal light reflex distance ("MRD 1": margin reflex distance 1, in millimetres) without taking compensatory frontalis overaction into account, the clinician may overlook upper lid ptosis that the patient is "concealing" by lifting his or her brows. This is seen in Fig. 5.9.

The Dry Eye Patient

The corollary of the patient with ptosis due to contralateral eyelid retraction is that of the patient with severe dysfunctional tear film syndrome [21].

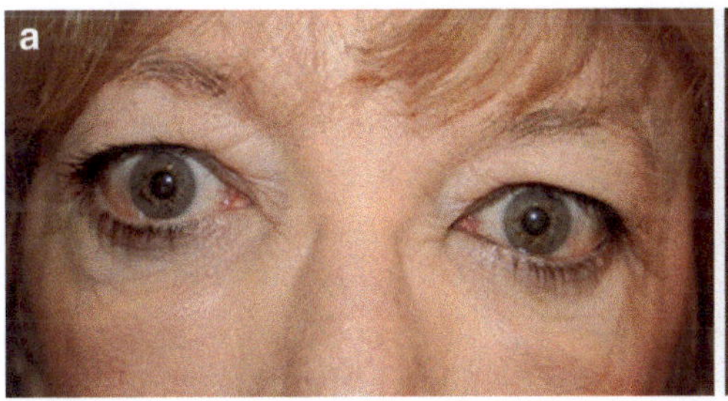

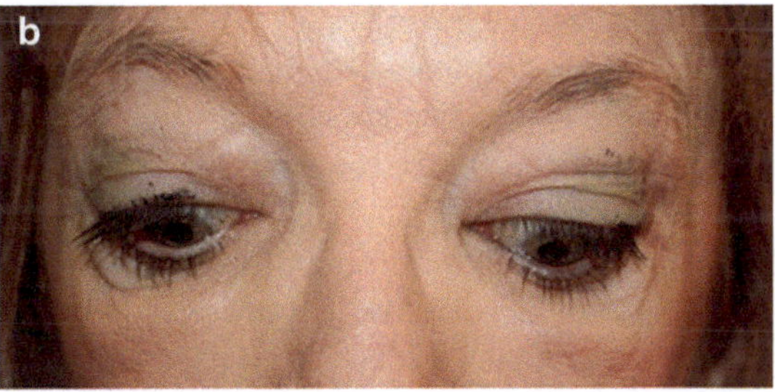

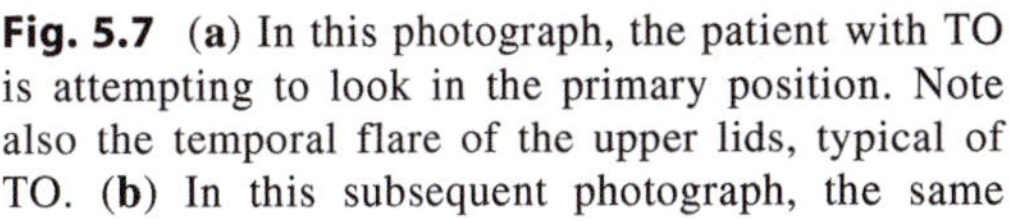

Fig. 5.7 (**a**) In this photograph, the patient with TO is attempting to look in the primary position. Note also the temporal flare of the upper lids, typical of TO. (**b**) In this subsequent photograph, the same patient is looking down. Note the bilaterally retracted upper lids. They appear higher than they were, because they have not moved down significantly on downgaze

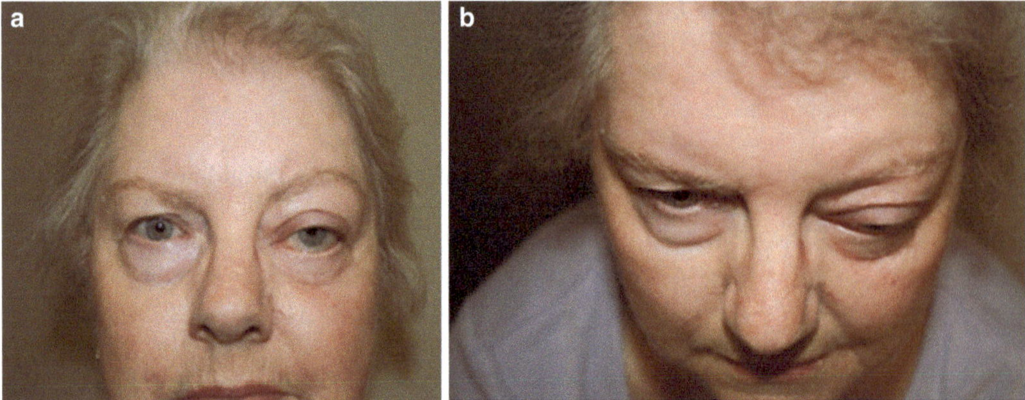

Fig.5.8 This patient with left proptosis had ipsilateral ptosis. (**a**) Frontal view. (**b**)O verheadvi ew

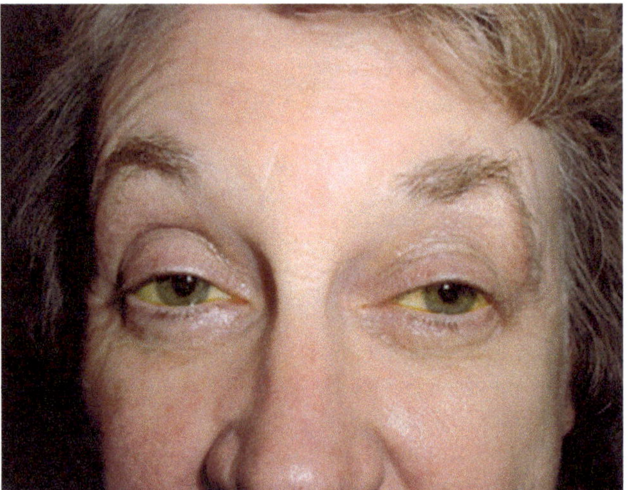

Fig.5.9 Frontalis overaction in a patient with bilateral upper lid ptosis

Patients with dry eyes may attempt to protect their ocular surface, and in particular their cornea, by voluntarily dropping one or both upper eyelids, i.e., "secondary blepharospasm."

This patient may unknowingly depress his or her brows to effect lowering of the upper lids to improve protection of the corneal surface. If this is not diagnosed preoperatively, the patient might undergo a surgically satisfactory browlift procedure only to appear worse postoperatively. This is because postoperatively the patient may further depress the brows to improve corneal protection.

Classification of Ptosis: The Key to Aetiology!!

It is important to classify ptosis not only for the facilitation of diagnosis but also for the selection of the most appropriate therapy, whether surgical or medical. Ptosis surgery can sometimes be unpredictable, and a straightforward method of classifying the aetiology of any ptosis can assist management.

The following discussion provides a framework for approaching the ptosis patient and establishing an aetiology.

The *history of the ptosis* is essential. This topic is covered in the History and Physical Examination chapter by Dr. David Silbert and has been mentioned above. However, some of the salient features may be worth mentioning again.

Duration of ptosis. If ptosis has been present since birth, this may suggest a benign cause. However, we saw a 23-year-old final year medical student who had been diagnosed with a variant of Duane's syndrome. In fact, on our assessment, the student clearly had a congenital, or at least an early-onset, third nerve palsy with aberrant regeneration. MRI and MRA of the brain and orbits were undertaken and were fortunately normal.

Congenital ptosis of the more common dystrophic type usually has lid "hangup" in downgaze. This is seen in Fig. 5.10a, b.

Variability of ptosis. Patients with ptosis of any aetiology almost always declare that it is somewhat worse in the afternoon and evening. Nevertheless, myasthenia gravis is an important consideration when there is significant variability and fatiguability.

All of these findings are discussed in greater detail above.

Definitive Examination of the Ptosis

We have suggested some clinical examination points above, and of course other chapters deal with this as well.

Special Diagnostic Tests for Ptosis

1. *Tensilon (edrophonium) test.* This is dealt with in more detail in the myogenic ptosis and myasthenia gravis chapters. In Australia, Tensilon is no longer commercially available, and Intensive care facilities are recommended when the Tensilon test is performed. However, having personally done Tensilon tests in the outpatient setting for many years, we suspect intensive care facilities may not always be necessary, particularly in younger, healthier patients.
2. *Blood tests.* Assays for acetylcholine receptor antibodies (AChR) and muscle-specific kinase (MUSK) antibodies will assist in the diagnosis of myasthenia gravis.
3. *Radiology.* Imaging is used primarily to evaluate for neurological and orbital causes of ptosis

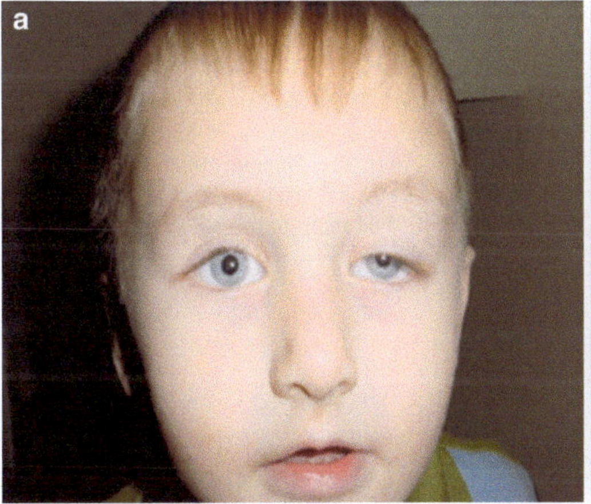

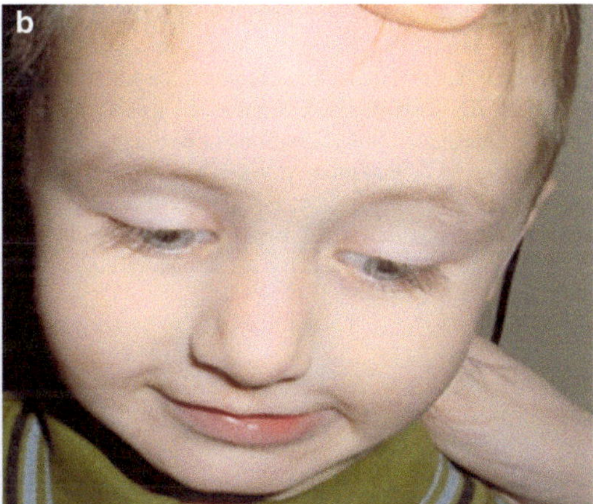

Fig. 5.10 This boy with a prominent left upper lid ptosis demonstrates the typical lid hangup in downgaze seen with congenital dystrophic ptosis. (**a**) Frontal view. (**b**)O verheadvi ew

and depends on the clinical scenario. The investigations include CT or MRI of the brain and orbits, preferably with contrast, and CT angiography (CTA), MRA, and MRV of the intracranial and orbital vessels when indicated.

4. *Single fibre electromyography*. Next to AChR antibodies, single fibre electromyography (SFEMG) is a very helpful test for myasthenia gravis. While acetylcholine receptor antibody assay is the most specific test for myasthenia gravis overall, SFEMG is said to be the most sensitive test for ocular myasthenia when the frontalis and orbicularis oculi muscles are evaluated.

References

1. Sandhu SS, Gnanaraj L, James A, Figueiredo FC. Unusual cause of visual symptoms after bilateral laser in situ keratomileusis. J Cataract Refract Surg. 2005;31:446–9.
2. Papalkar D, Francis IC. Unusual cause of visual symptoms after bilateral laser in situ keratomileusis. J Cataract Refract Surg. 2006;32:187.
3. Chaudhary N, Davagnanam I, Ansari SA, Pandey A, Thompson BG, Gemmete JJ. Imaging of intracranial aneurysms causing isolated third cranial nerve palsy. J Neuroophthalmol. 2009;2:238–44.
4. Saito R, Sugawara T, Mikawa S, Fukuda T, Kohama M, Seki H. Pupil-sparing oculomotor nerve paresis as an early symptom of unruptured internal carotid-posterior communicating artery aneurysms: three case reports. Neurol Med Chir (Tokyo). 2008;48:304–6.
5. Smith JB, Bishop VLM, Francis IC, Kos S, Kneale KA. Ophthalmic manifestations of perineural spread of facial skin malignancy. Aust N Z J Opthalmol. 1990;18:197–205.
6. McNab AA, Francis IC, Benger RS, Crompton JL. Perineural spread of cutaneous squamous cell carcinoma via the orbit. Clinical features and outcome in 21 cases. Ophthalmology. 1997;104:1457–14623.
7. Barton JJ, Jama A, Sharpe JA. Saccadic duration and intrasaccadic fatigue in myasthenic and nonmyasthenic ocular palsies. Neurology. 1995;45:2065–72.
8. Reitzen SD, Babb JS, Lalwani AK. Significance and reliability of the House–Brackmann grading system for regional facial nerve function. Otolaryngol Head Neck Surg. 2009;140:154–8.
9. Osher RH, Griggs RC. Orbicularis fatigue: the 'peek' sign of myasthenia gravis. Arch Ophthalmol. 1979;97:677–9.
10. Francis IC, Nicholson GA, Kappagoda MB. An evaluation of signs in ocular myasthenia gravis and correlation with acetylcholine receptor antibodies. Aust N Z J Ophthalmol. 1985;13:395–9.
11. Gorelick PB, Rosenberg M, Pagano RJ. Enhanced ptosis in myasthenia gravis. Arch Neurol. 1981;38:531.
12. Barton JJ, Fouladvand M. Ocular aspects of myasthenia gravis. Semin Neurol. 2000;20:7–20.
13. Francis IC, Loughhead JA. Bell's phenomenon: a study of 508 patients. Aust J Ophthalmol. 1984;12:15–21.
14. Francis IC. A tribute to Dr Medduma B. Kappagoda. Clin Exp Ophthalmol. 2005;33:414–6.
15. Kim JS. Pure lateral medullary infarction: clinical-radiological correlation of 130 acute, consecutive patients. Brain. 2003;126:1864–72.
16. Wan MK, Francis IC, Carter PR, Griffits R, van Rooijen ML, Coroneo MT. The spectrum of presentation of silent sinus syndrome. J Neuroophthalmol. 2000;3:207–12.
17. Carraway JH. The impact of Hering law on blepharoplasty and ptosis surgery. Aesthet Surg J. 2004;24:275.
18. Rootman J. Diseases of the orbit. Sydney: J. B. Lippincott Company; 1990. p. 241.
19. Ghabrial R, Francis IC, Fulcher GR. Transient retinal arterial compromise in Graves' orbitopathy. Eye. 1997;12:477–8.
20. Lee AG, Brazis PW. Clinical pathways in neuro-ophthalmology. An evidence-based approach. Re: "Lid retraction". Stuttgart: Thieme; 1998. p. 345–55.
21. Chen JJ, Rao K, Pflugfelder SC. Corneal epithelial opacity in dysfunctional tear syndrome. Am J Ophthalmol.2009; 148:376–82.

Chapter6
PreoperativeDec isionMak ingi nPt osisSur gery

Chris Thiagarajah and Robert Kersten

Abstract This chapter serves to instruct physicians to properly evaluate a patient with ptosis. This includes determining the etiology of the ptosis, proper medical and surgical intervention, and managing patient expectations.

Introduction

Evaluation of patients with blepharoptosis should be directed toward determining the etiology of the "drooping" eyelid and then selecting the preferred surgical approach. Assessment of ocular surface protective mechanisms should anticipate the patients who are more likely to tolerate ptosis correction. A discussion should be held with the patient to educate him or her about potential associated risks, benefits, and alternatives to the procedure and ascertain patient expectations to determine whether or not they are realistic.

History

Patient assessment starts with documenting the onset and progression of the ptosis, associated signs and symptoms, variability or pattern of diurnal variation and any factors that exacerbate or relieve the ptosis. Such information may help to distinguish ptosis caused by myasthenia gravis from levator dehiscence. Although ptosis that is worse in the evening may indicate myasthenia gravis, this diurnal variation can be observed in any ptotic patient. Many individuals with ptosis recruit the frontalis muscle in an attempt to lift the ptotic eyelid and clear the visual axis. This frontalis compensation often tends to "fatigue" late in the day (Fig. 6.1). Nevertheless, the degree of variability and fatigability in nonmyasthenic ptosis is generally much less than that in myasthenicpa tients.

It is important to inquire about past ocular or eyelid surgery as well as any history of previous periocular trauma, contact lens wear, and ocular allergy. Previous ocular surgery may lead to ptosis as a result of eyelid edema, anesthetic toxicity to the levator muscle, and mechanical stretching of the attachments of the levator aponeurosis. Most often this ptosis is transient; however, it can be permanent and require surgical repair [1]. Ptosis repair should be delayed for at least 6 months following ocular surgery to allow for possible spontaneous resolution.

A history of hard or soft contact lens wear is important. Soft contact lenses may cause papillary conjunctivitis with resultant ptosis. Rigid contact lens use may cause ptosis as a result of levator aponeurosis stretching due to repetitive lid trauma from lateral traction on the upper eyelid during contact lens insertion and removal [2]. Foreign body sensation or conjunctival discharge may direct attention toward papillary conjunctivitis,

C.T hiagarajah (✉)
The Eye Care and Surgery Center of New Jersey
Westfield, NJ, USA
e-mail:t hiaeyemd@aol.com

A.J. Cohen and D.A. Weinberg (eds.), *Evaluation and Management of Blepharoptosis*,
DOI 10.1007/978-0-387-92855-5_6, © Springer Science+Business Media, LLC 2011

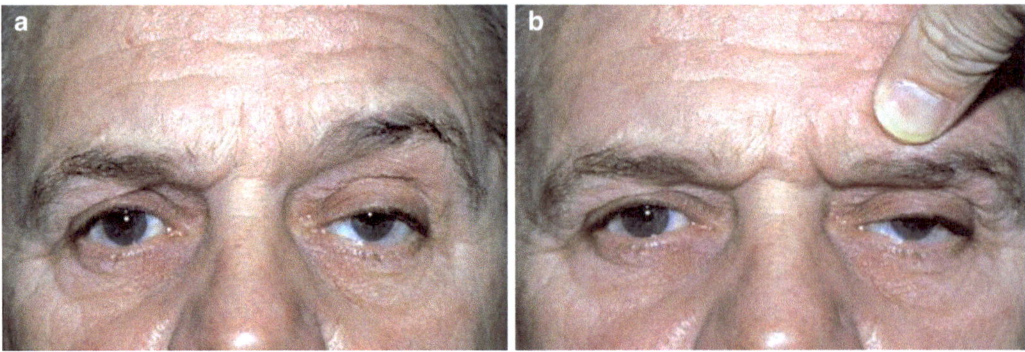

Fig. 6.1 (**a**) Patient with complaint of fatigable left ptosis with eyebrow compensation. (**b**) Manual depression of eyebrow shows a decreased marginal reflexdi stanceonl eft side

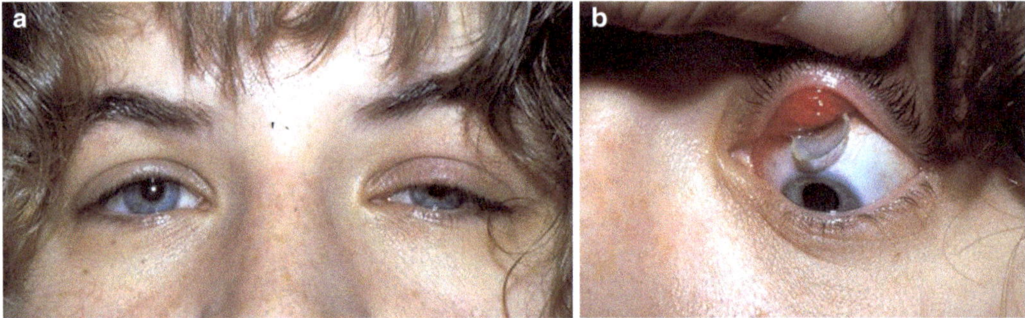

Fig.6.2 (**a**) New onset left ptosis in a young female patient. (**b**) Eversion of eyelid shows a displaced contact lens

displaced and retained contact lens in the superior fornix or embedded in the upper eyelid, or floppy eyelid syndrome (FES) (Fig. 6.2).

Problems with snoring, daytime somnolence, and restless sleep pattern may indicate obstructive sleep apnea, which often occurs in patients with FES. Patients with FES frequently display ocular inflammation and discharge upon awakening symptoms that may be confused with blepharitis.

Smoking cessation in the perioperative period should be stressed since it can impair wound healing. Systemic immunomodulatory drugs can delay wound healing and increase the risk of wound infection or suboptimal surgical results. One might wish to delay elective surgery until such immunosuppressive drugs are discontinued or their dosage is reduced.

PhysicalExam

A complete eye exam should be performed, including visual acuity testing. Pupillary exam may reveal anisocoria that is greater in dim lighting and dilation lag, suggesting Horner's syndrome, or a sluggishly responsive pupil with anisocoria that is greater in bright light, consistent with a third nerve palsy when accompanied by ptosis and the appropriate ocular motility disorder. A relative afferent pupillary defect (RAPD) may alert the clinician to an orbital process, such as an orbital apex syndrome, if there is an external ophthalmoplegia, visual loss, and proptosis. Ocular motility impairment associated with ptosis may be seen in myasthenia gravis, third nerve palsy, a myopathy such as chronic progressive external ophthalmoplegia, or an orbital disorder.

Slit lamp examination may reveal a decreased tear lake, rapid tear film breakup time, and punctate keratopathy, consistent with dry eye syndrome. Dry eyes should be addressed prior to surgery with tear supplements, possibly oral flax seed oil, topical cyclosporine and punctal occlusion, as needed. Corneal sensation may be tested with a cotton swab or tissue paper. Reduced corneal sensation markedly increases the risk of corneal "breakdown" if there is lagophthalmos and corneal exposure following ptosis repair. Upper eyelid eversion may reveal papillary conjunctivitis or evidence of prior surgery, such as a vertically shortened tarsal plate following a previous Fasanella-Servat procedure or Hughes' procedure. Excessive horizontal laxity of the upper eyelid and "spontaneous" eyelid eversion with superior traction may indicate FES, which is also associated with papillary conjunctivitis and eyelash ptosis. Severe eyelid laxity can make ptosis surgery more challenging and may need to be addressed surgically (by full-thickness wedge resection or lateral canthal tendon tightening) if ectropion or eyelid margin contour deformity is encountered during ptosis repair.

Four key elements of ptosis evaluation are margin-reflex distance in primary gaze, lid position in downgaze, levator function, and lid crease position. The margin-reflex distance in primary gaze (MRD1) is important in quantifying the degree of ptosis (Fig. 6.3). This is defined as the distance from the central corneal light reflex to the margin of the upper eyelid. The normal MRD1 in adults is approximately 4 mm. The position of the ptotic eyelid should be noted in primary position and in downgaze. With mechanical disinsertion of the levator aponeurosis as in involutional ptosis, the palpebral fissure tends to narrow even further in downgaze, which may cause difficulty reading. On the other hand, in congenital ptosis with reduced levator function, the levator muscle neither contracts nor relaxes well. This results in the ptotic eyelid appearing higher in downgaze, essentially lid lag, when compared to the contralateral (normal) side in cases of unilateral congenital ptosis.

The degree of levator function (LF) may help in determining if the ptosis is the result of levator aponeurosis disinsertion, where LF is usually good to excellent, or due to myogenic or neurogenic causes, where LF is commonly diminished. Levator function is primarily assessed by measuring the excursion of the upper eyelid margin from extreme downgaze to extreme upgaze without frontalis muscle recruitment. Although definitions vary, the authors classify LF as follows: "normal" (excellent) muscle function is 14–17 mm (Fig. 6.4a, b); "good" function, 10–13 mm; "fair" (intermediate) function is 6–10 mm; and "poor" function, 5 mm or less. LF is important in determining the most effective surgical procedure for correcting the ptosis. In addition to the measurement of upper eyelid excursion, one may further assess levator function by checking active force generation [5], which is a qualitative test since there are no commercially available instruments to quantitatively measure levator force generation.

The position of the upper eyelid crease is elevated in patients with involutional ptosis, while there tends to be a poor or absent crease patients

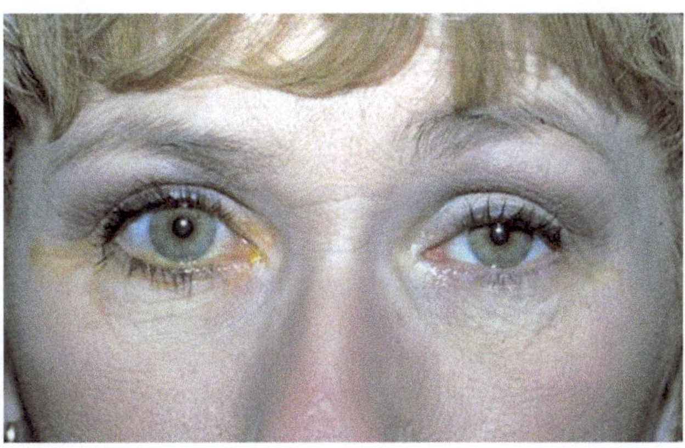

Fig.6.3 Marginalre flex distance (MRD_1) of 4 mm on the righta nd1m mont hel eft

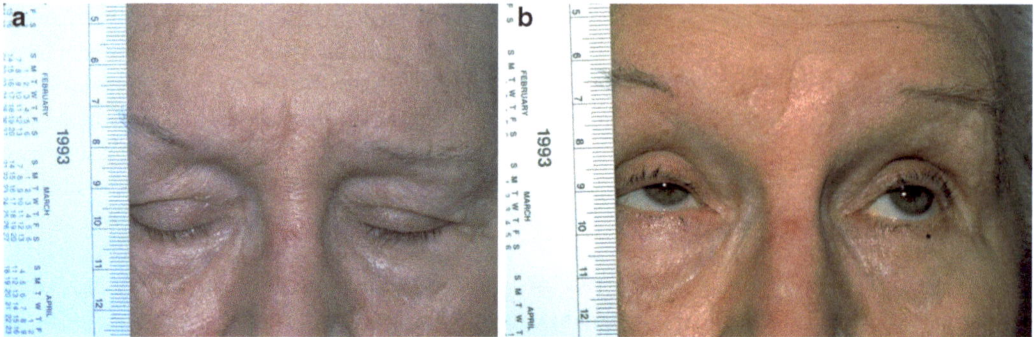

Fig.6.4 (**a**) Determination of levator function. First, have the patient look down. (**b**) Measurement of the amount of upper eyelid excursion after patient is asked to look up. This patient's levator function is approximately 12 mm

with severe congenital ptosis. However, this is not a reliable differentiating feature since patients with severe levator dehiscence or disinsertion may also display absence of the lid crease.

Tear film breakup time, lacrimal lake depth, and fluorescein or rose Bengal staining of the cornea should be assessed preoperatively. Tear production testing is not routinely performed before ptosis surgery. Any preoperative lagophthalmos, impairment of the Bell's phenomenon, and lower eyelid retraction should be noted since they may need to be surgically addressed, or less aggressive ptosis repair should be considered.

Ice and rest testing can be done if myasthenia gravis is suspected. Having the myasthenic patients rest their eyes for up to 15–30 min often shows improvement of their MRD1, i.e., a positive rest or sleep test. Alternatively placing a bag of ice over the ptotic eyelid for 2 min may show improvement in MRD1; a 2 mm increase in the MRD1 after ice application is highly suggestive of myasthenia gravis [3], i.e., a positive ice test (Fig. 6.5a–c). Myasthenic patients may show fatigability on sustained upward gaze, ocular motility impairment, orbicularis oculi muscle weakness and a Cogan lid twitch sign.

The opposite upper eyelid should be observed to see if it lowers after the ptotic eyelid is raised manually or with phenylephrine eye drops. This contralateral lid drop, which is due to Hering's law and is often labeled Hering's dependency, is important to note since it may indicate the need for bilateral ptosis repair in patients with ptosis that appears to be primarily unilateral. Another option in patients with a positive Hering's sign would be to lift the ptotic eyelid less, in anticipation of the opposite eyelid falling. This can be titrated on the operating table with an awake and alertpa tient.

Determinationo fPr ocedure

The most common procedures for ptosis repair are external levator resection, Müller's muscle-conjunctival resection (MMCR), frontalis sling, and full-thickness horizontal eyelid resection. There are many advocates of the Fasanella-Servat procedure as well. Determining the cause of the ptosis may help with the selection of the optimal procedure. Nevertheless, the choice of surgical procedure tends to be most dependent on the severity of the ptosis, levator function, response to phenylephrine, and surgeon preference.

It is important to understand the differences between acquired and congenital ptosis. The most common etiology of acquired ptosis is dehiscence or disinsertion of the levator aponeurosis from the tarsal plate, which is usually managed by reattachment of the levator muscle to the tarsal plate. Congenital ptosis typically results from dysgenesis of the levator palpebrae superioris muscle. Patients with congenital ptosis who have intermediate or good levator function may benefit from levator resection or MMCR.

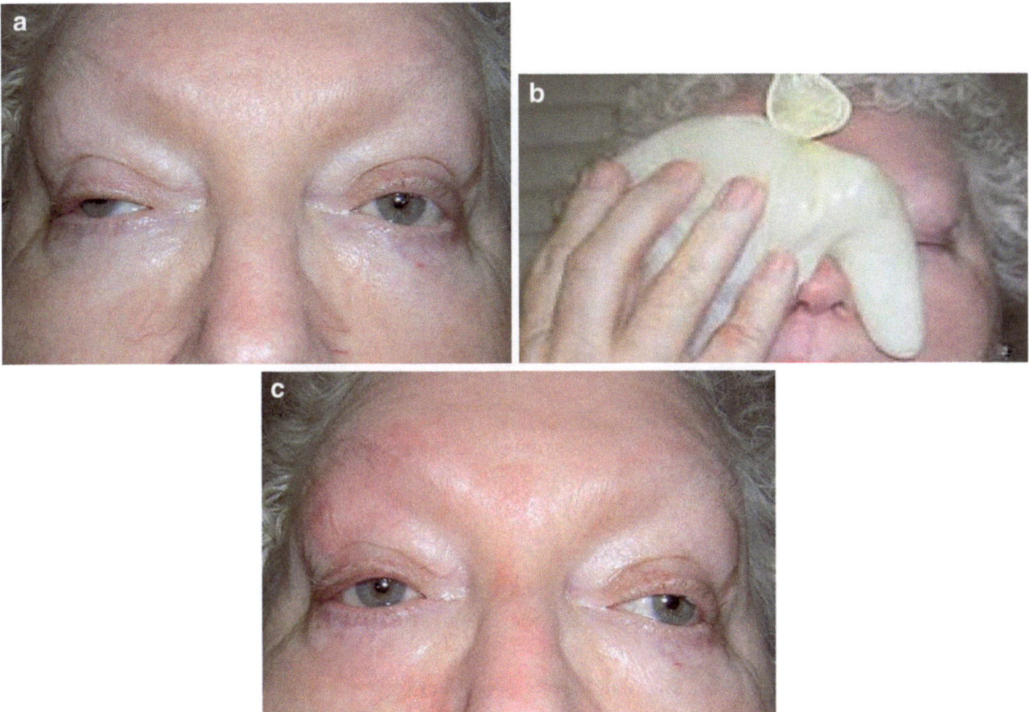

Fig. 6.5 (**a**) Patient with variable ptosis and diplopia. (Note MRD$_1$ on the right eyelid of −2.) (**b**) A bag of ice was placed over the right eye for 5 min. (**c**) Immediately after the application of ice. The MRD$_1$i mprovedt o1.5m m

However, in those with congenital ptosis and a poorly functioning levator muscle, even very aggressive surgical resection of the levator muscle may not adequately elevate the ptotic eyelid, and carries a significant risk of postoperative lagophthalmos. The same is true for patients with acquired ptosis and poor levator function. Most patients with severe ptosis recruit the ipsilateral frontalis muscle to elevate the eyelid. Attaching the frontalis muscle to the tarsal plate via various sling materials allows the frontalis action to more efficiently and effectively elevate the ptotic eyelid.

Most cases of ptosis with good to fair levator function can be corrected by levator aponeurosis advancement and reattachment to the anterior surface of the tarsal plate. This is done through a skin incision in the eyelid crease. The two approaches to external levator resection are the small incision approach, involving a 1 cm incision in the central lid crease, and the traditional approach, using an incision that extends the full width of the eyelid crease. It is the authors' preference to use the small incision approach unless the procedure is combined with blepharoplasty or the patient has had prior ptosis surgery or eyelid trauma. In the latter situations, altered anatomy and scarring can increase the difficulty of surgery warranting an incision across the entire lid in order to optimize surgical exposure.

Patients who have mild to moderate ptosis (3 mm or less) and good levator function may be appropriate candidates for MMCR. One or two drops of 2.5% phenylephrine solution are placed in the affected eye. Eyelid elevation to a satisfactory height 5 min after phenylephrine challenge points toward good Müller's muscle function and suggests that the patient may be a candidate for MMCR [4] (Fig. 6.6). MMCR works by tightening Müller's muscle, which may effectively plicate the levator muscle and/or aponeurosis. A transconjunctival approach is usually utilized, although an anterior approach has been described. Performing MMCR in patients who display

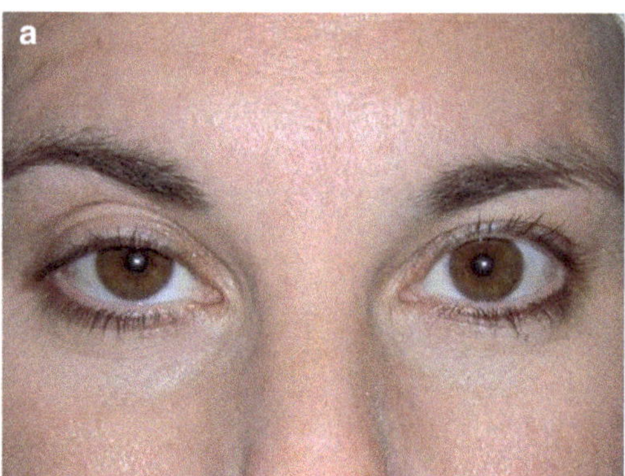

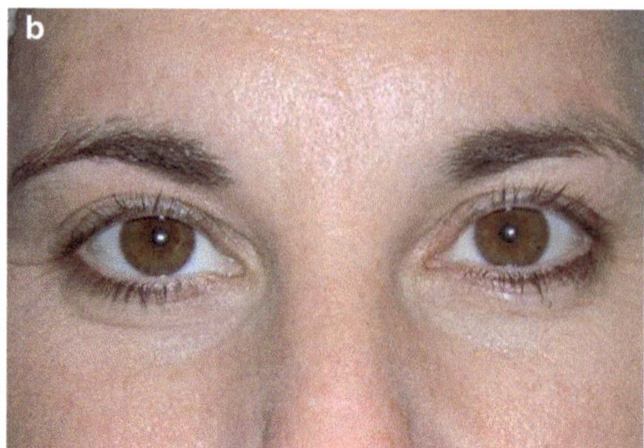

Fig.6.6 (**a**) Patient has mild ptosis of the right upper eyelid. (**b**) After placement of 2.5% phenylephrine solution in the right eye, there is resolution of the ptosis and good upper eyelid symmetry

suboptimal elevation with the phenylephrine test may produce disappointing results. These patients may benefit more from the Fasanella-Servat procedure or an external levator resection. That being said, a mild undercorrection on the phenylephrine test may be addressed by increasing the amount of tissue resection in the MMCR procedure. Furthermore, some colleagues have reported satisfactory ptosis correction with MMCR in patients with a negative phenylephrine test.

The frontalis sling procedure is most commonly used to correct ptosis with poor levator function, regardless of the etiology. Reduced levator function can be seen in patients with congenital ptosis, third nerve palsies, or myopathies, such as chronic progressive external ophthalmoplegia. The frontalis sling essentially works by providing more efficient transfer of brow elevation to the ptotic eyelid by directly coupling the lid margin to the frontalis muscle via the sling material. Some have reported success with maximal levator resection with superior tarsectomy in congenital ptosis [6], but the authors prefer to use the frontalis sling since lagophthalmos is usually less severe following this procedure. Frontalis suspension is often ineffective in patients with unilateral ptosis and ipsilateral amblyopia because they lack the visual drive to recruit the frontalis muscle on the amblyopic side.

A full-thickness horizontal eyelid resection can be used in patients who have undergone multiple previous failed surgeries or in thyroid patients who have had an overcorrection (ptosis) after upper eyelid retraction repair [7]. It lifts the eyelid quite well but carries a definite risk of lagophthalmos.

Finally, one must decide whether to perform a unilateral or bilateral procedure on a patient with unilateral ptosis. As discussed above, preoperative examination of a patient with ptosis should include the evaluation of Hering's dependency. Because the eyelids receive equal innervation, when one eyelid is ptotic, there is an increased stimulus to raise both upper eyelids. This is especially true when the ptotic eyelid is blocking the visual axis. When the ptotic eyelid is elevated (surgically or manually with a finger), the stimulus to raise both eyelids may be reduced and the height of the opposite eyelid may drop. Patients with unilateral ptosis and a marked Hering's dependency may develop ptosis on the contralateral side postoperatively, and the same is true for patients with bilateral asymmetric upper eyelid ptosis when the more ptotic side is lifted. These patients may require bilateral surgery for an optimal surgical outcome, i.e., symmetry.

BloodT hinners

Anticoagulants and platelet inhibitors are important to note. Excessive bleeding during and after surgery may interfere with optimal surgical outcomes. Intraoperative bleeding may create swelling of the upper eyelid, distorting the true eyelid contour and margin-reflex distance. A hematoma within or near the levator aponeurosis or muscle may impair the muscle function or mechanically restrict eyelid elevation. During surgery, it is common to make adjustments while the patient is awake, and these factors can interfere with reliable assessment of the true lid height and contour, reducing the accuracy of the procedure. Postoperative hemorrhage can rarely result in devastating visual consequences, such as blindness due to bleeding posterior to the orbital septum that can increase intraorbital pressure, i.e., orbital compartment syndrome, resulting ino pticne rveis chemiaa ndblindne ss [8].

Additionally, herbal medicines, such as garlic, ginkgo biloba, ginger, ginseng, willow bark, and vitamin E, have anticoagulative properties and may promote bleeding during surgery. These "alternative" medications should not be ignored and should be stopped before surgery. The risks of discontinuing blood thinners before surgery should be weighed against potential bleeding concerns.

While anticoagulant medications are usually stopped preoperatively, there are no universally accepted guidelines for discontinuing anticoagulants before elective eyelid surgery [9, 10, 11]. The length of time before surgery that these drugs should be held depends on the pharmacokinetics of the specific anticoagulant medication in question. Coordination with the patient's primary care physician or specialist, with discussion of the pros and cons of temporary discontinuation of anticoagulants, is prudent.

PatientExp ectations

Expectations after ptosis surgery vary widely from patient to patient. A young female patient who has asymmetrical bilateral ptosis secondary to hard contact lens use may have greater cosmetic concerns than an elderly male patient with a severely ptotic eyelid that is obstructing his vision and whose main concern is alleviating the visual impairment. Most patients reveal in their chief complaint a clue as to what they consider to be the problem. A patient who presents with "My eyelids aren't even" has different expectations from one who presents with the statement "My eyelid is blocking my vision." Before proceeding with surgery, a frank discussion should be held with the patient to ascertain the patient's expectations and determine whether or not they are "reasonable" and achievable, in order to reduce the likelihood of postoperative patient dissatisfaction.

Preoperative photos should be obtained for the insurance company and for medicolegal documentation, and can prove to be useful for review with patients before and after surgery. For example, patients may believe that an issue was caused by surgery when in fact it was present before surgery, which was evident on the preoperative photos. Other components of facial aging, such as dermatochalasis or brow ptosis, can be pointed with photographs or a mirror. This will allow the patient to make an informed decision as to whether or not to address these other issue with ptosis repair.

One may wish to discuss the difference between a cosmetic and a functional surgical outcome with the patient. An explanation of what exactly will be addressed and achieved during surgery, is helpful in aligning the patient's expectations with the likely outcome of surgery. Patients undergoing functional repair of upper eyelid ptosis for superior visual field improvement commonly have cosmetic concerns as well, and those can be addressed. Patients may assume that upper blepharoplasty is a natural component of ptosis surgery and may be greatly disappointed with a satisfactory outcome of ptosis repair if the dermatochalasis remains. When reviewing the risks of surgery during the informed consent process, it is important to notify the patient of the potential need for reoperation (7% of cases, in the authors' experience), as well as what to expect following surgery, including the time course for the resolution of bruising and swelling. "Managing" patient expectations is a critical component of surgery and increases the odds of having a satisfied patient.

When Not to Operate

The decision to not operate on a patient may be based on many factors. The patient may seem hostile, express discontent with multiple prior surgeons (even though they may praise *your* skills), indicate unreasonable expectations, balk at any mention of possible adverse outcomes, or the surgeon may simply sense a vague "red flag" during interactions with the patient. Some patients may have very complex medical issues or the inability to safely discontinue blood thinners for surgery, and it may be deemed preferable to defer *elective* eyelid surgery rather than risk potential serious adverse outcomes. On the other hand, if surgery is necessary to save the eye or protect vision, that is an entirely different scenario. However, that is seldom the case with blepharoptosis, i.e., ptosis surgery is an elective procedure.

Myasthenia gravis may produce unilateral or bilateral ptosis. Treatment of myasthenic ptosis is usually not surgical, except for a small subset of patients who are in sustained remission and have stable ptosis that is unresponsive to medical therapy.

Patients who have had ptosis surgery with a suboptimal result may request repeat surgery soon after the prior procedure. However, most surgeons prefer to wait 4–6 months before reoperating on these patients to allow for complete healing and resolution of the swelling. Early reoperation may produce yet another suboptimal result. An exception is overcorrection after ptosis repair. As opposed to the swollen, undercorrected upper eyelid that may elevate as the edema resolves, the overcorrected eyelid is much less likely to descend with time. Thus, in the scenario of overcorrection, early intervention may be appropriate, particularly if there is significant exposure keratopathy.

Patients with corneal hypesthesia or advanced dry eye disease are at increased risk for keratopathy following ptosis surgery. These patients may develop corneal decompensation, ulceration, or even perforation from severe exposure keratopathy. Along the same vein, patients with myogenic ptosis often have impaired eye closure secondary to orbicularis oculi muscle weakness, and ptosis repair is more likely to result in corneal exposure problems than in patients with involutional ptosis. Ptosis repair in myogenic patients can actually exacerbate the ptosis as a result of reflex blepharospasm due to lagophthalmos and exposure keratopathy. Patients who have any of these conditions require special consideration before deciding to proceed with surgery.

Patients with third cranial nerve palsy are at high risk for intractable diplopia after ptosis repair. While eye muscle surgery can be performed before or after ptosis surgery, it can be difficult to achieve single binocular vision in patients with severe third nerve palsy. Sometimes, it is simpler in these cases to leave the ptosis uncorrected, effectively providing a patch to prevent diplopia – not an optimal solution, but a practical one.

One major reason to not operate on a patient is when there is a large mismatch between the patient's and surgeon's expectations of the risks, benefits, and potential outcomes of the procedure. A decision to proceed with surgery in this situation can result in a dissatisfied patient regardlesso ft hes urgicalo utcome.

References

1. Bernardino CR, Rubin PA. Ptosis after cataract surgery. Semin Ophthalmol. 2002;17(3–4):144–8.
2. Kersten RC, de Condiliis C, Kulwin DR. Acquired ptosis in the young and middle aged adult population. Ophthalmology.1995; 102(6):924–8.
3. Golnik KC, Pena R, Lee AG, Eggenberger ER. An ice test for the diagnosis of myasthenia gravis. Ophthalmology.1999; 106:1282–6.
4. Ayala E, Galvez C, Gonzalez-Candial M, Medal R. Predictability of conjunctival-Müllerectomy for blepharoptosis repair. Orbit. 2007;26(4):217–21.
5. Frueh BR, Musch DC. Levator force generation in normal subjects. Trans Am Ophthalmol Soc. 1990;88: 109–19.
6. Mauriello JA, Wagner RS, Caputo AR, Natale B, Lister M. Treatment of congenital ptosis by maximal levator resection. Ophthalmology. 1986;93(4): 466–9.

7. Bassin RE, Putterman AM. Full-thickness eyelid resection in the treatment of secondary ptosis. Ophthal Plast Reconstr Surg. 2009;25(2):85–9.
8. Hass AN, Penne RB, Stefanyszyn MA, Flanagan JC. Incidence of postblepharoplasty orbital hemorrhage and associated visual loss. Ophthal Plast Reconstr Surg.2004;20(6):426–32.
9. Parkin B, Manners R. Aspirin and warfarin therapy in oculoplastic surgery. Br J Ophthalmol. 2000;84(12): 1426–7.
10. Bartley GB. Oculoplastic surgery in patients receiving warfarin: suggestions for management. Ophthal Plast Reconstr Surg. 1996;12(4): 229–30.
11. Linnemann B, Schwonberg J, Mani H, Prochnow S, Lindhoff-Last E. Standardization of light transmittance aggregometry for monitoring antiplatelet therapy: an adjustment for platelet count is not necessary. J Thromb Haemost. 2008;6(4):677–83. Epub 2008 Jan8.

PartI II
PtosisSub types

Chapter 7
Pseudoptosis

Adam J. Cohen and David A. Weinberg

Abstract Pseudoptosis is a "waste basket," or heterogeneous group, of miscellaneous disorders in which there is an illusion of ptosis rather than "true" ptosis. The condition creating the appearance of pseudoptosis may involve the eye in question or the opposite eye.

Pseudoptosis is a "waste basket," or heterogeneous group, of miscellaneous disorders in which there is an illusion of ptosis rather than "true" ptosis. The condition creating the appearance of pseudoptosis may involve the eye in question or the opposite eye, as is discussed below. It is critical to rule out pseudoptosis before undertaking ptosis surgery. This chapter reviews the most common etiologies of pseudoptosis.

Dermatochalasis is likely the most common eyelid condition that causes confusion when evaluating the patient with apparent ptosis. Excess upper eyelid skin may overhang the eyelashes and obstruct visualization of the eyelid margin, giving the impression of a low-lying eyelid (Fig. 7.1). One should also remember that severe dermatochalasis and/or eyebrow ptosis may produce a true mechanical ptosis, as opposed to pseudoptosis. Gentle elevation of the eyebrow and the excess eyelid skin allows for accurate measurement of the true eyelid margin position and should alleviate any potential component of mechanical ptosis. Obviously, if one were to lift the eyebrow and/or upper eyelid skin more vigorously, that traction might raise the eyelid margin and lead to a false measurement of eyelid position. The clinician should remember that if dermatochalasis and true ptosis coexist, blepharoplasty can unmask the ptosis, and it may appear to the patient that the blepharoplasty procedure caused the ptosis. In such cases, it is important to discuss these issues with the patient in advance and decide whether to correct both the dermatochalasis and the ptosis at the same time or to consider staged surgery, if needed.

Blepharochalasis syndrome, an uncommon form of hereditary, recurrent eyelid edema, often manifesting in early childhood or adolescence, may be mistaken for dermatochalasis [1]. This intermittent and painless, immunogenic eyelid swelling can result in ptosis. Once the swelling abates, the mechanical ptosis resolves. Any condition with upper eyelid edema may cause a droopy eyelid, but this is generally true mechanical ptosis rather than pseudoptosis.

Asymmetric upper eyelid creases (Fig. 7.2) are frequently found in patients presenting with pseudoptosis. On the side of the higher lid crease, more pretarsal skin is exposed compared with the opposite eye. This creates an illusion of ptosis in the eye with the higher lid crease. In these patients, surgery is directed toward creating symmetry between the eyelid creases, by either raising the lower crease or trying to lower the higher crease. It is generally much easier and more predictable to lift a crease, which involves excision of skin and/or fat, depending upon how much "extra" skin is present. Resecting preaponeurotic fat creates a higher line of adhesion between

A.J. Cohen (✉)
Private Practice, The Art of Eyes, Skokie, IL, USA
e-mail: acohen@theartofeyes.com

A.J. Cohen and D.A. Weinberg (eds.), *Evaluation and Management of Blepharoptosis*,
DOI 10.1007/978-0-387-92855-5_7, © Springer Science+Business Media, LLC 2011

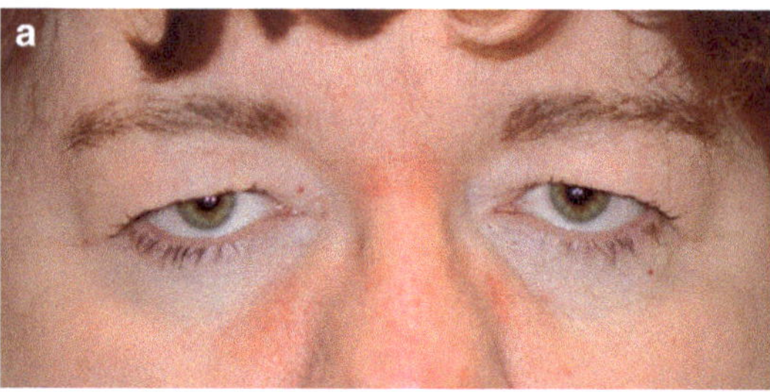

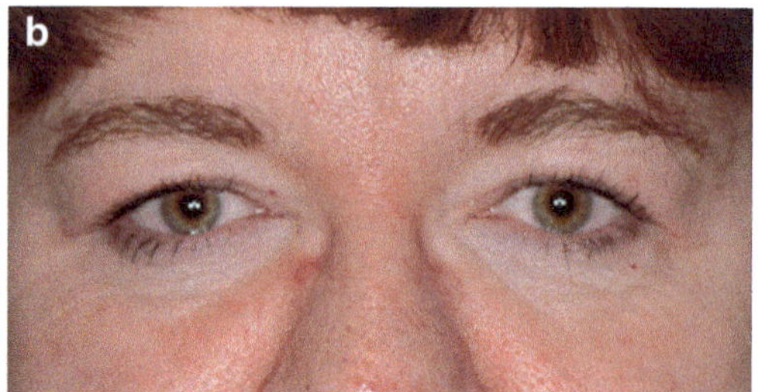

Fig. 7.1 Severe upper eyelid dermatochalasis before (**a**) and after (**b**) bilateral upper blepharoplasty. When the excess, overhanging skin of both upper eyelids was gently lifted preoperatively, it was noted that the upper eyelid margins were in satisfactory position, essentially in the samel ocationt heya ref oundpos toperatively

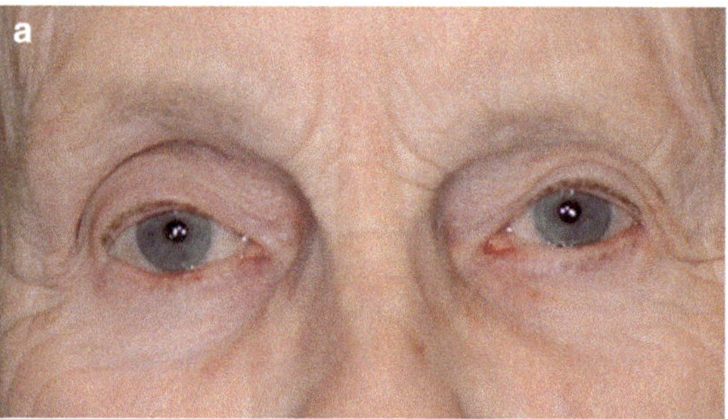

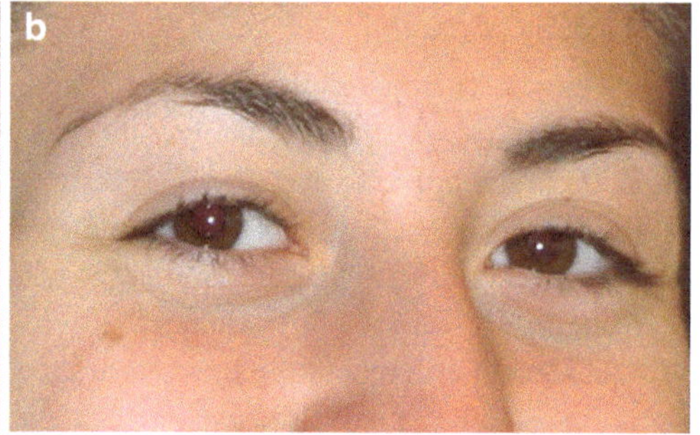

Fig. 7.2 Two patients with asymmetric upper eyelid creases. Although the MRD1 (margin-reflex distance to the upper eyelid margin) is virtually equal in the two eyes, there is the illusion of ptosis on the side with the higher lid crease

levator aponeurosis and skin, and it is the highest adhesion point between levator and skin that creates the lid crease. This adhesion may be facilitated with sutures placed between the incision edge and levator, often referred to as "lid crease sutures." In order to lower the height of the higher crease, it is usually necessary to place a spacer graft (commonly fat) between levator aponeurosis and skin/orbicularis muscle in order to preclude higher adhesions between these structures. This is a more involved procedure since there is another surgical site from which the fat is harvested, often the abdomen, and the grafted fat will usually "shrink" to some degree over the months following surgery, thus requiring an initial "overfill." Therefore, although the patient may prefer the appearance of the upper eyelid with the lower crease and thus initially opt for lowering the height of the higher lid crease, the surgeon usually encourages the patient to do the opposite, that is, to raise the lower crease. Raising an eyelid crease is much quicker, easier (for both the patient and the surgeon), carries less potential morbidity, and is much more predictable, inge neral.

Eyelid retraction, which produces a widened palpebral fissure, may result from thyroid eye disease, prior eyelid surgery or trauma, and a long list of other conditions [2]. The widening of the eyelid fissure, especially if it is the upper eyelid that is retracted, may create an illusion of contralateral ptosis (Fig. 7.3) [3]. Furthermore, some patients with eyelid retraction develop compensatory blepharospasm, possibly in response to corneal exposure, and this blepharospasm in the opposite eye may simulate blepharoptosis. Ipsilateral or asymmetric proptosis is often associated with eyelid retraction, and, in the same vein, may produce the illusion of ptosis in the contralateral eye with the narrower palpebral fissure.

Benign essential blepharospasm, Meige syndrome, hemifacial spasm (Fig. 7.4), and aberrant regeneration of the facial nerve may cause involuntary eyelid twitching or spasmodic eyelid

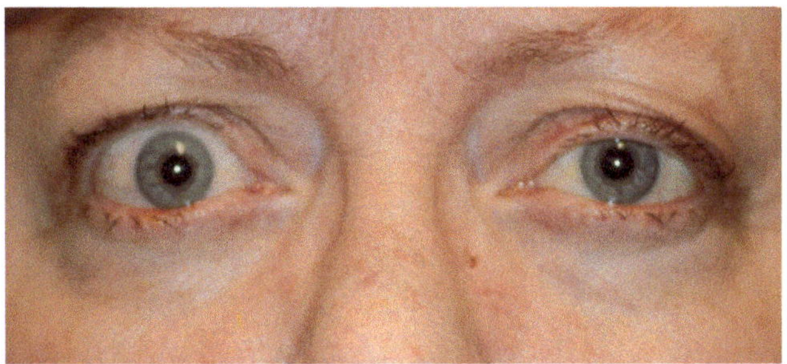

Fig. 7.3 Right upper eyelid retraction due to thyroid eye disease. Some patients with unilateral eyelid retraction present with the complaint of contralateral ptosis. In this case, there is obvious superior scleral show on the right, but that is not always the case, especially if the patient has compensatory blepharospasm. When the left upper eyelid was manually raised, the right upper eyelid did not lower, consistent with primary eyelid retraction on the right rather than compensatory retraction due to contralateralpt osis

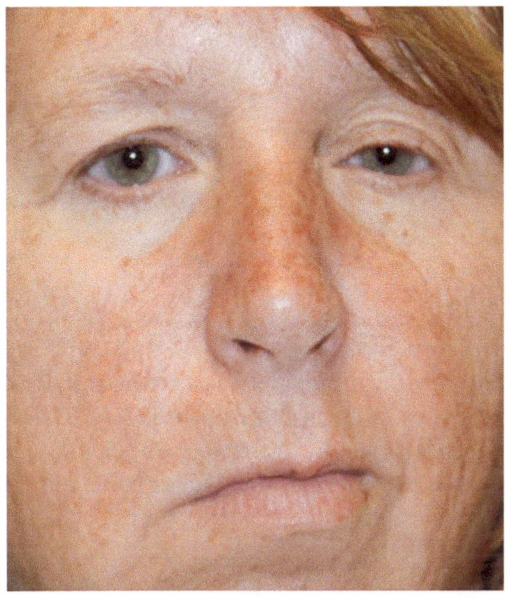

Fig. 7.4 Left hemifacial spasm producing apparent left upper eyelid ptosis. Note the "reverse ptosis" of the lower lid and the raised left corner of the mouth, which are cluest ot hepr esenceof he mifacials pasm

closure that may resemble ptosis. Although blepharospasm is often primary, secondary ocular causes include keratitis, uveitis, scleritis, and any condition that produces photophobia. Many patients with essential blepharospasm also have ocular surface disease that can contribute to the blepharospasm. Once these secondary conditions are eliminated or addressed, chemodenervation with botulinum toxin injections may be the treatment of choice. While blepharospasm and the other spastic disorders may produce a pseudoptosis, the botulinum toxin may inadvertently spread to the levator muscle and produce a temporary paralysis, causing true ptosis (Fig. 7.5). This resolves over the ensuing weeks, and apraclonidine eye drops may be helpful during this time. If a history of botulinum use exists, the clinician may wish to wait about 2 months following the last toxin injections to obtain accurate eyelid height measurements. That being said, it may be impossible in such patients to obtain completely reliable eyelid measurements without the influence of either the blepharospasm or the botulinum toxin, and judgment should be exercised in such cases. Some patients have coexistent blepharospasm and ptosis, and one may need to assess the upper eyelid position on a few separate occasions following botulinum toxin administration. The central upper eyelid should be avoided toxin injection and injection volume minimized to limit diffusion of the toxin. Ptosis surgery is sometimes indicated in blepharospasm patients, and orbicularis myectomy may be performed concurrently. Frontalis suspension, eyebrow elevation, and levator advancement surgery may be employed in patients with apraxia of eyelid opening [4, 5].

Vertical strabismus may cause pseudoptosis. When the hypertropic eye is the fixating eye, the opposite eye assumes a hypotropic position.

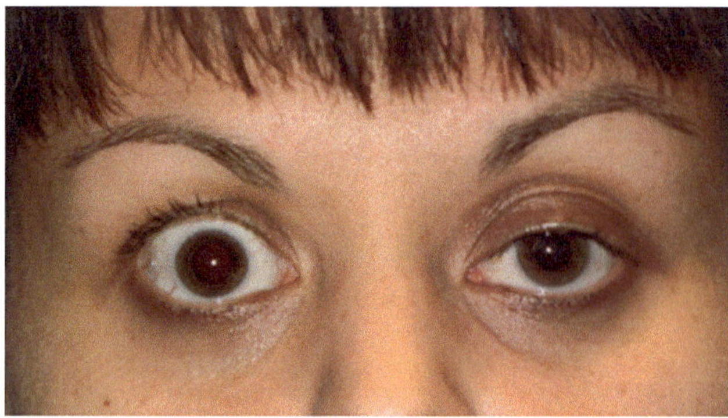

Fig.7.5 Leftuppe re yelid ptosis following glabellar botulinum toxin injections. Note the right upper eyelid retraction that is secondary to the left ptosis (via Hering's law). This was confirmed by a drop in the right upper eyelid height when the left upper eyelidw asm anuallyra ised

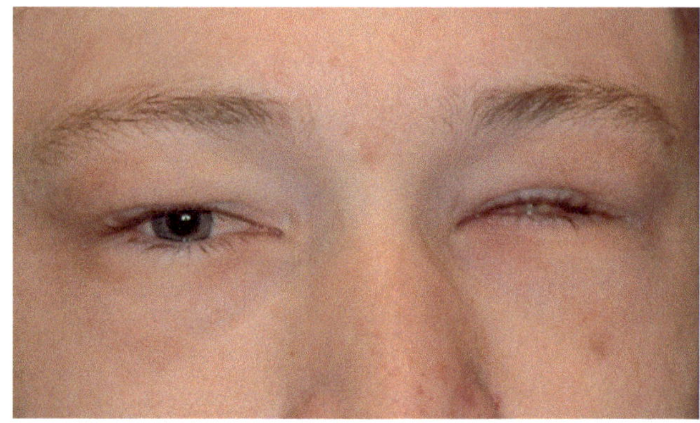

Fig.7.6 Leftuppe re yelid ptosis due to left phthisis bulbi, i.e., left enophthalmos. Placement of a scleral shell prosthesis or removal of the eye and insertion of an appropriate-sized implant and overlying prosthesis should correctt hept osis

The upper eyelid is lower in the hypotropic eye due to attachments between the superior rectus and levator palpebrae superioris [6], i.e., the upper eyelid follows the visual axis. No upper eyelid repositioning surgery should be undertaken until the ocular misalignment has been satisfactorily addressed. On a related note, correction of a vertical misalignment by resection of the inferior rectus muscle tends to elevate the lower eyelid ("reverse ptosis") due to attachments between the lower eyelid retractors and the inferior rectus muscle around Lockwood's ligament, and this narrows the palpebral fissure. This could be perceived by the patient as upper eyelid ptosis, although they more often just describe the eye as "looking smaller."

Lack of posterior eyelid support can result from abnormalities of the globe and socket, and this can produce true ptosis or the appearance of ptosis. Enophthalmos, anophthalmos, microphthalmos, and phthisis bulbi may produce a ptotic upper eyelid due to insufficient orbital soft tissue volume with the inability to adequately buttress the eyelid (Fig. 7.6). Therefore, the eyelids assume a more posterior position with a more vertical orientation, resulting in a narrower palpebral fissure. Following enucleation, an undersized orbital implant and/or a small prosthesis can result in a superior sulcus deformity and enophthalmos, with a narrowed palpebral fissure [4]. The solution is to add volume to the socket via a larger ocular prosthesis and/or an additional orbital implant. The added volume pushes the prosthesis, and hence the eyelids forward into their "proper" anatomic position, widening the palpebral fissure. There can also be a volume deficiency in the superior orbit due to the descent of the implant or the prosthesis (which can result from lower eyelid laxity), providing less support for the upper eyelid (Fig. 7.7). These issues can be corrected by horizontally tightening the lower eyelid and placing an implant along the orbital floor, below, and

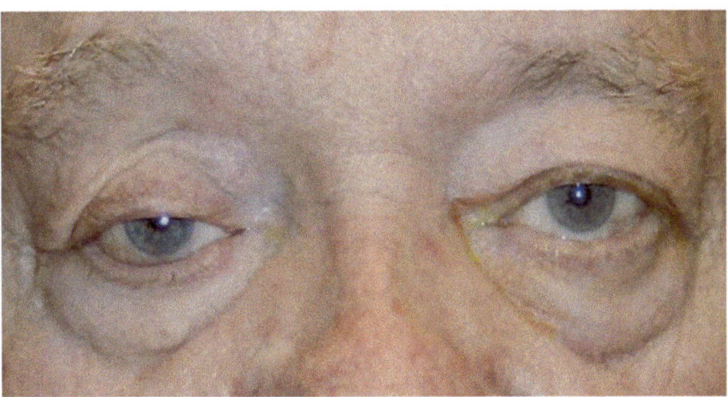

Fig.7.7 Rightuppe re yelid ptosis due to a combination of factors in this anophthalmic socket, including lower eyelid laxity resulting in an inferiorly positioned prosthesis and orbital soft tissue volume deficiency (note the superior sulcus deformity)

behind the intraconal sphere implant, which lifts the sphere implant and displaces fat into the superior sulcus. In general, the underlying orbital or socket abnormality, e.g., soft tissue deficiency or expanded orbital volume due to a blowout fracture, that is responsible for enophthalmos should be addressed before undertaking ptosis surgery. However, in certain cases, the patient may elect instead to only undergo ptosis repair that may simply camouflage the enophthalmos. In such cases, even though the upper eyelid malposition has been repaired, the enophthalmos may still be evident.

When the two eyes are positioned at a different vertical height, eyelid position can be affected. The resultant eyelid position depends on whether the entire orbit is "malpositioned," i.e., orbital dystopia or craniofacial syndromes, or whether the globe is malpositioned in the orbit, hyperglobus or hypoglobus. Hyperglobus or hypoglobus can produce an appearance of ptosis, ipsilateral to the higher globe. Hyperglobus may result from a space-occupying lesion beneath the globe, either in the orbit or the maxillary sinus, while hypoglobus may be produced by either loss of support beneath the globe (e.g., orbital floor defect or silent sinus syndrome [7]) or a mass above the globe pushing downward on the eye. Obviously, correction of the pseudoptosis in these cases involves addressing the underlying orbital and/or sinus pathology.

The mantra "Define the problem, then solve the problem" provides strong words of wisdom in oculofacial plastic surgery, hence the importance of a thorough examination and careful consideration when deciding on the best course of action when approaching surgical intervention. When a patient presents with a droopy eyelid, one must be certain to first rule out pseudoptosis before moving "full steam" ahead with ptosis surgery.

References

1. Koursch DM, Modjtahedi SP, Selva D, Leibovitch I. The blepharochalasis syndrome. Surv Ophthalmol. 2009;54(2):235–44.
2. Bartley GB. The differential diagnosis and classification of eyelid retraction. Ophthalmology. 1996; 103(1):168–76.
3. Amato MM, Monheit B, Shore JW. Ptosis surgery. In: Tasman W, Jaeger EA, editors. Duane's ophthalmology, 2007 edition. Philadelphia, PA: Lippincott Williams & Wilkins; 2007.
4. Kerty E, Eidal K. Apraxia of eyelid opening: clinical features and therapy. Eur J Ophthalmol. 2006;16(2): 204–8.
5. Nicoletti AG, Pereira IC, Matayoshi S. Browlifting as an alternative procedure for apraxia of eyelid opening. Ophthal Plast Reconstr Surg. 2009;25(1):46–7.
6. Mitchell PR, Parks MM. Third cranial nerve palsies, congenital. In: Tasman W, Jaeger EA, editors. Duane's ophthalmology, 2007 edition. Philadelphia, PA: Lippincott Williams & Wilkins; 2007.
7. Enophthalmos. www.emedicine.medscape.com/article/ 1218658.A ccessed07D ec2009.

Chapter8
CongenitalPt osis

Edward J. Wladis and Dale R. Meyer

Abstract Multiple etiologies have been implicated in the pathogenesis of congenital ptosis (Kersten, Bartley, Nerad, et al. eds. Orbit, eyelids, and lacrimal system. Basic and clinical science course. 2001). In light of the wide array of mechanisms by which this problem arises, the management of congenital ptosis has traditionally proven somewhat difficult, and its repair necessitates accurate preoperative diagnostic assessment, careful consideration of one's operative plan, and meticulous surgical technique. In this chapter, we review a variety of causes of congenital ptosis, discuss several hallmark diagnostic features, and outline a management strategy. A more extensive discussion of the individual steps inherent to each surgery can be found in greater detail in the "Surgical Treatment" section of this book.

Pathogenesis

Myogenic Causes

The most common etiology of congenital ptosis is an embryonic dysgenesis of the levator palpebrae muscle [1]. Whereas the normal levator muscle contains striated muscle fibers, cases of myogenic ptosis are marked by infiltration of fibroadipose tissue, thereby inhibiting the normal contracting and relaxing functions of the muscle. As such, the ptotic eyelid in these cases has a reduced levator function and – secondary to decreased muscular compliance – may also demonstrate reduced movement on downgaze ("eyelid lag") and lagophthalmos.

Dysgenesis of the levator muscle may also be associated with a maldevelopment of the superior rectus muscle, in light of their common embryologic origin. In this situation, the patient may display myogenic ptosis superimposed on a vertical strabismus or a limited Bell's phenomenon ("double elevator palsy").

In cases of myogenic congenital ptosis, special consideration should be given to the patient's external appearance, as it may yield clues as to a possible underlying cause [2]. Specifically, the blepharophimosis syndrome is characterized by severe ptosis, telecanthus, epicanthus inversus, horizontal eyelid shortening, nasal hypoplasia, and a flattened orbital rim. This disorder may be inherited in an autosomal dominant fashion.

Congenital orbital fibrosis is another syndromic cause of myogenic congenital ptosis. In this autosomal dominant problem, patients present with ptosis and limitations of extraocular motility. While any (and all) of the extraocular muscles may be involved, the inferior rectus is most commonly implicated in this disorder, and patients often experience poor downgaze excursions and a chin-up posture.

E.J.W ladis (✉)
Departmentof Ophthalmology, AlbanyM edicalC enter
Albany, NY, USA
e-mail:te dwladis@hotmail.com

A.J. Cohen and D.A. Weinberg (eds.), *Evaluation and Management of Blepharoptosis*,
DOI 10.1007/978-0-387-92855-5_8, © Springer Science+Business Media, LLC 2011

Aponeurotic Causes

Because the levator aponeurosis conveys force for the elevation of the eyelid, a disturbance in the normal aponeurotic anatomy yields a ptotic eyelid [3]. Aponeurotic ptosis is a rare congenital problem, in which the aponeurosis fails to insert in its normal position on the tarsus. Consequently, the ptotic eyelid has a high eyelid crease with normal levator function (as the muscle itself remains healthy), due to an elevation from the normal interdigitation of the levator fibers with the skin. Cases of congenital aponeurotic ptosis may be associated with birth trauma.

Mechanical Causes

The eyelid descent seen in cases of mechanical ptosis is due to a weight essentially "pulling down" the eyelid. Specifically, while the levator muscle is healthy, it must work to overcome the burden of the eyelid mass, and the eyelid thus droops. Edema, congenital abnormalities, and neoplastic disease have all been implicated in mechanicalptos is [1].

Neurogenic Causes

Whereas the aforementioned causes of congenital ptosis are marked by infiltration weakening the muscle (myogenic), anatomic disruption (aponeurotic), and overburdening a healthy muscle (mechanical), neurogenic causes are secondary to innervational defects. While this subset of congenital ptosis represents a relatively rare finding, the diagnosis and management of neurogenicptos isis e xceptionallyimporta nt [2].

Congenital cranial nerve III (oculomotor) palsy is a potential cause of neurogenic congenital ptosis. While the nerve palsy may be partial or complete, isolated ptosis is an exceptionally rare finding in an oculomotor palsy, and clinicians should carefully look for any associated findings. Specifically, the combination of ptosis and an inability to elevate, depress, and adduct the globe strongly suggests a cranial nerve III palsy. Furthermore, pupillary dilatation should encourage one to consider this diagnosis. While a greater discussion of this diagnosis can be found elsewhere in this book, the presence of congenital cranial nerve III palsy necessitates immediate neuroimaging.

Horner syndrome is an additional neurogenic cause of congenital ptosis. The ptosis in this disease is due to an interruption in sympathetic nervous system input to Müller's muscle on the affected side, and generally results in a mild ptosis, with associated miosis and anhydrosis. Furthermore, the iris may appear lighter on the affected side. Cases of suspected Horner syndrome can be confirmed by the absence of dilation or asymmetric dilation after instillation of 10% cocaine solution into the affected eye. Hydroxyamphetamine drops can then be used to distinguish between pre and postganglionic etiologies. An appropriate systemic workup is performed, based on the results of the pharmacological testing.

Cases of misdirected innervation to the levator muscle are termed "synkinetic." The most common variant of synkinetic congenital ptosis is Marcus-Gunn jaw-winking syndrome. In this condition, the synkinesis is usually due to an abnormal connection between the levator muscle and the motor division of cranial nerve V that innervates the external pterygoid muscle, which is involved in mastication. As such, the eyelid is ptotic in a resting position, and the patient has weak levator function. However, with the movement of the patient's jaw (most commonly, lateral mandibular movement), the eyelid opens. Often, this condition is initially noticed by nursing mothers, as infants are able to raise their ptotic eyelids with feeding. More rarely, the synkinesis may occur as a result of a misdirected cranialne rveIII.

Pseudoptosis

Finally, consideration should be given to the appearance of a drooping upper eyelid in the absence of a true eyelid descent; eyelids may appear to be spuriously low in a variety of conditions. Contralateral eyelid retraction may give the false appearance of ptosis, and careful marginal reflex distance measurements should be taken to guard against this possibility. Furthermore, a lack of mechanical support may result in a mistaken diagnosis of ptosis, as occurs in enophthalmos, phthisis bulbi, microphthalmos, anophthalmos, and a superior sulcus defect. Finally, hypertropia can result in a low marginal reflex distance measurement, although the eyelid itself is well-positioned; correlation with the contralateral globe may help to guard against misdiagnosis [1, 2].

Examination

Several features distinguish between congenital and acquired variants of ptosis, and a thorough history is often useful to determine etiology. Often, the history is acquired from a parent or caregiver, and should start with an antenatal review. Careful consideration should be paid to any history of birth trauma, known syndromes, systemic disease, and developmental concerns. Furthermore, clinicians should inquire about any family history of ptosis. The age of onset of the ptosis can be ascertained from a thorough history and a review of old photographs. Eyelid lag is more typically a feature of congenital ptosis than acquired ptosis, and may thus be used to support a diagnosis of myopathic ptosis, as opposed to involutional ptosis, where the ptosis is greater in downgaze; the opposite is typically true in congenital ptosis, i.e., the ptosis is less evident in downgaze.

A comprehensive ophthalmic examination is critical when evaluating congenital ptosis. In addition to assessing visual acuity, a cycloplegic refraction should be performed to evaluate for possible anisometropia and amblyopia. Evaluation of ocular motility is needed to assess for strabismus and for the possibility of decreased ductional amplitude. Pupillary size and reaction should be measured to exclude potential neurogenic causes.

In planning for surgical intervention, the ocular surface should be studied. Given the risk of fibrosis and weakness in congenital ptosis, lagophthalmos should be assessed. The degree of impaired closure may be exacerbated by surgical correction of congenital ptosis, meaning that ocular surface dryness and irritation should be evaluated and treated prior to surgery.

As with any ptosis evaluation, the upper and lower marginal reflex distances should be measured in a patient facing directly forward without the recruitment of frontalis to spuriously elevate the eyelids. The eyelid crease should be measured, and its distinctness (or absence) should be documented, as an elevated eyelid crease may indicate an aponeurotic etiology whereas an absent crease may be suggestive of a neurogenic or myogenic source. Furthermore, the eyelid shape should be evaluated, and any contour abnormality, phimosis, or telecanthus necessitates further investigation.

Most critically, the levator function should be assessed. While normal levator function is 12–17 mm, a wide range of levator strengths can be encountered among congenital ptosis patients, and the degree of levator function can be used to determine the approach for surgical correction. While there is some variation in definitions of levator function by different clinicians, levator function can be broadly classified as "poor" (less than 4 mm), "fair" (5–7 mm), and "good" (greater than 8 mm).

External photographs are exceptionally useful in surgical planning and should be taken on all ptosispa tients.

PreoperativeC onsiderations

While the specific nature of each surgery performed for the repair of congenital ptosis is presented elsewhere in this book, careful consideration should be given to the steps necessary to determine the proper approach for each variant. By carefully matching preoperative findings and measurements to the benefits and limitations of each type of surgery, clinicians can optimize their results. Through meticulous measurement of preoperative levator function and upper marginal reflex distance, surgeons can choose the procedure that affords maximum benefit to patients with congenital ptosis. In addition, careful consideration of the patient's preoperative amount of lagophthalmos may temper the robustness of surgical attempts to lift the eyelid, and exacerbating the patient's inability to close his or her eyes may result in worsening of ocular surface dryness. As a general rule, we define "poor" levator function as less than 4 mm of excursion, "moderate" function as 5–7 mm, and "normal" functiona sa tle ast8mm [1, 2].

Preoperative considerations necessitate a careful informed consent process with the patient, the patient's family, and – where appropriate – with the patient's pediatrician or ancillary physicians who may care for the patient. Essentially, the limitations inherent to ptosis repair should be reviewed in detail. All parties involved should be intimately aware of the preoperative findings and their significance, and any systemic or ophthalmic syndromes that have been unearthed in the preoperative phase should be discussed in depth. Furthermore, because preoperative ocular surface disease and lagophthalmos necessitate a conservative surgical approach, the possibility of undercorrection and postoperative dry eye should be addressed. Contour defects merit specific consideration, as they may not be completely repaired in the surgical process.

SurgicalR epair

Surgical interventions for repair of congenital ptosis fall into three categories. Patients with fair or good levator function are candidates for levator resection surgery. In cases of 1–2 mm of ptosis, a Müllerectomy can be considered in patients who respond favorably to provocative testing with phenylephrine eye drops. Finally, patients who have poor levator function and significant ptosis should be treated with frontalis suspension techniques. In order to provide general guidelines for the selection of a specific surgical technique, the severity of ptosis is juxtaposed against the amount of levator function. Please see Fig. 8.1 for a potential management strategy. In light of more extensive details regarding the technical aspects of these procedures that can be found elsewhere in this book, our discussion of the various surgeries that can be employed in congenital ptosis centers on their clinical utility and application.

Müllerectomy

The usefulness of posterior ptosis repair is somewhat limited in cases of congenital ptosis. Specifically, Müllerectomy procedures are best employed in cases of minimal ptosis (1–2 mm) with good levator function, and these patients represent a very small portion of cases of congenital ptosis. However, when appropriate, patients can be tested for candidacy with provocative testing with phenylephrine drops. After instillation of such drops, Müller's muscle is selectively stimulated, and the ptosis may reverse. As such, the patient may undergo repair via Müllerectomy, in which Müller's muscle is resected in a transconjunctival fashion, thereby increasingits s trength [4].

LevatorR esection

Assuming that it is employed appropriately, levator resection surgery is highly effective in cases of congenital ptosis. Essentially, this surgery advances and plicates the levator muscle, thus increasing its effect. Nonetheless, the relationship between the amount of levator advancement and eyelid elevation is nonlinear; as such, rough guidelines have previously been developed to determine the amount of levator to resect during surgery, but these strategies should be adapted to each surgeon's experience.

Historically, Beard developed an algorithm in which the surgeon preoperatively determines the amount of levator for intraoperative resection. Alternatively, Burke advocated for intraoperative adjustment of the resection, based on the upper marginal reflex distance. In either case, the

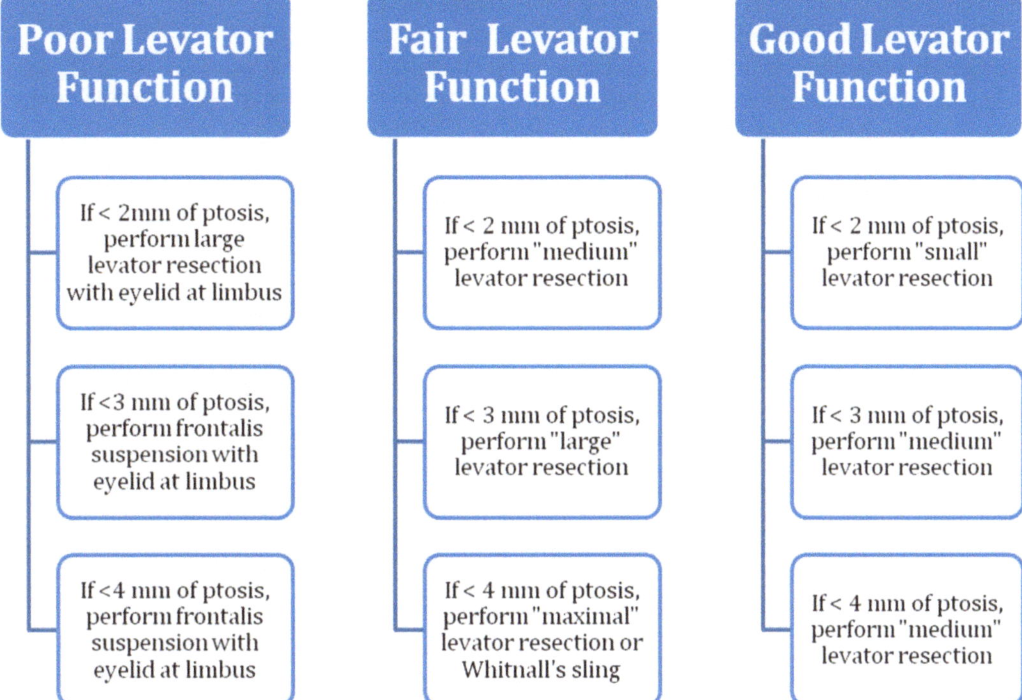

Fig.8.1 Potentialma nagements trategyf orc ongenitalpt osis

aponeurosis is advanced and apposed to the tarsal plate with interrupted sutures.

While the amount of levator muscle resected during surgery varies by patient, the levator can truly only be resected to the level of Whitnall's ligament. Alternatively, a Whitnall's sling procedure is performed by plicating the levator muscle deep to Whitnall's ligament to the tarsus. For additional advancement, some surgeons advocatc a "supramaximal" levator resection or a "Whitnall's sling plus" procedure, in which the levator muscle that lies superior to Whitnall's ligament is surgically advanced to the tarsus [1, 5].

Frontalis Suspension

The aforementioned techniques of ptosis repair generally serve those patients with fair to good levator function and modest ptosis. In more severe cases, a frontalis suspension technique must be employed to elevate the eyelid. In this technique, the eyelid is "hooked" to the eyebrow so that the stronger frontalis muscle is recruited to raise the eyelid. A variety of materials have been used for the sling that links the eyelid to the frontalis, including autogenous or banked fascia lata, silicone, polytetrafluoroethylene, and other synthetic supplies. As discussed in the surgical techniques portion of this textbook, a variety of approaches have been employed to perform frontaliss uspensions urgery.

Conclusions

Given the variations in the degree of ptosis and health of the levator muscle encountered in the management of congenital ptosis, this disorder can be a demanding entity, and meticulous evaluation and planning are essential to optimal results. Careful consideration of the patient's preoperative examination enables clinicians to diagnose syndromes and comorbid conditions, identify potential etiologies, choose a surgical approach, and execute repair of the ptotic eyelid. However, unlike typically acquired levator aponeurosis dehiscence, most cases of congenital myogenic ptosis are marked by functional and anatomic defects within the levator muscle, and surgical interventions are designed to mask these problems. Future directions might target alternative, more molecular advances to restore the normal anatomy and function of these eyelids.

References

1. Meyer DR. Congenital ptosis. In: Nerad JA, editor. Focal points. San Francisco, CA: American Academy of Ophthalmology; 2001.
2. Kersten RC, Bartley GB, Nerad JA, et al., editors. Orbit, eyelids, and lacrimal system. Basic and clinical science course. San Francisco, CA: American Academy of Ophthalmology; 2001.
3. Kersten RC, de Conciliis C, Kulwin DR. Acquired ptosis in the young and middle-aged adult population. Ophthalmology.1995; 102:924–8.
4. Putterman AM, Urist MJ. Müller muscle-conjunctiva resection. Arch Ophthalmol. 1975;93:619–23.
5. Holds JB, McLeish WM, Anderson RL. Whitnall's sling with superior tarsectomy for the correction of severe unilateral blepharoptosis. Arch Ophthalmol. 1993;111:1285–91.

Chapter 9
Involutional Ptosis

Jose Luis Tovilla

Abstract Aponeurotic ptosis, previously called senile or involutional ptosis, is the most common type of acquired ptosis. It is caused by a disinsertion or dehiscence of the levator aponeurosis from the tarsus. Clinical examination reveals a high lid crease, generally good levator function, and typically worsening of the ptosis on downgaze. These patients tend to do well with surgical correction, which involves advancement and reattachment of the levator aponeurosis to the anterior tarsal surface.

Introduction

Blepharoptosis results from underaction of the eyelid retractors relative to the eyelid protractors, causing the upper eyelid to be lower than its normal anatomic position. Ptosis may be classified into different categories (such as myogenic, involutional/aponeurotic, neurogenic, and mechanical), which may be differentiated by various clinical features and associated findings on clinical examination.

This chapter will discuss aponeurotic ptosis, the most common type of acquired ptosis [1–3]. This entity was previously called "senile ptosis" because it occurs most often in the elderly as an involutional disorder. However, the term "senile" is synonymous with advanced age, and we believe that this term is inappropriate since younger patients may develop aponeurotic ptosis associated with contact lens use or ocular trauma [2–6]. In addition, many patients found the term "senile" offensive since it implied dementia.

Background

Aponeurotic, or aponeurogenic, ptosis was first described by Jones, Quickert, and Wobig, in 1975, who demonstrated that the levator aponeurosis appeared dehisced or disinserted from the tarsus [7]. Since then, multiple studies have provided a better understanding of the pathophysiological aspects of this type of ptosis [3–8].

The levator aponeurosis normally inserts onto the upper two-thirds of the anterior surface of the tarsus and transmits force from the levator muscle to the eyelid, resulting in eyelid elevation and formation of the eyelid crease. The lid crease is a very important landmark for function and cosmesis.

Etiology

Disinsertion of the levator aponeurosis from the tarsal plate may be congenital or acquired. Congenital aponeurotic ptosis is uncommon and

J.L. Tovilla (✉)
Department of Ophthalmology, Clínica Florida Satelite, Naucalpán, Mexico
e-mail: jltovilla@yahoo.com

A.J. Cohen and D.A. Weinberg (eds.), *Evaluation and Management of Blepharoptosis*, DOI 10.1007/978-0-387-92855-5_9, © Springer Science+Business Media, LLC 2011

may be caused by birth trauma, especially in children born by forceps delivery. On the other hand, acquired aponeurotic ptosis tends to show gradual onset and progression. There are multiple factors that can cause disinsertion of the levator aponeurosis, such as continuous rubbing of the eye, chronic use of contact lenses, inflammatory diseases, or trauma (including eyelid or intraoculars urgery) [2–10].

ClinicalFi ndings

The patient with aponeurotic ptosis presents with drooping of the upper eyelid, which may be unilateral or bilateral (symmetric or asymmetric). Because the fibers of the levator aponeurosis are disinserted from their attachment to the septa between the orbicularis fibers [11], the eyelid crease may be displaced upward or may be absent. The levator dehiscence results in thinning of the eyelid, and sometimes the cornea may be visualized through the skin. Levator excursion is generally normal (12 mm or greater) becauset hem usclei tselfi sh ealthy [1–11].

A frequent complaint of patients with aponeurotic ptosis is worsening of the ptosis when they look down because the eyelid has no opposition on downgaze. This may limit the patient's ability to read [12]. Patients tend to compensate for this phenomenon with hyperfunction of the frontalis muscle. Persistent brow elevation may lead to frontalisf atigueore venc ephalgia [12].

OphthalmicExam

Evaluation of the patient with aponeurotic ptosis should include a complete ophthalmic exam. Preoperative visual acuity testing is mandatory for medicolegal documentation in case of any postoperative complications.

Visual acuity and refraction (astigmatism and axis) may change after ptosis surgery. This occurs because the weight of the upper eyelid on the cornea may affect the shape of the cornea, and hence refractive error may change after surgical repositioning of the eyelid. Corneal topography has usually demonstrated an increase in "against-the-rule" astigmatism in patients 6 weeks after surgical correction of ptosis [13]. These changes tend to be temporary, with a decrease in refractive shift by 12 months after surgery [13]. For this reason, one should avoid prescribing glasses to patients prior to and up to 3 months following ptosis surgery.

Determination of the dominant eye is very important when dealing with ptosis that is unilateral or asymmetric. Due to Hering's law ptosis may be masked in the contralateral (less ptotic) eye when the more ptotic eyelid is on the side of the dominant eye [3]. The agonist muscles (levator and frontalis muscles) generate an increased effort to keep the more ptotic eyelid open to uncover the patient's dominant eye. Since Hering's law dictates that equal innervational stimulus is delivered to yoke muscles, i.e., the two levator muscles in this case, the increased effort on the more ptotic side is transmitted to the levator in the contralateral eyelid. Hence, the less ptotic eyelid may be found in a normal or retracted position on examination. When one manually elevates or surgically repairs the more ptotic eyelid, the contralateral eye may then fall, unmasking the previously inapparent ptosis on that side. This is an important issue to consider before proceeding with ptosis repair.

In patients with aponeurotic ptosis, ocular motility should be normal, and it should be tested to confirm that one is not dealing with another type of ptosis, e.g., neurogenic or myogenic. The presence or absence of Bell's phenomenon should be evaluated. Myasthenia gravis should be considered in all patients with ptosis, and one may check for levator fatigability by asking the patient to alternate between upgaze and downgaze repeatedly, or by asking the patient to look in extreme upgaze for up to 1–2 min. The ice test may be very helpful [14]. If the ptosis shows evidence of fatiguing (worsening) with repeated or sustained use, or improvement with the ice test, further testing for myasthenia gravis should be performed (see chapter on myasthenia gravis). When evaluating the anterior surface of the globe, fluorescein dye test should be done because of the risk of postoperative worsening of pre-existing dry eye syndrome or other keratopathies. Fundoscopic examination may be important when considering certain conditions such as the mitochondrial genetic disorder, Kearns–Sayre syndrome (see chapter on myogenic ptosis).

Many cases of involutional ptosis occur in elderly patients who have excess upper eyelid skin (dermatochalasis). It is then very important to carefully assess if the lower position of the eyelid is a mechanical effect of the redundant skin and/or due to an aponeurotic defect. In many cases, these two findings (dermatochalasis and aponeurotic ptosis) exist concurrently, and each needs to be addressed surgically. The same is true regarding a ptotic brow, which may also contribute to mechanical ptosis. The eyelid position (margin reflex distance) may be observed when one manually gently lifts the eyebrow (hence eliminating the weight of the overlying excess skin from the eyelid), with care to avoid lifting the eyelid margin. This will indicate whether blepharoplasty and/or browlift alone will be sufficient to address the droopy eyelid (in the case of "pure" mechanical ptosis), or whether levator advancement surgery will also be necessary. It is also important to establish whether eyelid ptosis is being masked by compensatory brow elevation; therefore, upper eyelid position should be evaluated when the brow is returned to its normal anatomic position, either by having the patient relax his/her forehead or by gently pushing the brow down if necessary.

The eyelid crease is one of the most important defining structures of the eyelid, and it should be carefully evaluated and addressed. Eyelid crease features include its presence or absence, position (height), contour, and continuity (some patients have a partial or discontinuous crease), and in some cases, there are multiple creases. Manual elevation of overlying redundant skin may be required to observe the crease position. The normal distance from the crease to the eyelid margin in men is usually about 1 mm lower than that in women. Since the crease is formed by the attachments and action of the levator muscle, any asymmetry in the eyelid crease between the two eyelids may indicate the presence of levator aponeurosisdis insertion [11].

Finally, application of phenylephrine eye drops may be very helpful in determining which ptosis procedure should be performed. Phenylephrine stimulates Müller's muscle, causing the upper eyelid to elevate in most patients [2–4, 14–18]. Ptosis responding to phenylephrine can be corrected by a posterior approach, i.e., Müller's muscle-conjunctival resection [15, 18–20] (Fig. 9.1a–d).

AnatomicandHi stopathological Changes

Anatomic findings in acquired involutional blepharoptosis include dehiscence or disinsertion of the levator aponeurosis from the tarsus [2–10] and dehiscence of the medial limb of Whitnall's ligament [7]. The disinserted aponeurosis is usually visualized at the distal end of the orbital septum [4]. Histopathological studies in some patients have revealed a normal levator aponeurosis [4] but a myogenic degeneration of the muscle itself, characterized by a fatty degeneration in the area of the Whitnall's ligament [7, 16]. In most of these studies, Müller's muscle appeared to be grossly intact [3, 12, 13], but microscopic fibrosis with plentiful collagen fibers was observed in Müller's muscles of patients with acquired blepharoptosis induced byprolonge dha rdc ontactle nsw ear [6].

During surgery through an external approach, Müller's muscle can be identified in the space between the superior border of the tarsus and the disinserted levator aponeurosis. An anatomic landmark is the peripheral vascular arcade on the anterior surface of Müller's muscle. Identification of this structure is helpful when repositioning the aponeurosis, especially in patients with involutional blepharoptosis that may show prominent fatty infiltration of the levator muscle and Müller's muscle. This fatty infiltration has been confirmed by light microscopy and appears to be a degenerative change found in adults with acquired ptosis [15]. Clinical findings in patients

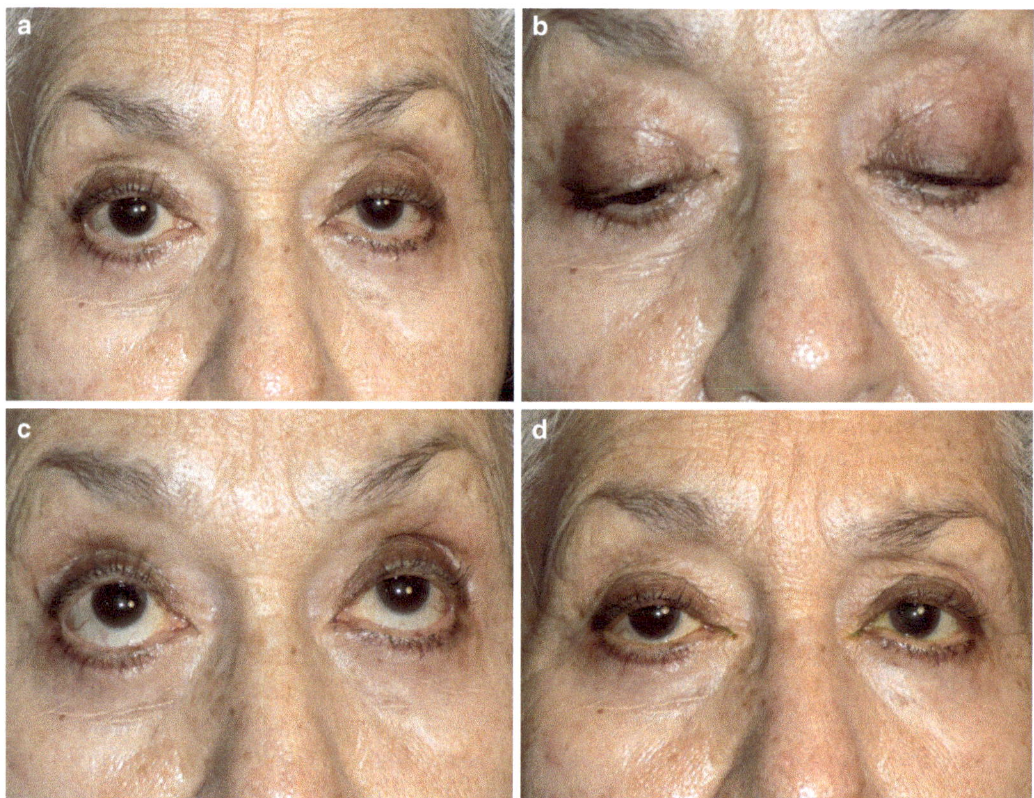

Fig. 9.1 Clinical photograph of a patient with aponeurotic ptosis. (**a**) The left upper eyelid is in an abnormal low position. Note the high crease and the elevated left eyebrow to compensate for the ptosis. (**b**) Worsening of ptosis in downgaze with significant obstruction of the visual axis on the left side ("downgaze ptosis"). (**c**) Good levator muscle function. (**d**) Good response and ptosis correction after instillation of phenylephrine drops in the left eye. The eyelid crease and height improved. Due to the law of equal innervation (Hering's law), the right upper eyelid is now ptotic, and the right eyebrow is raised involuntarily. On the other hand, the left eyebrow does not need to be elevated anymore. This patient needs ptosis surgery on both eyelids in order to achieve an optimal result

with fatty infiltration of the aponeurosis are essentially the same as those in patients with involutional ptosis with a "noninfiltrated" levatora poneurosis.

Treatment

Once the diagnosis of involutional ptosis is made, different surgical options are available, and these surgical techniques are discussed in detail elsewhere in this book. Briefly, the goal of surgery is to reattach a disinserted or dehisced aponeurosis to the superior anterior surface of the tarsus, or simply shorten and tighten a weak levator muscle, most frequently through an external approach. In some cases, superior tarsectomy may be performed, before reattaching the aponeurosis, to augment the effect of the levator advancement surgery. The external approach allows for surgical correction of the ptosis and resection of the redundant skin (dermatochalasis), if present. Ptosis surgery is usually done under local anesthesia, with or without IV sedation, in adults. Traditionally, the incision is made at the level of the eyelid crease, or, when the crease is absent, at the preferred position of the new eyelid crease [2–4, 15–18]. Although a small incision technique has been described, with favorable results [17], the traditional approach has been to open the eyelid in its entire length [18] because it allows for optimal surgical access and visualization.

Since the pathophysiology of involutional ptosis is generally presumed to be disinsertion or attenuation of the levator aponeurosis, the goal of surgery is to reattach the aponeurosis to the tarsal plate.

Sometimes the aponeurosis may be very thin or, as mentioned above, fatty infiltrated, making the procedure more technically challenging [16–18]. Having the patient awake allows for more precise eyelid positioning and may assist in identifying the levator aponeurosis and muscle in cases in which the anatomy is significantly altered, e.g., by prior trauma or surgery.

If a patient has a mild ptosis, with good response to phenylephrine eye drops, a posterior approach procedure can be performed. This can be accomplished either with the Fasanella–Servat procedure (conjunctiva-tarso–Müllerectomy) [19] or with Müller's muscle-conjunctival resection,a sde scribedb yPutte rman [20].

My personal algorithm for the Müller's muscle-conjunctival resection procedure is very straightforward. During the preoperative exam, if the ptotic eyelid elevates more than the contralateral upper eyelid on the phenylephrine test, 8 mm of conjunctiva and Müller's muscle is resected. If the ptotic eyelid elevates to a height equal to the other eye, 9 mm of tissue is excised. If the eyelid does not reach the opposite eyelid's height, 10 mm of tissue is removed. Other algorithms for amount of tissue resection have been described. Putterman and Urist resected 8.25 mm of Müller muscle and conjunctiva when the eyelid achieved a "normal" height after 10% phenylephrine testing [20]. The resection amount varied if the height was lower or higher than the desired eyelid position. A further modification of the technique was described by Dresner which also depended on the response to phenylephrine testing [21]. When phenylephrine testing resulted in at least 2 mm of eyelid elevation, the author applied 4 mm of resection for 1 mm of ptosis, 6 mm of resection for 1.5 mm of ptosis, 10 mm of resection for 2 mm of ptosis, and 12 mm of resection for 3 mm or more of ptosis.

Conclusions

In conclusion, involutional, or aponeurotic, ptosis is the most common type of ptosis and is usually an acquired disorder. It is characterized by a droopy eyelid, good to excellent levator function, a higher eyelid crease, thinning of the eyelid with corneal show-through, and worsening of the ptosis on downgaze.

Preoperative evaluation should include a complete eye and adnexal examination, and it is very important to rule out Hering's law dependency on the contralateral side. The primary surgical techniques include levator advancement surgery, with or without superior tarsectomy, Müller's muscle-conjunctival resection, and the Fasanella–Servatproc edure.

References

1. Clauser L, Tieghi R, Galiè M. Palpebral ptosis: clinical classification, differential diagnosis, and surgical guidelines: an overview. J Craniofac Surg. 2006;17(2): 246–54.
2. Morax S. Involutional ptosis. J Fr Ophtalmol. 2006; 29(6):703–11.
3. Rathbun JE. Blepharoptosis. In: Rathbun JE, editor. Eyelid surgery. Boston, MA: Little, Brown and Company; 1983. p. 201–57.
4. Dortzbach RK, Sutula FC. Involutional blepharoptosis. A histopathological study. Arch Ophthalmol. 1980;98:2045–9.
5. Kersten RC, de Concilis C, Kulwin DR. Acquired ptosis in the young and middle-aged adult population. Ophthalmology. 1995;102:924–8.
6. Watanabe A, Araki B, Noso K, Kakizaki H, Kinoshita S. Histopathology of blepharoptosis induced by prolonged hard contact lens wear. Am J Ophthalmol. 2006;141:1092–6.
7. Shore JW, McCord Jr CD. Anatomic changes in involutional blepharoptosis. Am J Ophthalmol. 1984;98: 2045–9.
8. Jones LT, Quickert MH, Wobig JL. The cure of ptosis by aponeurotic repair. Arch Ophthalmol. 1975;93:629–34.
9. Sutula FC. Histological changes in congenital and acquired blepharoptosis. Eye. 1988;2:179–84.
10. Berke RN, Wadsworth JA. Histology of levator muscle in congenital and acquired ptosis. Arch Ophthalmol.1955; 53:413–28.
11. Collin JRO, Beard C, Wood I. Experimental and clinical data on the insertion of the levator palpebrae superioris muscle. Am J Ophthalmol. 1978;85:792–801.

12. Wojno TH. Downgaze ptosis. Ophthal Plast Reconstr Surg.1993;9:83–9.
13. Holck DE, Dutton JJ, Wehrly SR. Changes in astigmatism after ptosis surgery measured by corneal topography. Ophthal Plast Reconstr Surg. 1998;14: 151–8.
14. Jacobson D. The "ice pack test". Ophthalmology. 1999;106:1282–6.
15. Ben Simon GJ, Lee S, Schwarcz RM, McCann JD, Goldberg RA. External levator advancement vs Müller's muscle-conjunctival resection for correction of upper eyelid involutional ptosis. Am J Ophthalmol. 2005;140(3):426–32.
16. Cahill K, Buerger G, Johnson B. Ptosis associated with fatty infiltration of Müller's muscle and levator muscle. Ophthal Plast Reconstr Surg. 1986;2(4):213–7.
17. Frueh BR, Musch DC, McDonald HM. Efficacy and efficiency of a small-incision, minimal dissection procedure versus a traditional approach for correcting aponeurotic ptosis. Ophthalmology. 2004;111(12): 2158–63.
18. Shovlin JP. The aponeurotic approach for the correction of blepharoptosis. Int Ophthalmol Clin. 1997; 37(3):133–5.
19. Fasanella RM, Servat J. Levator resection for minimal ptosis: another simplified operation. Arch Ophthalmol.1961; 65:493.
20. Putterman AM, Urist MJ. Müller's muscle-conjunctival resection. Arch Ophthalmol. 1975;93:619–23.
21. Dresner SC. Further modifications of Müller's muscle conjunctival resection procedure for blepharoptosis.O phthalP lastR econstrS urg.1991; 7:114–22.

Chapter 10
Myogenic Ptosis

Natan D. Kahn and David A. Weinberg

Abstract Myogenic ptosis may present in children or adults. There is commonly reduced levator function and associated weakness of the extraocular, orbicularis oculi, and facial muscles. In some cases, one may find bulbar, limb, and respiratory muscle weakness, as well as a variety of other associated findings, such as frontal balding and polychromatophilic cataracts in myotonic dystrophy. Myogenic ptosis can frequently be diagnosed via muscle biopsy or genetic testing. Ptosis surgery may be quite effective, although frontalis slings are often ultimately necessary due to the progressive nature of myopathic ptosis in many or most cases.

Introduction

Myogenic ptosis is drooping of the upper eyelid on the basis of muscle dysfunction. The myopathy may be secondary to congenital maldevelopment, acquired dystrophic or myopathic changes, neuromuscular junction blockade, trauma, or a number of other miscellaneous causes (see Table 10.1). Myogenic ptosis tends to be more difficult to treat than involutional ptosis because the myopathy impairs levator function. This typically requires either more aggressive levator resection, which carries certain associated risks and disadvantages, or frontalis suspension ptosis repair.

Congenital Myogenic Ptosis

Congenital ptosis is one of the more common forms of myogenic ptosis and is characterized by drooping of one or both upper lids at birth, with a diminished or absent lid crease, and lid lag on downgaze due to a tethering effect of the abnormal muscle. Although congenital ptosis can be quite variable in its severity, histopathologic evaluation generally demonstrates fibrofatty infiltration and dysgenesis of the levator muscle [1]. Determination of levator function by measuring the upper eyelid excursion between extreme downgaze and upgaze, while maintaining a stable brow position, is critical in ptosis surgical decision making. Other factors important to consider in congenital ptosis are: associated extraocular muscle impairment; facial anomalies; variation in eyelid position with jaw movement (Marcus Gunn jaw winking syndrome); contralateral lid position when manually lifting the ptotic lid in unilateral, or asymmetric, cases (Hering's law dependency); Bell's phenomenon; lagophthalmos; tear production; and orbicularis oculi and frontalis muscle function [2].

N.D. Kahn (✉)
Maine Eye Center, Portland, ME, USA
e-mail: nkahn@maineeyecenter.com

A.J. Cohen and D.A. Weinberg (eds.), *Evaluation and Management of Blepharoptosis*,
DOI 10.1007/978-0-387-92855-5_10, © Springer Science+Business Media, LLC 2011

Table 10.1 Myogenic ptosis – general overview of conditions, causes, and clinical features

Condition	Incidence	Usual age at presentation	Etiology	Clinical features	Inheritance	Diagnosis	Treatment	Prognosis
Congenital ptosis (heterogeneous collection of disorders)	Unknown	Birth or occasionally shortly thereafter	Usually a developmental myopathy – histopathology may show decreased striated muscle fibers, hyaline degeneration, fatty replacement, increased endomysial collagen, and loss of cross-striations	Ptosis, decreased levator function, often a reduced or absent upper lid crease, lid lag on downgaze; Bilateral in ~20% of patients; may be isolated or associated with other ocular findings, e.g., amblyopia, astigmatism, anisometropia, or other organ anomalies; concurrent superior rectus muscle maldevelopment will manifest as "double elevator palsy"	~15% have a positive family history of congenital ptosis – variable reported inheritance	Clinical, based on age at onset and clinical findings – there are a number of distinct syndromes, e.g., congenital blepharophimosis syndrome and congenital fibrosis syndrome	Surgery – type of ptosis repair depends on degree of levator function and any associated anomalies, e.g., epicanthal folds	Nonprogressive
Congenital myopathies (see below)	Overall ~6/100,000 live births						No cure for any of the congenital myopathies	
Central core myopathy (Shy–Magee syndrome, muscle core disease, central fibrillar myopathy)	Rare	Birth, but may progress and become more noticeable later	Mutation in the skeletal muscle ryanodine receptor gene (RYR1), which encodes a protein that functions as a calcium release channel in the sarcoplasmic reticulum and connects the sarcoplasmic reticulum with the transverse tubule	Usually mild floppiness, delayed milestones, moderate limb weakness and may have ptosis; risk of malignant hyperthermia with some anesthetic agents	Autosomal dominant	Muscle biopsy shows presence of central or eccentric cores within muscle fibers; genetic testing	The drug salbutamol may significantly help the weakness	Variable severity and progression, but often nonprogressive

Condition	Incidence	Usual age at presentation	Etiology	Clinical features	Inheritance	Diagnosis	Treatment	Prognosis
Multiminicore myopathy	Rare	Usually at birth or during infancy	Due to mutations in the RYR1 and SEPN1 genes in ~50% of cases (SEPN1 codes for a glycoprotein in the endoplasmic reticulum)	Different subtypes; usually severe limb weakness and scoliosis and breathing difficulty; external ophthalmoplegia in the ophthalmoplegic form; risk of malignant hyperthermia with some anesthetic agents (with the RYR1 mutation)	Typically autosomal recessive	Muscle biopsy displays multiple "minicores" (small zones of sarcomeric disorganization and/or diminished oxidative activity that correlate with lack of mitochondria); genetic testing	Supportive care	May die from respiratory failure or pneumonia
Nemaline myopathy	Most common congenital myopathy	Early childhood	Causative mutations have been found in 6 different genes (ACTA1, CFL2, NEB, TNNT1, TPM2, and TPM3) that encode protein components of the muscle thin filament	Trouble breathing and feeding; skeletal issues; ptosis and ophthalmoparesis are very rare	Autosomal dominant or recessive	Muscle biopsy reveals aggregates of rod-shaped structures (nemaline bodies); genetic testing	Supportive care	Typically nonprogressive
Congenital fiber-type disproportion	Rare	Birth	Mutation in ACTA1, SEPN1, or TPM3 (ACTA1 is the gene for skeletal muscle alpha-actin)	Floppiness, limb and facial weakness, and breathing difficulty; ptosis, ophthalmoplegia, and facial or bulbar weakness with severe limb or respiratory weakness portend a poor prognosis	Autosomal dominant, recessive or X-linked	Muscle biopsy shows type 1 fiber atrophy; genetic testing	Supportive care	Usually nonprogressive or may show improvement over time; may die from respiratory failure or pneumonia

(continued)

Table 10.1 (continued)

Condition	Incidence	Usual age at presentation	Etiology	Clinical features	Inheritance	Diagnosis	Treatment	Prognosis
Myotubular myopathy (severe infantile form of centronuclear myopathy)	Rare (1/50,000)	Birth to childhood – decreased fetal movements may even be noted prenatally by mother	Defect in MTM1 gene, which encodes for myotubularin	Severe weakness and floppiness – usually affects ocular, facial, and neck muscles, breathing and swallowing; there may be generalized muscle weakness, involvement of the heart and respiratory muscles, osteopenia	X-linked (most severe form), autosomal dominant (least severe and usually does not affect eyes) or autosomal recessive	Muscle biopsy displays small muscle fibers with centrally located nuclei with peri-nuclear halos, resembling fetal myotubes; genetic testing	Supportive care	Frequently fatal in childhood (average life expectancy, 5 months)
Centronuclear myopathy	Rare	Infancy or early childhood	Mutation in DNM2 (dynamin 2) gene (autosomal dominant form) or BIN1 (amphiphysin 2) gene (autosomal recessive form)	Ocular (ptosis, ophthalmoparesis), facial and neck muscle weakness; may show limb weakness, involvement of the heart and respiratory muscles	X-linked, autosomal dominant or recessive	Muscle biopsy shows characteristic centrally located nuclei in many muscle fibers; genetic testing	Supportive care	Often progressive

Myotonia congenita	1:23,000 (autosomal dominant), 1:50,000 (autosomal recessive); higher incidence (1:10,000) in northern Scandanavia	Variable	Two major forms – Thomsen disease (milder) and Becker disease (more common); mutation in CLCN1 gene, which alters structure or function of chloride channels, thus impairing chloride ion flow and triggering prolonged muscle contraction	Intermittent episodes of myotonia (sustained muscle contraction); may affect any skeletal muscle, including the ocular muscles; stiffness relieved by repeated contractions of the muscle (the "warm-up" phenomenon)	Autosomal dominant (Thomsen disease) and autosomal recessive (Becker disease) forms	Clinical, based on myotonic episodes starting in early childhood, improvement in stiffness with brief exercise, myotonic contraction elicited by percussion of muscles; EMG shows myotonic bursts; elevated creatine kinase; genetic testing	Muscle stiffness may improve with mexiletine, tocainide, procainamide, quinine, or phenytoin, as well as some other medications	Nonprogressive, and symptoms may improve later in life
Congenital myasthenic syndromes	Rare	Infancy usually, but occasionally a decade or two later	Heterogeneous group of genetic disorders of neuromuscular transmission – multiple mutations have been reported (RAPSN, COLQ, CHRNE, DOK7, CHRNA1, and CHAT)	Feeding difficulties, hypotonia with or without limb weakness, ptosis, facial and bulbar weakness, impaired gait, respiratory insufficiency, contractures, stridor. Fatiguability usually present.	Autosomal recessive or dominant (less common)	Diagnosis made by EMG (RNS or single fiber). Often initially misdiagnosed as congenital muscular dystrophy or myopathy.	Supportive care; may improve with pyridostigmine, 3,4-diaminopyridine and/or ephedrine	Generally nonprogressive

(continued)

Table 10.1 (continued)

Condition	Incidence	Usual age at presentation	Etiology	Clinical features	Inheritance	Diagnosis	Treatment	Prognosis
Myasthenia gravis (MG)	2/1,000,000	May present at any age, but female incidence peaks in the third decade of life, whereas male incidence peaks in the sixth or seventh decade; mean age of onset is 28 years in females and 42 years in males	Impaired neuromuscular transmission usually due to antibodies that destroy, alter, or block acetylcholine (ACh) receptors on the postsynaptic muscle membrane (which are found in 80–90% of patients with generalized MG); up to 50% of seronegative patients (those without identifiable ACh receptor antibodies) display antibodies to muscle-specific kinase (MuSK); numerous drugs have been reported to cause MG	Weakness of any skeletal (voluntary) muscle; ptosis and/or ophthalmoparesis are present initially in ~50% and eventually in up to 90% of patients; in those presenting with purely ocular myasthenia, ~84% develop generalized myasthenia, usually within 1–2 years of onset	Not typically inherited, although there are rare reports of MG in more than one family member; neonatal myasthenia results from maternal transmission of antibodies to the fetus; congenital myasthenic syndromes are rare disorders caused by defective genes that produce proteins in the acetylcholine receptor or in acetylcholinesterase; certain human leukocyte antigen (HLA) haplotypes are associated with MG, but these vary per ethnic group	Ice test, sleep test, edrophonium test, acetylcholine receptor and MuSK antibody assays, repetitive nerve stimulation, single fiber EMG	Anticholinesterases, systemic immunomodulatory therapy, thymectomy; ptosis surgery and extraocular muscle surgery may be indicated in a select population of patients with chronic stable ("burnt out") disease	Very favorable prognosis with treatment; only 3–4% mortality rate currently

Condition	Incidence	Usual age at presentation	Etiology	Clinical features	Inheritance	Diagnosis	Treatment	Prognosis
Lambert–Eaton myasthenic syndrome (LEMS)	Incidence unknown; ~3% of patients with small cell lung cancer, but also associated with a variety of other cancers; ~50–70% of patients with LEMS have an identifiable cancer	Typically middle age or older, but has been reported in children	Impaired neuromuscular transmission due to impaired presynaptic release of acetylcholine resulting from autoimmune (antibody-mediated) attack directed against the voltage-gated calcium channels on the presynaptic motor nerve terminal; this affects parasympathetic, sympathetic, and enteric neurons	Limb weakness (especially involving proximal leg muscles), ptosis, diplopia, dysarthria, dysphagia, decreased deep tendon reflexes, facilitation (improved strength after exercise), autonomic dysfunction (often dry mouth); rapid, repetitive muscle use increases strength (allows accumulation of more acetylcholine in the synapse)	None known	EMG displays: (1) Low-amplitude CMAP (compound muscle action potential) after a single, supramaximal stimulus; (2) Postexercise potentiation of CMAP; (3) Decremental response at lower rates of stimulation after repetitive nerve stimulation and incremental response at higher rates of stimulation; Identification of underlying malignancy; Test for acetylcholine receptor antibodies to rule out myasthenia gravis	Cholinesterase inhibitor; potassium channel blocker; plasmapheresis; high-dose IVIG; immunosuppressive drugs; treatment of the underlying malignancy, if identified	Life expectancy impacted by the underlying malignancy and not usually by LEMS; respiratory failure is rare

(continued)

Table 10.1 (continued)

Condition	Incidence	Usual age at presentation	Etiology	Clinical features	Inheritance	Diagnosis	Treatment	Prognosis
Botulism	~145 cases per year in the U.S. (15% foodborne, 65% infant botulism, 20% wound botulism)	Any age	Paralytic illness caused by a neurotoxin produced by the bacterium *Clostridium botulinum*; toxin causes a peripheral cholinergic blockade by inhibiting exocytotic release of acetylcholine from the presynaptic nerve terminal	Food-borne and wound botulism – facial weakness, diplopia, ptosis, dysarthria, dysphagia, difficulty breathing, autonomic effects (dilated pupils, blurred vision, dry mouth, nausea, vomiting, abdominal cramps, bradycardia, hypotension, urinary retention), decreased tendon reflexes, paralysis; Infant botulism – constipation, floppy movements, and trouble controlling the head due to muscle weakness, weak cry, ptosis, lethargy, difficulty sucking or feeding, paralysis	None known	Based on clinical presentation; EMG or single fiber EMG is highly diagnostic; send serum, feces, gastric aspirate, suspected contaminated food for toxin assay, culture and mouse bioassay; PCR-based detection of clostridial genes; ELISA identification of toxin (not widely available)	Medical emergency since this condition is potentially fatal; trivalent equine antitoxin (most effective within first 24 h, so it should be given empirically if adequate clinical suspicion); Wound botulism – wound debridement, penicillin G or metronidazole; Foodborne botulism – emetics (no magnesium), gastric lavage, enemas; Infant botulism – human botulinum immune globulin (costs $45,000 per patient!), antitoxin and antibiotics not effective; supportive care – may require mechanical ventilation if respiratory failure (which occurs in 1/3 of patients); prevention – avoid potentially contaminated foods	Prognosis is usually good with early detection, early antitoxin administration, and intensive supportive therapy. Potentially fatal; mortality rate now 3–10%; full recovery may take weeks to months

Condition	Incidence	Usual age at presentation	Etiology	Clinical features	Inheritance	Diagnosis	Treatment	Prognosis
Chronic progressive external ophthal-moplegia	Rare	Typically in young adulthood	Mitochondrial cytopathy (mitochondrial DNA deletions)	Progressive bilateral and usually symmetric ptosis, impaired ocular motility and orbicularis weakness; may have generalized skeletal muscle weakness; ptosis often precedes ophthalmoparesis; diplopia uncommon; pupils not affected	Sporadic or maternal transmission, as with all mitochondrial DNA disorders	Biopsy of affected muscles demonstrates dark red staining of the muscle fibers ("ragged red fibers"); genetic testing	Supportive care	Typically progressive
Kearns–Sayre syndrome	Rare	Before the age of 20	Mitochondrial cytopathy (deletions or rear-rangements in mitochondrial DNA)	CPEO (progressive bilateral and usually symmetric ptosis, impaired ocular motility, and orbicularis weakness) plus pigmentary ("salt and pepper") retinopathy that may be accompanied by cardiac conduction defects (heart block), generalized skeletal muscle weakness, increased CSF protein (>100 mg/dl), cognitive impair-ment, hearing loss, short stature (38%), hypogonadism (20%), cerebellar ataxia, diabetes, seizures; ptosis often precedes ophthalmo-paresis; diplopia uncommon; pupils not affected	Usually sporadic (with de novo mitochon-drial DNA deletions, often between positions 8,469 and 13,147 on the mitochondrial genome); rarely maternal inheritance or autosomal recessive due to nuclear DNA mutation; variable expressivity; clinical presentation often depends on the proportions of normal and rearranged mtDNA molecules (heteroplasmy), the type of tissue affected, and the sensitivity of the tissue to abnormal mtDNA	Muscle biopsy may show ragged red fibers; genetic testing for mitochondrial defects (will not detect rare nuclear DNA mutations)	Symptomatic and supportive therapy; generally requires cardiac drugs or pacemaker for heart block	Progressive disorder; severity and clinical spectrum varies widely from patient to patient; life expectancy may be reduced, particularly if the cardiac issues are not addressed proactively (may progress to complete heart block)

(continued)

Table 10.1 (continued)

Condition	Incidence	Usual age at presentation	Etiology	Clinical features	Inheritance	Diagnosis	Treatment	Prognosis
Oculo-pharyngeal dystrophy	1:1,000 in French Canadians in Quebec; variable incidence in other populations	Usually after age 45 (in the 60s for the recessive form)	Defective gene for polyadenylate binding protein nuclear 1 (PABPN1) on chromosome 14	Ptosis, dysphagia, and often proximal limb weakness; ophthalmoparesis is common	Usually autosomal dominant	Genetic testing for GCN trinucleotide repeat in the first exon of PABPN1 (12–17 GCN repeats in autosomal dominant form; 11 GCN repeats in autosomal recessive form); if genetic testing is negative, consider muscle biopsy, which shows fiber size variability, increased endomysial fibrosis, and cytoplasmic basophilic rimmed vacuoles, and characteristic filamentous nuclear inclusions; EMG consistent with myopathic process	Surgical management of the ptosis and the dysphagia (if indicated)	Progressive disorder that is currently untreatable

Condition	Incidence	Usual age at presentation	Etiology	Clinical features	Inheritance	Diagnosis	Treatment	Prognosis
Myotonic dystrophy type 1 (the "classic" form)	~1:20,000; more common in Iceland and Quebec; most common form of muscular dystrophy in adults	Usually in the second or third decade of life; onset at birth or soon thereafter in the congenital form	Expansion of the CTG trinucleotide repeat in the gene *DMPK*	The classic form displays generalized muscle weakness and wasting, including facial weakness and ptosis, myotonia (sustained muscle contraction), polychromatophilic PSC cataracts, balding and often cardiac conduction defects, as well as other multisystem involvement; infantile hypotonia, respiratory deficits, and mental retardation in the congenital form	Autosomal dominant with variable expressivity	Genetic testing; EMG shows myopathic changes and myotonic discharges; muscle biopsy may show myopathy	Symptomatic and supportive therapy; genetic counseling; ptosis surgery	Slowly progressive; may reduce life expectancy (often due to cardiac arrhythmia)
Familial periodic paralysis	Rare	Hypokalemic form – attacks usually begin in adoles-cence; hyperkalemic form – attacks typically begin in infancy or early childhood	Group of inherited neurologic disorders caused by mutations in genes that regulate sodium and calcium channels in nerve cells	Characterized by episodes in which the affected muscles become slack, weak, and unable to contract. Between attacks, the affected muscles usually function normally. Limbs are most commonly affected, but may cause eyelid and facial weakness, muscle pain, cardiac dysrhythmia, difficulty in breathing or swallowing; may be at increased risk for malignant hyperthermia	Autosomal dominant	Family history; genetic testing: Hypokalemic form – 55–70% have mutations in CACNA1S; Hyperkalemic form type 1 – caused by point mutations in SCN4A, encoding the voltage-gated skeletal muscle sodium channel. Targeted mutation analysis for nine common mutations detects a mutation in ~55% of affected individuals	Avoiding carbohy-drate-rich meals and strenuous exercise, and taking acetazol-amide daily may prevent hypokalemic attacks. Attacks can be managed with IV or PO potassium. Eating carbohydrate-rich, low-potassium foods and avoiding strenuous exercise and fasting can help prevent hyperkalemic attacks	Repeated attacks may eventually lead to chronic weakness

(continued)

Table 10.1 (continued)

Condition	Incidence	Usual age at presentation	Etiology	Clinical features	Inheritance	Diagnosis	Treatment	Prognosis
Statin myopathy	Rare (~0.1%) – the risk appears to be dose-dependent – patients with preexisting nonmetabolic myopathy are at greater risk	Any age	Several proposed mechanisms – autoimmune muscle injury; metabolic muscle defects (including reduced levels of small proteins involved in myocyte maintenance); rhabdomyolysis; impaired cholesterol synthesis impacting myocyte membrane behavior	Muscle pain, tenderness, fatigue, cramping – ptosis is very rare, and the association with statin use is unclear	None known	Diagnosis is presumptive, based upon clinical history of statin usage	Discontinuation of the statin (HMG CoA reductase inhibitor) medication	The myopathy usually resolves after stopping the statin
Corticosteroid myopathy	Unknown	Any age	With systemic corticosteroids, muscle fiber atrophy involving type II > type I fibers; With periocular and topical corticosteroids, myopathic changes have been observed in some cases, but not consistently	With systemic corticosteroids, usually proximal muscle weakness and wasting, especially in the legs, and may cause glaucoma; Topical and periocular corticosteroids may cause ptosis, mydriasis and glaucoma	None known	Diagnosis is presumptive, based upon clinical history of corticosteroid administration	Discontinuation of the corticosteroid medication; ptosis surgery is sometimes required	Ptosis may improve after discontinuation of the medication

Condition	Incidence	Usual age at presentation	Etiology	Clinical features	Inheritance	Diagnosis	Treatment	Prognosis
Highly active antiretroviral therapy (HAART) myopathy	Myopathy seen in up to 20% of patients on zidovudine for at least 1 year	Any age	Nucleoside-analogue reverse-transcriptase inhibitors in HAART for HIV appear to cause mitochondrial toxicity (possibly via mitochondrial DNA depletion due to inhibition of DNA polymerase gamma, oxidative stress, inhibition of mitochondrial bioenergetic machinery, mitochondrial depletion of l-carnitine, apoptosis)	Ptosis, ophthalmoplegia	None known	Diagnosis is presumptive, based upon clinical history of HAART therapy for HIV infection, particularly usage of zidovudine (azidothymidine, AZT)	Discontinuation of zidovudine often leads to significant recovery	Myopathy has fairly good prognosis
Trauma (accidental, surgical, myotoxicity from local anesthetic injection)	Unknown	Any age	Damage to the muscle fibers and/or their neurovascular supply	Clinical features depend on the location and extent of the trauma; may cause paresis and restriction	None	Diagnosis based on clinical history; forced ductions and active force generation testing may help differentiate paretic from restrictive process	Observe for at least several months for spontaneous improvement and then consider eye muscle surgery to achieve single binocular vision in primary gaze	Prognosis depends upon the nature and extent of the injury
Inflammatory	Not uncommon	Any age	Myositis that interferes with muscle function	Orbital inflammation may be characterized by a wide range of clinical presentations which depend upon the location and extent of orbital involvement; pain is usually a prominent feature, and often see inflammatory signs (lid erythema and edema, conjunctival injection and chemosis)	None known	Diagnosis based on clinical presentation and orbital imaging	Systemic or periocular anti-inflammatory drugs, e.g. corticosteroids	Usually excellent with appropriate anti-inflammatory therapy, although the prognosis ultimately impacted by any associated or causative local or systemic disorders

(continued)

Table 10.1 (continued)

Condition	Incidence	Usual age at presentation	Etiology	Clinical features	Inheritance	Diagnosis	Treatment	Prognosis
Infiltrative (neoplastic, sarcoid, amyloid)	Rare	Any age	Infiltration of the muscle which impairs muscle function by damaging the muscle fibers or altering the muscle compliance	Varied clinical presentation, depending upon extent of orbital involvement and the nature of the underlying condition	Diverse category with potential genetic susceptibility in certain disorders	Diagnosis based upon orbital biopsy, bloodwork, imaging	Treatment depends upon the specific underlying etiology	Prognosis depends upon the underlying etiology

Suggested Reading for Myogenic Ptosis Table:

Brais B. Oculopharyngeal muscular dystrophy: a polyalanine myopathy. Curr Neurol Neurosci Rep. 2009;9:76–82.

Cherington M. Botulism: update and review. Semin Neurol. 2004;24:155–63.

D'Amico A, Bertini E. Congenital myopathies. Curr Neurol Neurosci Rep. 2008;8:73–9.

Dinges WL, Witherspoon SR, Itani KM, Garg A, Peterson DM. Blepharoptosis and external ophthalmoplegia associated with long-term antiretroviral therapy. Clin Infect Dis. 2008;47:845–52.

Edmond JC. Mitochondrial disorders. Int Ophthalmol Clin. 2009;49:27–33.

Elrod RD, Weinberg DA. Ocular myasthenia gravis. Ophthalmol Clin North Am. 2004;17:275–309.

Fontaine B. Periodic paralysis. Adv Genet. 2008;63:3–23.

Fraunfelder FW, Richards AB. Diplopia, blepharoptosis, and ophthalmoplegia and 3-hydroxy-3-methyl-glutaryl-CoA reductase inhibitor use. Ophthalmology. 2008;115:2282–5.

Kinali M, Beeson D, Pitt MC, Jungbluth H, Simonds AK, Aloysius A, et al. Congenital myasthenic syndromes in childhood: diagnosis and management challenges. J Neuroimmunol. 2008;201–202:6–12. Epub 2008 Aug 15.

Lehmann-Horn F, Jurkat-Rott K, Rudel R. Diagnostics and therapy of muscle channelopathies – Guidelines of the Ulm Muscle Centre. Acta Myol. 2008;27:98–113.

National Institute of Neurological Disorders and Stroke/National Institutes of Health. NINDS congenital myopathy information page. http://www.ninds.nih.gov/disorders/myopathy_congenital/myopathy_congenital.htm

Pfeffer G, Cote HC, Montaner JS, Li CC, Jitratkosol M, Mezel MM. Ophthalmoplegia and ptosis: mitochondrial toxicity in patients receiving HIV therapy. Neurology. 2009;73:71–2.

Pourmand R. Lambert–Eaton myasthenic syndrome. Front Neurol Neurosci. 2009;26:120–5. Epub 2009 Apr 6.

Silkiss RZ, Lee H, Gills Ray VL. Highly active antiretroviral therapy-associated ptosis in patients with human immunodeficiency virus. Arch Ophthalmol. 2009;127:345–6.

Song A, Carter KD, Nerad JA, Boldt C, Folk J. Steroid-induced ptosis: case studies and histopathologic analysis. Eye. 2008;22:491–5.

Weimer MB, Wong J. Lambert–Eaton myasthenic syndrome. Curr Treat Options Neurol. 2009;11:77–84.

Wheeler TM, Thornton CA. Myotonic dystrophy: RNA-mediated muscle disease. Curr Opin Neurol. 2007;20:572–6.

Double elevator palsy is a form of congenital ptosis in which the superior rectus muscle is also involved, thereby limiting upgaze in addition to the ptosis. This can be seen as an isolated condition or as part of a familial congenital fibrosis syndrome(Fig. 10.1) [3].

Several congenital syndromes include ptosis as one of the characteristic findings on physical examination. Blepharophimosis syndrome (Fig. 10.2) is an autosomal dominant disorder characterized by congenital ptosis associated with epicanthus inversus, telecanthus, and blepharophimosis, i.e., horizontal shortening of the palpebral fissure. One form is associated with female infertility [4]. Other syndromes associated with congenital ptosis include Michels, Noonan, Schwartz–Jampel, Marden–Walker, Dubowitz, and Smith–Lemli–Opitz syndromes [5].

The type of ptosis procedure performed for congenital ptosis, as with acquired ptosis, depends upon the severity of the ptosis and the degree of levator function (Figs. 10.3–10.5). In patients with synkinetic ptosis, as in Marcus Gunn jaw winking syndrome, the only way to eliminate the synkinetic upper eyelid movements is to "sacrifice" the levator muscle and do a frontalis suspension ptosis repair. However, the synkinesisma yre cur.

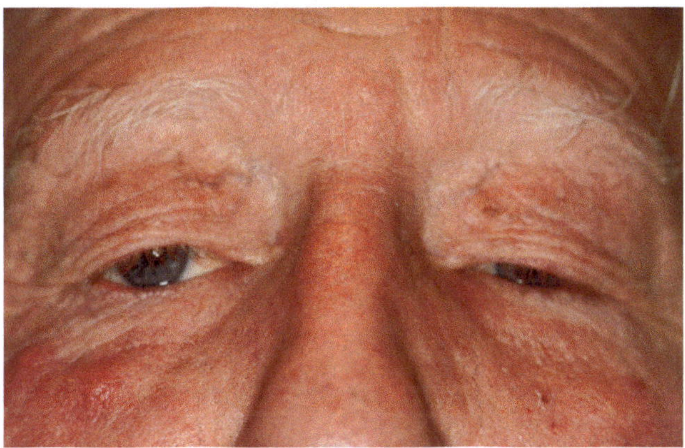

Fig. 10.1 Bilateral asymmetric ptosis with no measurable levator function associated with autosomal dominant congenital orbital fibrosis syndrome. Following strabismus surgery, the patient has single binocular vision with his eyes fixed in a direction of gaze down and slightly to the right. Since he has essentially no ocular motility in any direction bilaterally, his levator function by upper eyelid excursioni sz ero

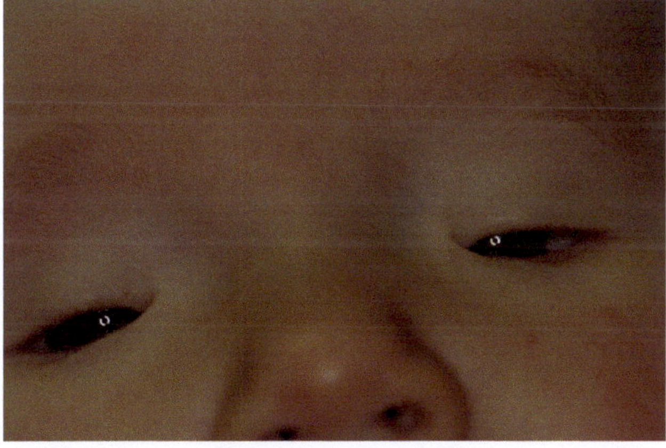

Fig. 10.2 Blepharophimosis syndrome. Note bilateral ptosis, blepharophimosis, telecanthus, and epicanthus inversus

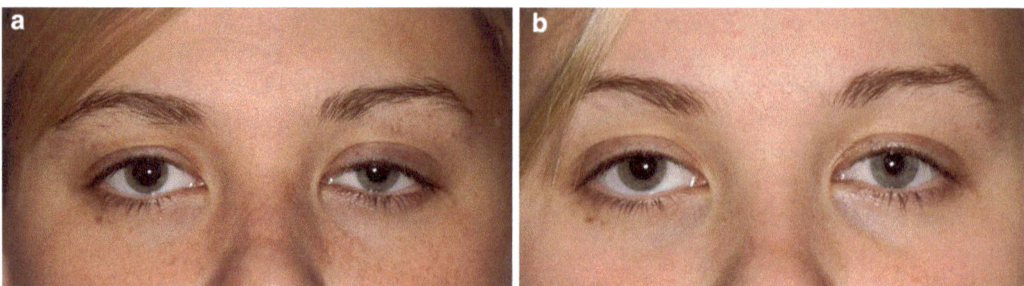

Fig. 10.3 Left congenital ptosis with fair levator function before (**a**) and after (**b**) Müller's muscle-conjunctival resection (MMCR). A favorable response to topical phenylephrine was noted preoperatively

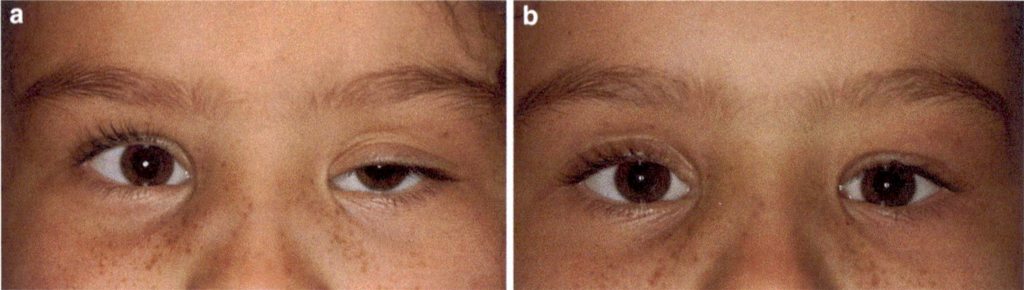

Fig. 10.4 Congenital left upper eyelid ptosis with fair levator function before (**a**) and after (**b**) unilateral levator resection

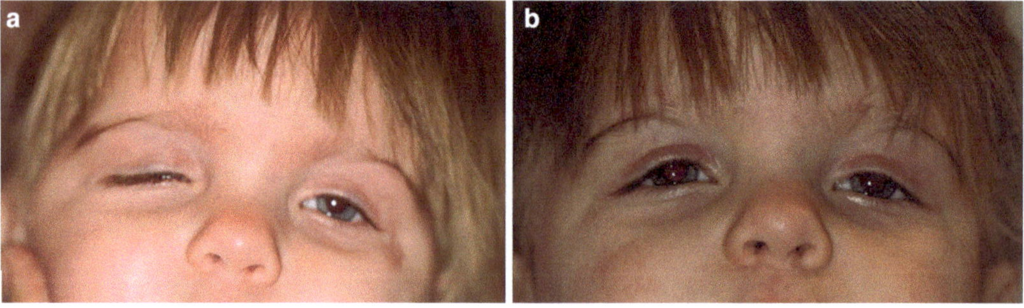

Fig. 10.5 Bilateral asymmetric congenital ptosis (associated with spina bifida) with poor levator function before (**a**) and after (**a**) frontalis slings using cadaveric fascia lata

AcquiredMyo genicPt osis

Chronic progressive external ophthalmoplegia (CPEO) (Fig. 10.6) typically refers to a mitochondrial myopathy characterized by the gradual development of bilateral and usually symmetric ptosis and generally impaired extraocular movements [6]. This results from a mitochondrial genetic defect, such as a DNA deletion. This condition may be associated with other ocular and systemic manifestations, in which case the designations "CPEO plus" and "Kearns–Sayre syndrome" are often applied [7]. Kearns–Sayre syndrome is the eponymous designation of CPEO associated with atypical retinitis pigmentosa [8] and cardiac conduction defects – the latter of which can cause complete heart block and death [9]. Ptosis surgery in CPEO, which typically involves a frontalis suspension procedure (Fig. 10.7), is frequently complicated by

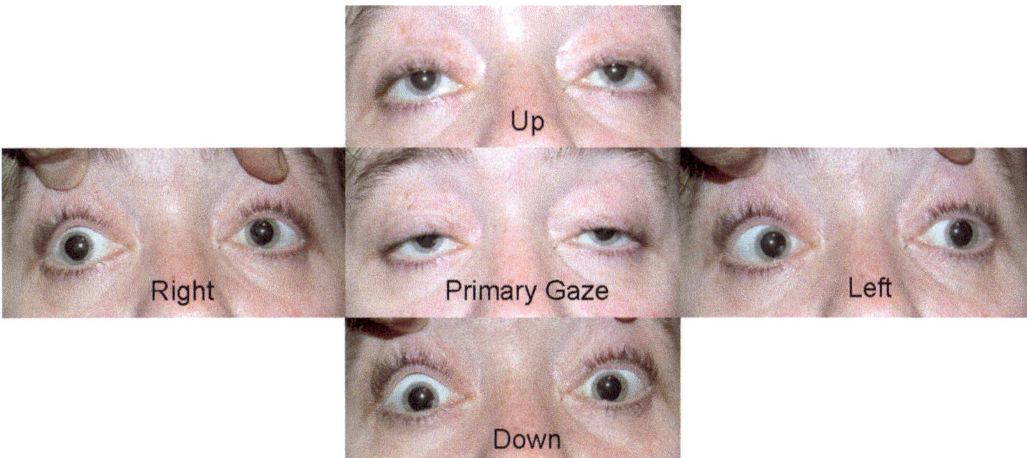

Fig. 10.6 Chronic progressive external ophthalmoplegia (CPEO). Note severe bilateral upper eyelid ptosis (levator function was poor) and severe generalized ophthalmoparesis that was symmetric bilaterally

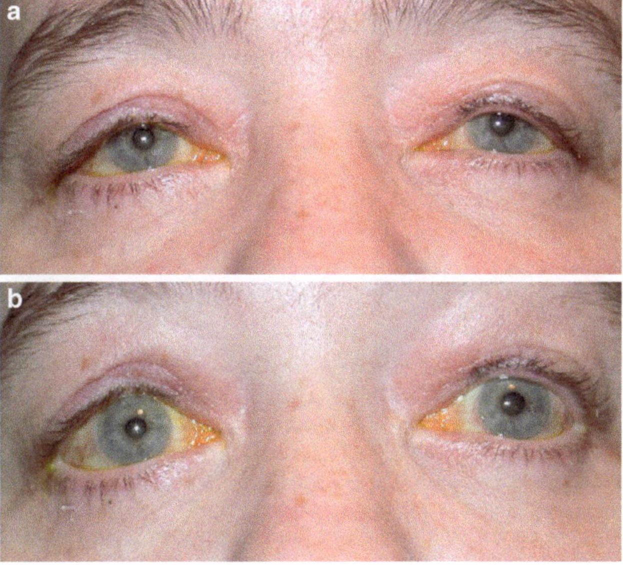

Fig. 10.7 Same CPEO patient as in Fig. 10.4 following placement of silicone frontalis slings, with brows relaxed (**a**) and brows elevated (**b**)

exposure keratopathy, as there is usually postoperative lagophthalmos (due to orbicularis muscle weakness) and a poor Bell's phenomenon. For that reason, one should generally be conservative with ptosis surgery in these patients. If there is any coexisting lower lid malposition, such as lower eyelid retraction or ectropion, it should certainly be corrected either prior to or at the time of ptosis repair. Complications associated with the use of general anesthesia may be higher in these patients because of impaired skeletal muscle metabolism of anesthetic agents [10]. Histologically, "ragged red fibers" are the *sine qua non* of CPEO and result from the absence of cytochrome oxidase staining in some of the muscle fibers. As with all diseases involving mitochondrial DNA defects, transmission to children is primarily maternal since the vast majority of the cytoplasm (containing the mitochondria) in the fertilized egg originates from the ovum and not the sperm [11]. However, rare cases of autosomal dominant inheritance have been documented [12]. Treatment with coenzyme Q10 has been reported to alleviate some of the clinical findings in the mitochondrial myopathies [13].

The muscular dystrophies are well recognized as a cause of myogenic ptosis. Myotonic muscular dystrophy (Figs. 10.8 and 10.9) is characterized by autosomal dominant inheritance; progressive ptosis; myotonia (slow relaxation of muscles after contraction); iridescent, round, polychromatic lens opacities ("Christmas tree cataracts"); frontal alopecia; distal limb weakness; and temporal wasting with weakness of the muscles of mastication, resulting in a long, thin face with a lax jaw and "hang-dog" expression [14, 15]. In addition to levator weakness, there is usually frontalis muscle weakness, which can limit the effectiveness of a frontalis sling for correction of the ptosis. In patients with severe weakness of the levator, orbicularis, and frontalis muscles (Fig. 10.10), there may be no satisfactory surgical option, and ptosis crutches and other nonsurgical treatments, such as latex eyelid makeup, may be the best way to effectively alleviate the ptosis without high risk of severe exposure keratopathy [16] (see chapter on nonsurgical treatment of ptosis).

Oculopharyngeal muscular dystrophy (OPMD) is an autosomal dominant progressive disorder with late onset, usually in the fifth or sixth decades. It is characterized by ptosis, dysphagia, and proximal limb weakness. It was first recognized in patients of French-Canadian heritage [17], although a number of other clusters have been identified throughout the world with different genetic mutations [18]. Nevertheless,

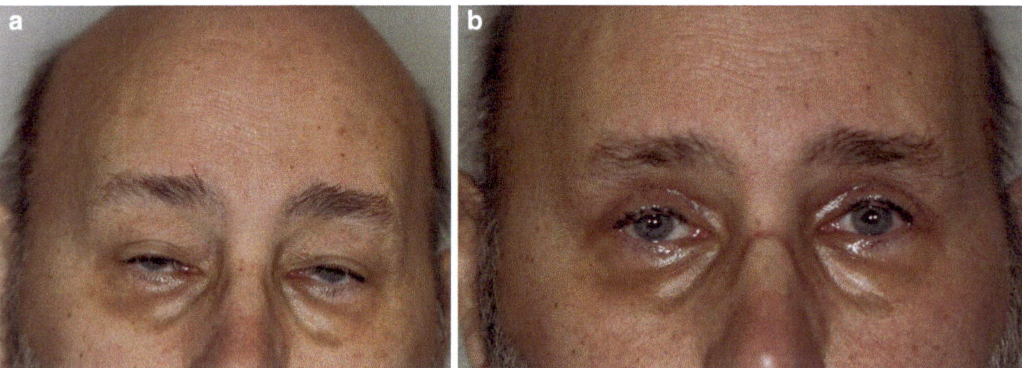

Fig. 10.8 Myotonic dystrophy patient with fair levator function ptosis before (**a**) and after (**b**) bilateral external levatorr esection

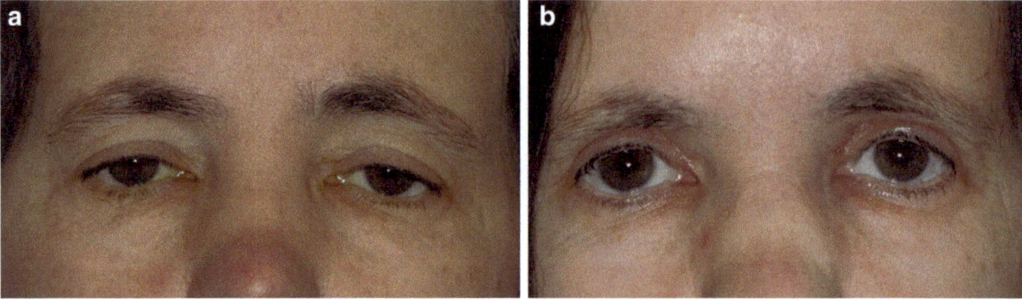

Fig.10.9 Myotonic dystrophy patient with intermediate levator function before (**a**) and after (**b**) bilateral external levatorr esection

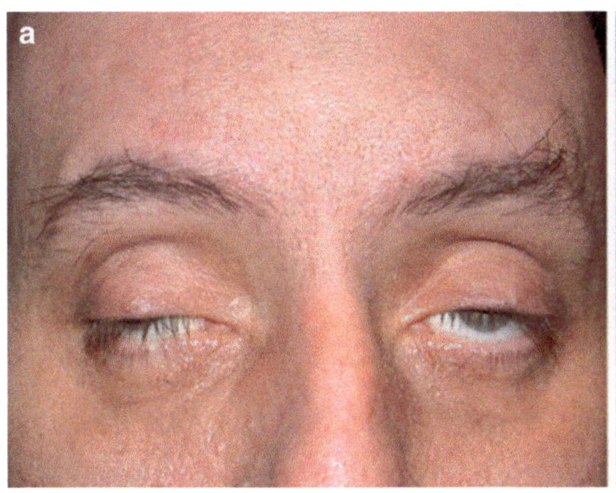
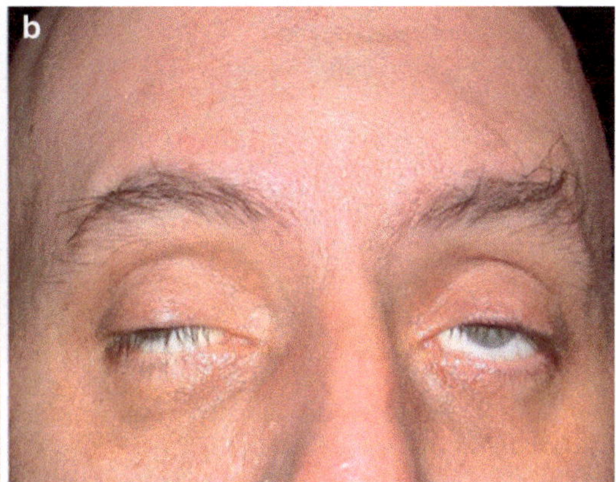

Fig. 10.10 Bilateral severe ptosis with poor levator function, associated with generalized ophthalmoparesis and severe orbicularis and frontalis muscle weakness, in a patient with myotonic dystrophy. There was barely any brow elevation with maximal frontalis contraction (notice the minimal change in brow position and the absence of any horizontal forehead rhytids). (**a**) Brows relaxed. (**b**) Maximal effort to raise brows. Moderate lagophthalmos was noted bilaterally. This patient was a poor surgical candidate and was therefore sent for ptosis crutches

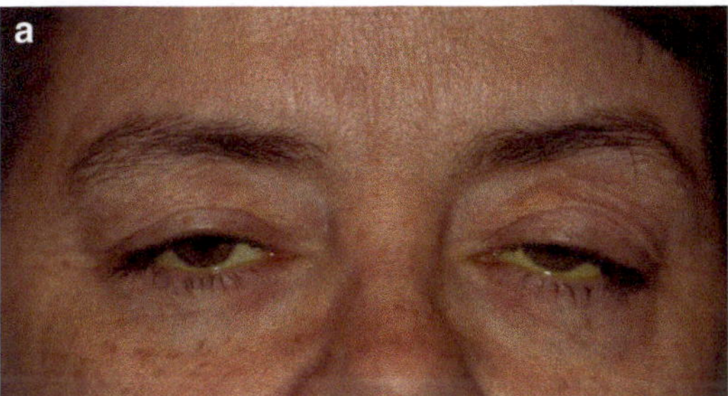
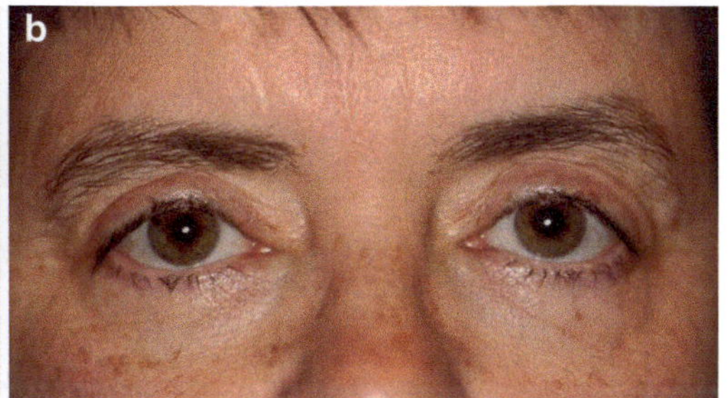

Fig.10.11 Oculopharyngeal muscular dystrophy patient with fair levator function before (**a**) and after (**b**)bi lateral externall evatorr esection

French Canadians remain one of the predominant populations with this disease. Histologically, intranuclear skeletal muscle aggregates are usually seen [19], and recent research has focused on medications [20, 21] and antibodies [22] that may diminish the collection of these nuclear polyA-binding protein 1 (PAPBN1) aggregates [23]. Early in the course of the disease, levator function is usually sufficient to perform standard external levator advancement surgery (Figs. 10.11 and 10.12). However, patients need to be warned that with disease progression, the ptosis is likely to recur, and frontalis slings may be necessary in the future (Figs. 10.13 and 10.14) [24]. It has been observed that the ptosis and compensatory retroflexed (chin up) head position (Fig. 10.15) may aggravate the swallowing difficulty. OPMD patients may benefit simply from adopting a slightly forward flexed head position while eating and drinking to reduce the likelihood of aspiration [25]. Cricopharyngeal myotomy has been found to be at least temporarily efficacious for thedys phagia [26].

Myasthenia gravis (MG) may cause ptosis (Fig. 10.16) on the basis of autoimmune antibody blockade or destruction of acetylcholine receptors on the involved muscle (see supplemental section on MG immediately following this chapter). The ptosis is usually more pronounced later in the day because of fatigability, which is a prominent component of MG. In addition to the variable and fatigable ptosis, incomitant and variable diplopia is often also seen, and sometimes weak eye closure. The

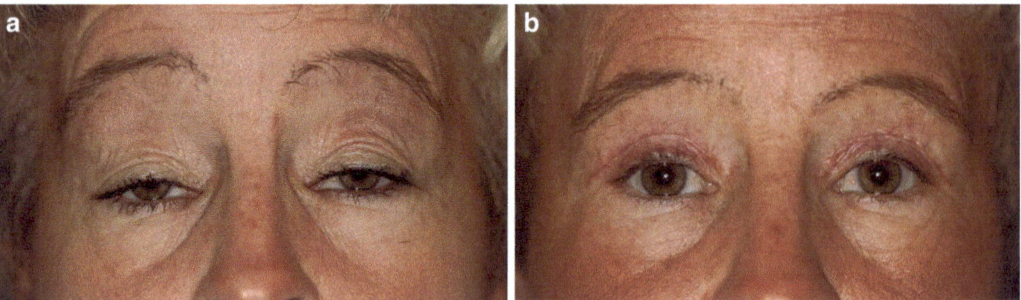

Fig. 10.12 Oculopharyngeal muscular dystrophy patient with fair levator function before (**a**) and after (**b**) bilateral externalle vatora dvancements urgery

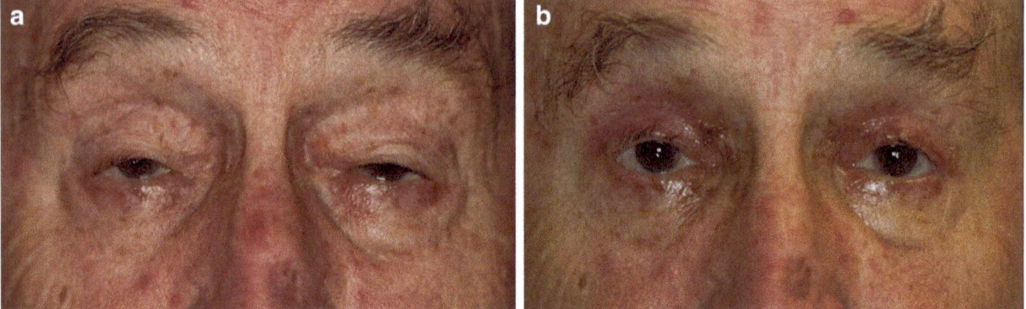

Fig. 10.13 Oculopharyngeal dystrophy patient with poor levator function before (**a**) and after (**b**) frontalis suspension ptosisr epairw iths iliconer ods

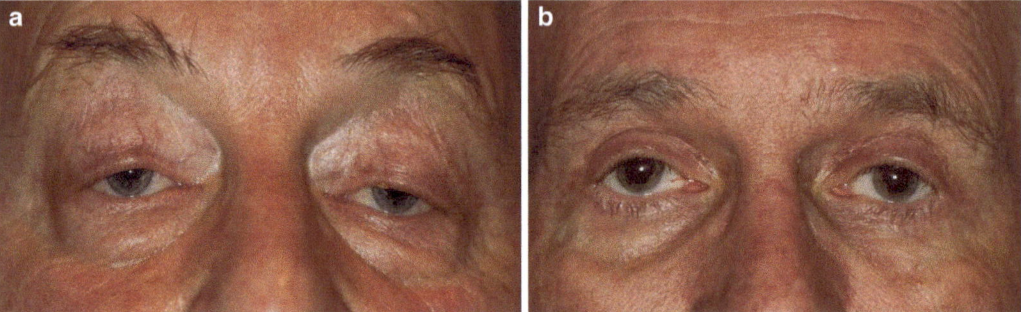

Fig. 10.14 Oculopharyngeal dystrophy patient with poor levator function before (**a**) and after (**b**) frontalis suspension ptosisr epairw iths iliconer ods

symptoms may be limited to the levator and extraocular muscles in ocular myasthenia or may be more widespread in generalized myasthenia, in which there may be facial, bulbar, limb, and/or respiratory muscle weakness. The Cogan lid twitch sign, in which the upper eyelid retracts momentarily due to an overshoot following an upward saccade from downgaze, is most commonly seen with MG, although its presence is not considered pathognomonic for MG [27]. Rest and the application of ice to the affected eye can temporarily alleviate ptosis and/or diplopia and may be helpful in clarifying the diagnosis. The presence of acetylcholine receptor antibodies in the blood, a significant response to intravenous Tensilon (edrophonium), a decremental

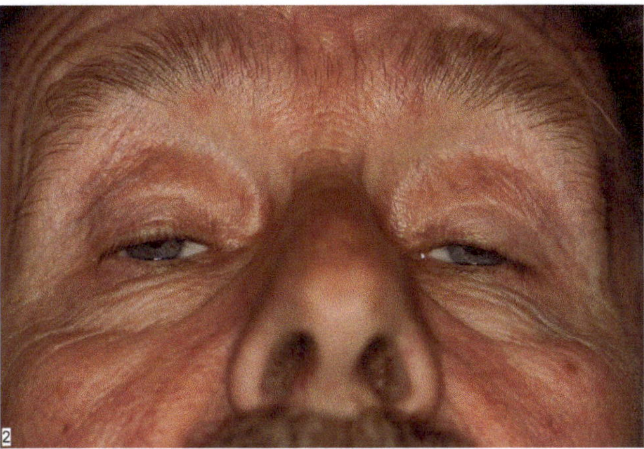

Fig. 10.15 Compensatory chin-up head position in patient with severe ptosis due to oculopharyngeal dystrophy

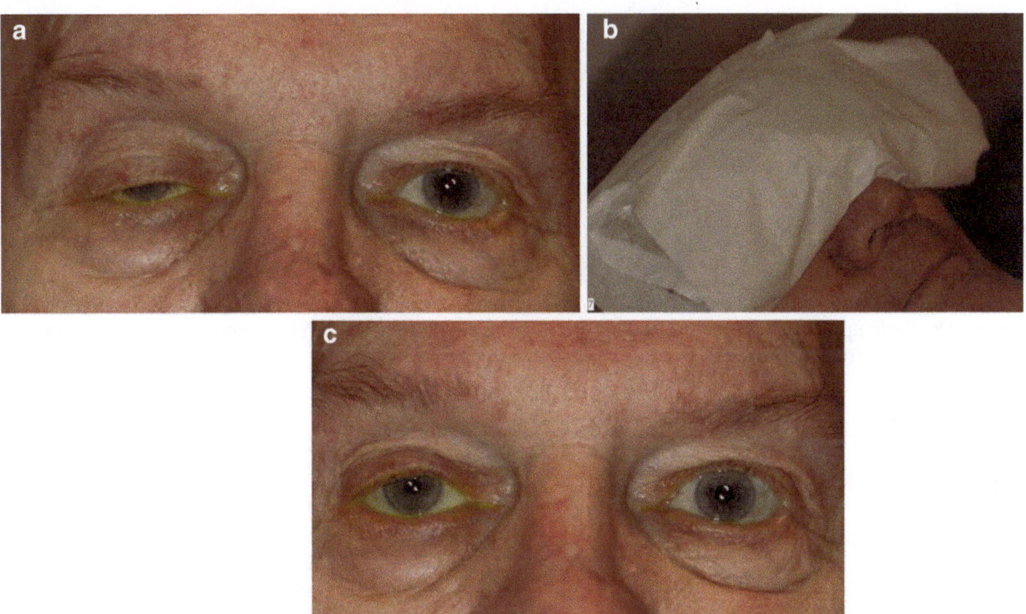

Fig. 10.16 Ptosis due to generalized myasthenia (associated with a thymoma) before (**a**), during (**b**) and after (**c**) a 2-min ice test. Patient presented with variable ptosis and diplopia. Note marked improvement in the ptosis, especially in the right eye, after the application of ice

response on repetitive nerve stimulation and "jitter" on single fiber electromyography (EMG) testing of the frontalis or orbicularis oculi muscle are other methods of making the diagnosis [28]. Mediastinal CT should be performed since thymomas are found in 12% of myasthenia gravis patients [29]. Up to 8% of Graves patients may have concurrent MG, and this disorder should be strongly considered in Graves patients with variable ptosis rather than the usual lid retraction [30]. Many patients with ocular myasthenia gravis have more clinical improvement with systemic steroids or immune-modulating drugs (such as azathioprine and rituximab) than with cholinesterase inhibitors such as pyridostigmine [31]. Only myasthenics in remission with chronic

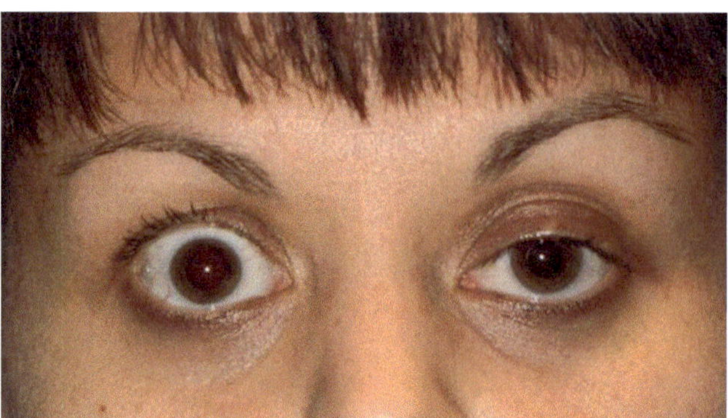

Fig. 10.17 Left upper eyelid ptosis, with compensatory right upper eyelid retraction, following glabellar botulinum toxininje ctionsforfro wnl ines

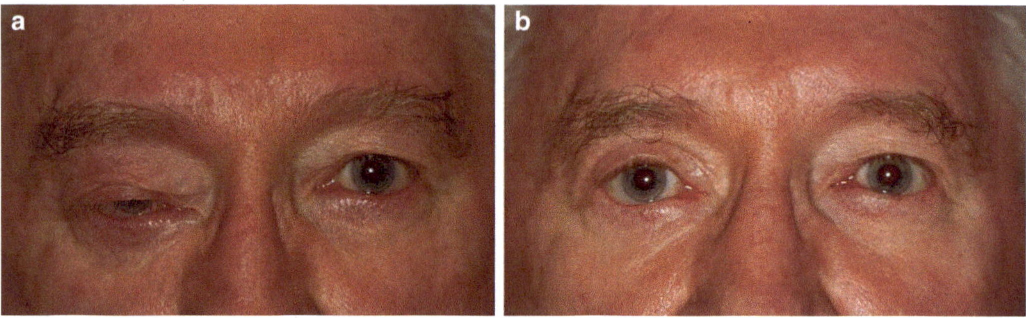

Fig. 10.18 Right upper eyelid ptosis following remote penetrating trauma with poor levator function before (**a**) and after (**b**) unilateral frontalis suspension ptosis repair with a silicone rod sling

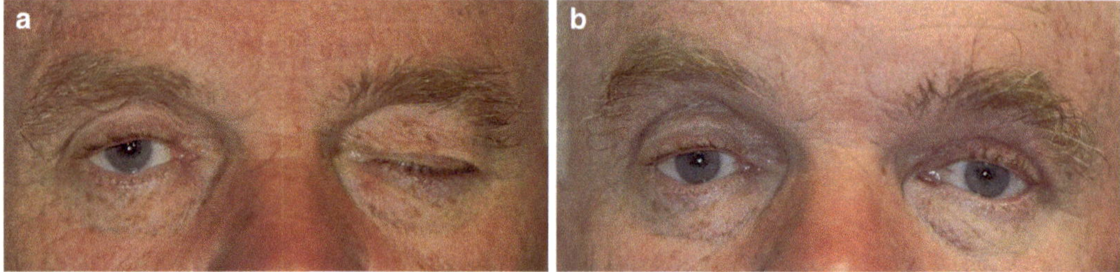

Fig. 10.19 Left upper eyelid ptosis due to remote blunt trauma before (**a**) and after (**b**) left external levator resection. Note incidental involutional ptosis on the right

stable ptosis are appropriate candidates for ptosis surgery [32].

Clinical findings resembling MG can be found in the Lambert–Eaton myasthenic syndrome (LEMS) and with various toxins. LEMS is a paraneoplastic syndrome, most frequently associated with small cell lung cancer, and usually affects large muscle groups that impact gait more often than ocular muscles. Hence, ptosis and diplopia are less common in this condition. The antibodies are directed against voltage-gated calcium channels, and the muscle weakness actually improves with sustained exertion, i.e., there is an "incremental response" with repetitive muscle activity in LEMS as opposed to the "decremental response" seen in MG, which can be demonstrated on EMG [33].

Botulinum toxin, either iatrogenically administered or released by a *Clostridium botulinum* infection, may cause ptosis (Fig. 10.17) and diplopia. The toxins of certain reptiles may also cause acetylcholine receptor blockade resulting in ptosis, diplopia, dysphagia, and respiratory failure, requiring treatment similar to thatofa mya sthenicc risis [27].

Blunt or sharp trauma may cause ptosis on the basis of levator muscle damage (Figs. 10.18 and 10.19). It is generally best to wait at least several months for spontaneous improvement, as early surgical intervention may ultimately result in overcorrection if the traumatic levator myopathy improves or resolves. Nevertheless, if there is no significant improvement, or the mechanism of injury makes it obvious that the levator muscle has been severed or separated from its attachment to the tarsal plate, early surgical exploration and repair may be considered. Certainly, if there is an eyelid laceration with evident involvement of the levator, the levator should be repaired primarily, taking care to avoid suturing the orbital septum. If the orbital septum is inadvertently incorporated into the repair, cicatricial lagophthalmos may result and may need to be surgically addressed if it is symptomatic. Iatrogenic injury to the levator muscle may result from orbital surgery or radiotherapy (Figs. 10.20 and 10.21).

There are a number of other miscellaneous causes of myogenic ptosis. These include medications such as corticosteroids, antiretroviral [34] (Fig. 10.22) and HMG co-A reductase drugs (statins) [35], radiation therapy, and pregnancy. Corticosteroid ophthalmic medications are well-known precipitants of ptosis, which typically reverses when the medication is discontinued [36]. Orbital inflammation (idiopathic or related to an identifiable cause such as sarcoidosis) and infiltrating tumors with involvement of the levator–superior rectus complex may produceptos is.

Evaluation of the Patient

While the history and physical exam of the ptosis patient is covered earlier in this text, it is worth reviewing at this point, with an emphasis on the myogenic ptosis patient. The diagnostic evaluation of the ptotic patient should include a detailed history documenting the duration, progression, and variability of symptoms, family history, medical and surgical history, and any medications taken. One should inquire regarding any particular signs or symptoms that may shed light on the etiology, such as concurrent diplopia, pain, decreased vision, proptosis, dysphagia, or limb weakness. Review of old photographs may be helpful in determining the onset and progression of the ptosis. The physical examination should ascertain best-corrected visual acuity in the ptotic eye. Decreased vision in a child may represent amblyopia, which could be due to the ptosis, and may indicate the need to accelerate the surgical intervention and contralateral patching

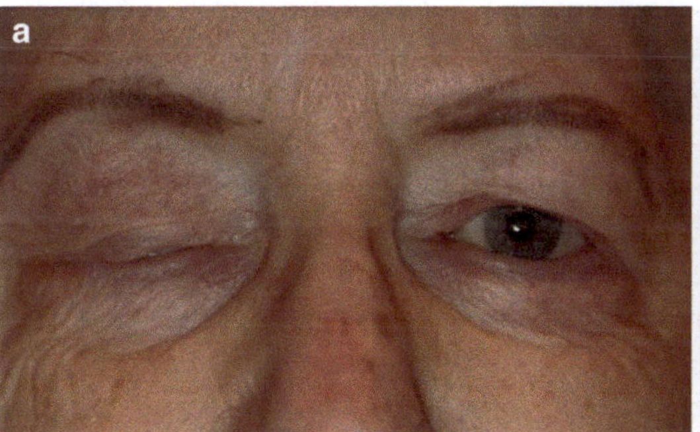

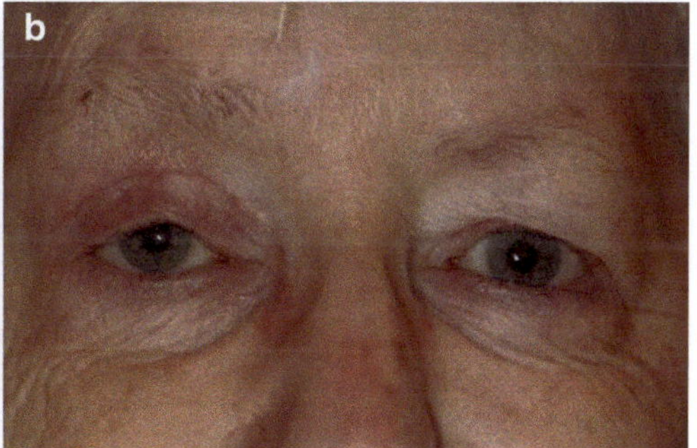

Fig. 10.20 Right upper eyelid ptosis following orbital radiotherapy to the right superior orbit for metastatic breast cancer before (**a**) and after (**b**) placement of a right frontalis sling. Prior right external levator resection was unsuccessful

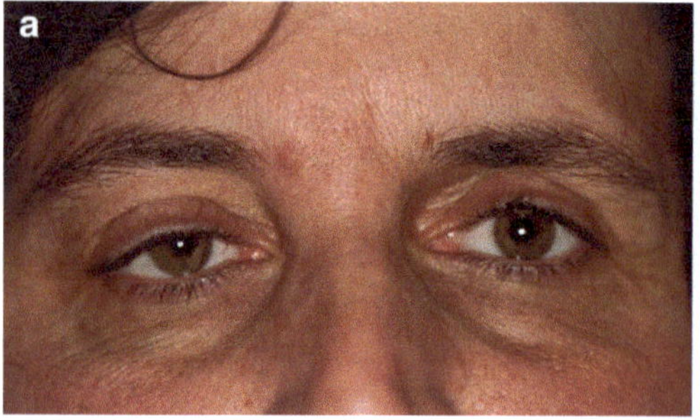

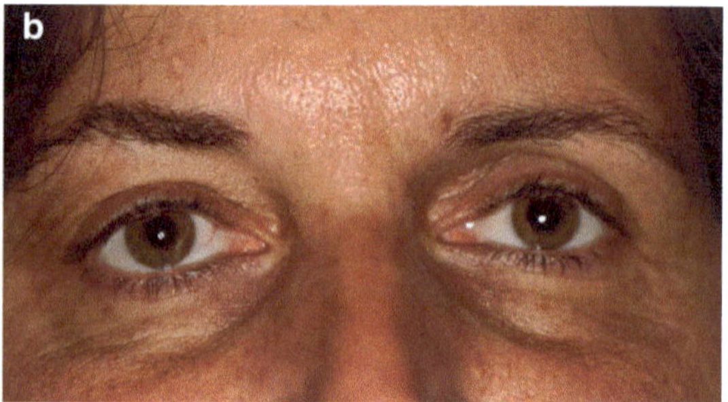

Fig. 10.21 Right upper eyelid ptosis with good levator function following orbital radiotherapy for a right sphenoid wing meningioma before (**a**) and after (**b**) right Müller's muscle-conjunctival resection. This was probably not due to a third nerve palsy, since pupils and extraocularm otility werenor mal

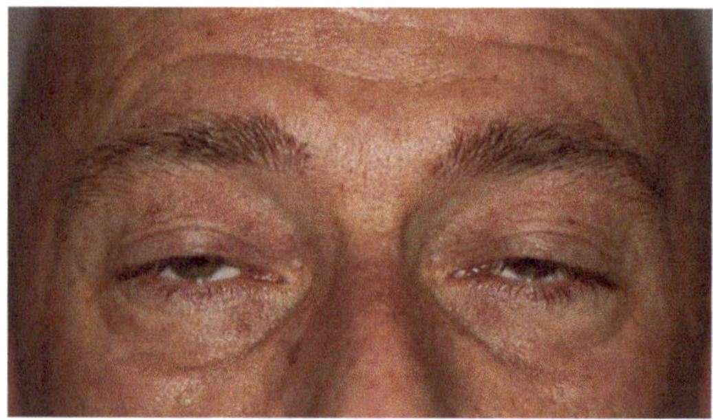

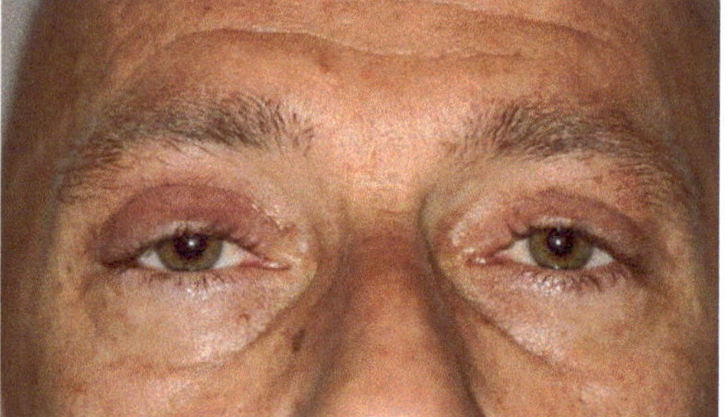

Fig.10.22 Bilateral ptosis due to antiretroviral therapy in an HIV-positive patient before (**a**) and after (**b**)bi lateral externall evatorr esection

therapy. The margin–reflex distance (MRD$_1$, distance from the corneal light reflex to the upper eyelid margin) and levator function (upper eyelid excursion from extreme downgaze to upgaze) should be measured. Severity of the ptosis and the degree of levator function weigh heavily in the decision regarding which approach to ptosis surgery should be pursued. Extraocular, frontalis, and orbicularis oculi muscle functions, in addition to facial nerve function, are important to assess, as weakness of any of those muscles may provide clues to a potential underlying disorder and may also complicate surgical intervention. It may be necessary to tighten and reposition the lower eyelid, do a lateral tarsorrhaphy, or surgically realign the eyes, for example. Noting the lid crease presence and position, or absence, may be helpful in determining the cause of the ptosis, in addition to decision making regarding maintaining, altering, or creating the lid crease. The presence of a poor Bell's phenomenon, lagophthalmos, dry eye, and lower eyelid laxity preoperatively may indicate a greater risk of postoperative exposure keratopathy and may alter the surgical plan. One should determine if the contralateral upper eyelid height drops with manual elevation of the ptotic lid, indicating Hering's law dependency. The ptotic child should be checked for a Marcus Gunn jaw wink as well as amblyopia. One should evaluate the patient for levator fatigue on sustained upgaze and a Cogan lid twitch, which may prompt the need for an ice or rest test, as well as additional testing for myasthenia gravis. Identification of any eyelid mass, inflammation, infection, or mechanical device (such as a gold weight) that could be contributing to the ptosis should be considered. Exophthalmometry may reveal proptosis or enophthalmos that heralds the presence of an occult orbital disorder.

If there is suspicion of a specific etiology, then the diagnostic evaluation should be directed accordingly. Examples of this include: variability and fatigability prompting a workup for myasthenia gravis; severe ophthalmoplegia with pigmented retinopathy may elicit bloodwork for a mitochondrial genetic disorder and cardiac consultation for possible Kearns–Sayre-associated heart block; slow release of a tight hand squeeze with frontal alopecia and typical facies - genetic testing for myotonic dystrophy; dysphagia and some proximal limb weakness with French–Canadian ancestry and a positive family history of ptosis – genetic testing and ENT consultation for oculopharyngeal dystrophy.

Treatment

The approach to treatment of myogenic ptosis is conceptually similar to management of any other type of ptosis, although myogenic patients tend to have more severe ptosis with poorer levator function plus a greater tendency to progress and higher risk of postoperative lagophthalmos (Fig. 10.23) than those with simple involutional ptosis. Nonsurgical management may be considered in patients who are not surgical candidates or those who are not interested in surgery. Nonsurgical options include simple compensatory strategies, such as recruitment of the frontalis muscle and maintaining a chin-up head position; eyelid crutches (which are attached to the back of the patient's spectacle frame); sympathomimetic eye drops (such as apraclonidine); or adhesives to temporarily adhere the lid skin to the brow skin, which carries the risk of exposure keratopathy unless this is done carefully and conservatively (see chapter on the nonsurgical treatment of ptosis).

As with other forms of ptosis, surgical treatment depends primarily on the severity of the ptosis and the levator muscle function. For patients with levator function greater than 10 mm, such as those with early or mild myopathy, standard external or internal levator resection, Müller's muscle-conjunctival resection (MMCR) or the Fasanella–Servat procedure may suffice [37]. When the levator function is between 5 and 10 mm, maximal levator advancement to the level of Whitnall's ligament (Whitnall's suspension), with or without concurrent superior tarsectomy,ma ybe s uccessful [38].

With levator function of 5 mm or less, most patients will require a frontalis sling procedure, in which the upper eyelid is linked to the brow subcutaneously, to successfully lift the severely ptotic eyelids. This may be performed utilizing

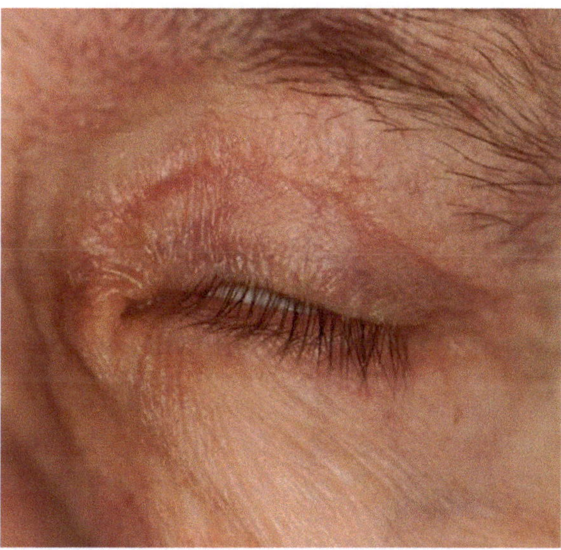

Fig. 10.23 Lagophthalmos, which was fortunately mild and asymptomatic, following frontalis suspension ptosis repair in a patient with oculopharyngeal muscular dystrophy

autologous, homologous, or heterologous tissue such as fascia lata [39], palmaris longus tendon [40], pericardium, or advancement of a frontalis muscle flap [41] for the sling. Synthetic (alloplastic) materials such as polyester suture or mesh, silicone rods [42], or polytetrafluoroethylene may also be used as slings. Various geometric configurations have been fashioned to optimize the eyelid elevation and contour, but the authors have found that in most cases, a simple pentagon, or even a single triangle, frontalis sling, works well with less bulk within the lid and brow area and may be more cosmetically acceptable [43]. Patients who also have poor frontalis muscle function, e.g., those with severe myotonic dystrophy, may not derive as much benefit from a sling. Alternatives to frontalis sling procedures in cases of poor levator function include aggressive blepharoplasty, full-thickness upper eyelid resection, or maximal levator advancement with superior tarsectomy.

In cases of myogenic ptosis that appear to be unilateral, there is frequently some degree of ptosis present on the contralateral side, which may be camouflaged by Hering's law eyelid retraction. Unilateral ptosis surgery [44] may result in unmasking of the contralateral ptosis, potentially necessitating subsequent surgical repair. One must be certain to test for Hering's law dependency during the preoperative exam. Additionally, instilling 2.5% phenylephrine ophthalmic solution in the more ptotic eye may contract Müller's muscle enough to elevate that lid and expose latent contralateral ptosis. Should the upper eyelids be in a symmetric, or nearly symmetric, position after phenylephrine eye drops, then one may choose to perform a MMCR solely on the more ptotic side – even if the levator function is less than 10 mm.

With myogenic ptosis, surgical decision making should take into account the increased risk of exposure keratopathy due to lagophthalmos in patients with concurrent orbicularis oculi muscle weakness, poor Bell's phenomenon due to ocular motility dysfunction, lower eyelid laxity and/or retraction, and preexisting dry eye syndrome. While aggressive levator advancement might be required to lift the upper eyelid to a "normal" position, undercorrection of the ptosis may be better tolerated, offering a compromise solution to the ptosis and poor eye closure and reduced ocular protective mechanisms. If exposure keratopathy is encountered postoperatively, this may be treated with aggressive ocular lubrication, punctal occlusion, taping the eyelids shut at bedtime, a moisture chamber, temporary or permanent tarsorrhaphy, and correcting lower lid laxity and retraction. When necessary to address severe, intractable exposure keratopathy, the upper lid position may be surgically lowered to improve eye closure. One may also supraplace the lower eyelid, sometimes employing a rigid spacer graft, to limit widening of the palpebral fissure when the upper eyelid is raised.

There are a myriad of potential complications of ptosis repair, which will be covered in detail elsewhere in this book, including hemorrhage, infection, corneal abrasion from an exposed suture on the inside of the eyelid, eyelid margin contour irregularities, entropion, chemosis or conjunctival prolapse, and suture/foreign body reactions. Most of these may be prevented by meticulous surgical technique and managed by appropriate early postoperative intervention, when necessary. For example, the standard Crawford frontalis sling procedure involves placement of the sling material through puncture holes in the lid just anterior to the tarsal plate. Depending on the vector of pull, the lashes may turn inward due to skin override. This can be avoided by tarsal or supratarsal fixation of the pretarsal skin at the time of surgery or Pang sutures placed postoperatively. Ensuring adequate surgical "pocket" creation and satisfactory depth of foreign or autologous material placement may help in avoiding extrusion or overlying skin reaction, such as pyogenic granuloma formation. Everting the lid during tarsal fixation to confirm the suture is not full-thickness may decrease the risk of corneal abrasion. Utilizing an eye shield when passing slings through the upper eyelid is strongly recommended to protect the globe during the procedure. Having the patient sit upright to evaluate eyelid position during the procedure may increase the possibility of a more symmetric outcome. Vitamin E oil, topical steroids, and other therapeutic modalities are purported to help diminish cutaneous scar formation, although this remains unproven.

Myogenic ptosis is unfortunately progressive in most cases, and therefore, patients need to be forewarned that they may need to undergo additional surgery in the future, with potentially more complex procedures as their disease advances. Nevertheless, they should be reassured that many therapeutic modalities are available and they should be tailored to their specific needs. Unfortunately, at this time, there is no specific therapy for the underlying genetic defect causing many of these myopathies, but rather supportive and symptomatic treatment for the clinical manifestations of their disease. As opposed to many other patients commonly encountered in an oculoplastics practice, those with myogenic ptosis will require regular and life-long follow-up due to the chronic progressive nature of their underlying disorder.

References

1. Hornblass A, Adachi M, Wolintz A, Smith B. Clinical and ultrastructural correlation in congenital and acquired ptosis. Ophthalmic Surg. 1976;7(1):69–76.
2. Frueh BR. The mechanistic classification of ptosis. Ophthalmology.19 80;87(10):1019–21.
3. Heidary G, Engle EC, Hunter DG. Congenital fibrosis of the extraocular muscles. Semin Ophthalmol. 2008;23(1):3–8.
4. Allen CE, Rubin PA. Blepharophimosis-ptosis-epicanthus inversus syndrome (BPES): clinical manifestation and treatment. Int Ophthalmol Clin. 2008;48(2):15–23.
5. De Baere E. Blepharophimosis, ptosis and epicanthus inversus. Gene Reviews. Initial posting 8 July 2004. Last revised 15 Feb 2006. Online at www.ncbi.nlm.nih.gov/bookshelf
6. Kearns TP, Sayre GP. Retinitis pigmentosa, external ophthalmoplegia, and complete heart block: unusual syndrome with histologic study in one of two cases. AMA Arch Ophthalmol. 1958;60(2):280–9.
7. Berenberg RA, Pellock JM, DiMauro S, Schotland DL, Bonilla E, Eastwood A, et al. Lumping or splitting? "Ophthalmoplegia-plus" or Kearns-Sayre syndrome? Ann Neurol. 1977;1(1):37–54.
8. Eagle Jr RC, Hedges TR, Yanoff M. The atypical pigmentary retinopathy of Kearns-Sayre syndrome. A light and electron microscopic study. Ophthalmology. 1982;89(12):1433–40.
9. Young TJ, Shah AK, Lee MH, Hayes DL. Kearns-Sayre syndrome: a case report and review of cardiovascular complications. Pacing Clin Electrophysiol. 2005; 28(5):454–7.
10. Lauwers MH, Van Lersberghe C, Camu F. Inhalation anaesthesia and the Kearns-Sayre syndrome. Anaesthesia.1994; 49(10):876–8.
11. Egger J, Wilson J. Mitochondrial inheritance in a mitochondrially mediated disease. N Engl J Med. 1983;309(3):142–6.
12. Leveille AS, Newell FW. Autosomal dominant Kearns-Sayre syndrome. Ophthalmology. 1980;87(2):99–108.
13. Ogasahara S, Yorifuji S, Nishikawa Y, Takahashi M, Wada K, Hazama T, et al. Improvement of abnormal pyruvate metabolism and cardiac conduction defect with coenzyme Q10 in Kearns-Sayre syndrome. Neurology.1985; 35(3):372–7.
14. Thornton C. The myotonic dystrophies. Semin Neurol.1999; 19(1):25–33.
15. Meola G, Moxley 3rd RT. Myotonic dystrophy type 2 and related myotonic disorders. J Neurol. 2004;251(10):1173–82.
16. Oya Y, Yoshida H, Takeshima M, Toyama J, Shigeto H, Ogawa M, et al. Beneficial effect of eyelid makeup (natural rubber latex) to induce a new fold in the treatment of blepharoptosis in myotonic dystrophy. Rinsho Shinkeigaku. 2000;40(5):483–6.
17. Codere F, Brais B, Rouleau G, Lafontaine E. Oculopharyngeal muscular dystrophy: what's new? Orbit.2001; 20(4):259–66.
18. Blumen SC, Korczyn AD, Lavoie H, Medynski S, Chapman J, Asherov A, et al. Oculopharyngeal MD among Bukhara Jews is due to a founder (GCG)9 mutation in the PABP2 gene. Neurology. 2000;55(9):1267–70.
19. Tome FM, Chateau D, Helbling-Leclerc A, Fardeau M. Morphological changes in muscular fibers in oculopharyngeal muscular dystrophy. Neuromuscul Disord. 1997;7 Suppl 1:S63–9.
20. Davies JE, Wang L, Garcia-Oroz L, Cook LJ, Vacher C, O'Donovan DG, et al. Doxycycline attenuates and delays toxicity of the oculopharyngeal muscular dystrophy mutation in transgenic mice. Nat Med. 2005;11(6):672–7.
21. Davies JE, Sarkar S, Rubinsztein DC. Trehalose reduces aggregate formation and delays pathology in a transgenic mouse model of oculopharyngeal muscular dystrophy. Hum Mol Genet. 2006;15(1): 23–31.
22. Chartier A, Raz V, Sterrenburg E, Verrips CT, van der Maarel SM, Simonelig M. Prevention of oculopharyngeal muscular dystrophy by muscular expression of Llama single-chain intrabodies in vivo. Hum Mol Genet.2009; 18(10):1849–59.
23. Verheesen P, de Kluijver A, van Koningsbruggen S, de Brij M, de Haard HJ, van Ommen GJ, et al. Prevention of oculopharyngeal muscular dystrophy-associated aggregation of nuclear polyA-binding protein with a single-domain intracellular antibody. Hum Mol Genet. 2006;15(1):105–11.

24. Molgat YM, Rodrigue D. Correction of blepharoptosis in oculopharyngeal muscular dystrophy: review of 91 cases. Can J Ophthalmol. 1993;28(1):11–4.
25. De Swart BJ, van der Sluijs BM, Vos AM, Kalf JG, Knuijt S, Cruysberg JR, et al. Ptosis aggravates dysphagia in oculopharyngeal muscular dystrophy. J Neurol Neurosurg Psychiatry. 2006;77(22):266–8.
26. Coiffier L, Perie S, Laforet P, Eymard B, St Guily JL. Long-term results of cricopharyngeal myotomy in oculopharyngeal muscular dystrophy. Otolaryngol Head Neck Surg. 2006;135(2):218–22.
27. Burde RM, Savino PJ, Trobe JD. Eyelid disturbances in clinical decisions in neuro-ophthalmology. 3rd ed. St. Louis: Mosby Publishers; 2002.
28. Benatar M. A systematic review of diagnostic studies in myasthenia gravis. Neuromuscul Disord. 2006;16(7):459–67.
29. Tormoehlen LM, Pascuzzi RM. Thymoma, myasthenia gravis, and other paraneoplastic syndromes. Hematol Oncol Clin North Am. 2008;22(3):509–26.
30. Marino M, Barbesino G, Pinchera A, Manetti L, Ricciardi R, Rossi B, et al. Increased frequency of euthyroid ophthalmopathy in patients with Graves' disease associated with myasthenia gravis. Thyroid. 2000;10(9):799–802.
31. Antonio-Santos AA, Eggenberger ER. Medical treatment options for ocular myasthenia gravis. Curr Opin Ophthalmol.2008 ;19(6):468–78.
32. Bradley EA, Bartley GB, Chapman KL, Waller RR. Surgical correction of blepharoptosis in patients with myasthenia gravis. Ophthal Plast Reconstr Surg. 2001;17(2):103–10.
33. Chan JW. Paraneoplastic retinopathies and optic neuropathies. Surv Ophthalmol. 2003;48(1):12–38.
34. Dinges WL, Witherspoon SR, Itani KM, Garg A, Peterson DM. Blepharoptosis and external ophthalmoplegia associated with long-term antiretroviral therapy. Clin Infect Dis. 2008;47(6):845–52.
35. Fraunfelder FW, Richards AB. Diplopia, blepharoptosis and ophthalmoplegia and 3-hydroxy-3-methyl-glutaryl-CoA reductase inhibitor use. Ophthalmology. 2008; 115(12):2282–5.
36. Song A, Carter KD, Nerad JA, Boldt C, Folk J. Steroid-induced ptosis: case studies and histopathologic analysis. Eye (Lond). 2008;22(4):491–5.
37. Wong VA, Beckingsale PS, Oley CA, Sulivan TJ. Management of myogenic ptosis. Ophthalmology. 2002;109(5):1023–31.
38. Patel SM, Linberg JV, Sivak-Callcott JA, Gunel E. Modified tarsal resection operation for congenital ptosis with fair levator function. Ophthal Plast Reconstr Surg. 2008;24(1):1–6.
39. Esmaeli B, Chung H, Pashby RC. Long-term results of frontalis suspension using irradiated, banked fascia lata. Ophthal Plast Reconstr Surg. 1998;14(3): 159–63.
40. Salvi SM, Currie ZI. Frontalis suspension sling using palmaris longus tendon in chronic progressive external ophthalmoplegia. Ophthal Plast Reconstr Surg. 2009;25(2):140–1.
41. Goldey SH, Baylis HI, Goldberg RA, Shorr N. Frontalis muscle flap advancement for correction of blepharoptosis. Ophthal Plast Reconstr Surg. 2000;16(2): 83–93.
42. Carter SR, Meecham WJ, Seiff SR. Silicone frontalis slings for the correction of blepharoptosis: indications and efficacy. Ophthalmology. 1996;103(4): 623–30.
43. Bagheri A, Aletaha M, Saloor H, Yazdani S. A randomized clinical trial of two methods of fascia lata suspension in congenital ptosis. Ophthal Plast Reconstr Surg. 2007;23(3):217–21.
44. Kersten RC, Bernardini FP, Khouri L, Moin M, Roumeliotis AA, Kulwin DR. Unilateral frontalis sling for the correction of unilateral poor-function ptosis. Ophthal Plast Reconstr Surg. 2005;21(6):412–6.

Chapter 11
Myasthenia Gravis

Ippolit C. A. Matjucha

Abstract Myasthenia gravis is a rare, auto-immune disease marked by fatigable weakness of striated muscles. Both ocular and systemic forms of myasthenia are seen, so that intermittent, variable ptosis, diplopia, proximal muscle weakness, poor deglutition, and dyspnea are all encountered; however, as some myasthenics present (at least initially) with ptosis alone, the disease remains a diagnostic consideration in nearly all patients with ptosis who present for oculoplastic assessment. Diagnosis is aided by a history of diurnal, fatigable symptoms; characteristic examination findings; serological assays for myasthenia-related auto-antibodies; electromyography; and response to trial treatment. Diagnostic imaging, both to look for thymoma and to rule out neurosurgical disease, is commonly performed. Usual treatment options are acetylcholine potentiators and immunosuppression. Some patients, however, may require thymectomy, plasmapheresis, or respiratory support.

Overview

Myasthenia Gravis (MG) is considered a rare disease in the USA, with a prevalence of perhaps 1 out of 5,000 patients. It is nevertheless an oft-encountered cause of ptosis, and is a diagnostic consideration, at least initially, in nearly all patients presenting with ptosis [1]. A full review discussion of the diagnostic and therapeutic considerations regarding MG is beyond the scope of this chapter; however, a brief review of considerations regarding MG when evaluating a patient with ptosis, and of therapeutic options, is presented.

MG is an auto-immune disease, with auto-antibodies most commonly directed against the postsynaptic, nicotinic acetylcholine receptor (AChR), so that the acetylcholine (ACh) released into the synaptic cleft is eventually blocked from the receptor; several additional pathogenic auto-antibodies have been described. *The clinical picture is one of intermittent or variable muscle weakness with fatigability.* The proximal muscles (moving the neck, upper arm, and thigh) are most commonly affected in generalized MG, but the disease can become lethal when the bulbar musculature (protecting the airway) and the muscles of respiration (diaphragm and intercostals) become involved.

The eyes can be affected by MG, either in its generalized form or by an eyes-only variant, *ocular MG.* The predominant ocular symptoms are variable, binocular diplopia and variable, unilateral or bilateral ptosis; symptoms typically improve with rest, and can be minimal on first awakening. Ocular MG may not be pathophysiologically distinct from generalized MG; instead, it may be that the high neuron-to-muscle-fiber ratio present in the extra-ocular muscles (1:12, up to 10 times higher than that in other striate

I.C.A. Matjucha (✉)
Neuro-opthalmologist, Comprehensive Surgical Ophthalmologist, Private Practice, Sudbury, MA, USA
e-mail: icmatjucha@verizon.net

A.J. Cohen and D.A. Weinberg (eds.), *Evaluation and Management of Blepharoptosis*,
DOI 10.1007/978-0-387-92855-5_11, © Springer Science+Business Media, LLC 2011

muscle [2]), and the need for exquisite muscle control to precisely align the eyes, makes it possible to have ocular symptoms from MG with antibody titers or affinities too low to produce more generalized symptoms [3]. Retrospective data suggest that perhaps one-third of patients with ocular myasthenina go on to develop generalized disease within 2 years, although the incidence of generalization may be lower in children [4, 5].

Diagnosis:C linical

The ophthalmologist is most likely to be involved in the diagnosis of MG patients who have purely or predominantly ocular symptoms. A patient presenting for the evaluation of isolated unilateral or bilateral ptosis should be questioned regarding variability of the ptosis and the presence of binocular diplopia. In concert with inquiring about the presence of fluctuating proximal or bulbar muscle weakness, and about fatigability with improvement of symptoms after rest, these questions will serve to implicate MG in most cases where it is present [6].

There is a large differential diagnosis for a patient presenting with ptosis and diplopia: remembering that *myasthenia never produces anisocoria, sensory loss, or aberrant regeneration* can prevent misdiagnosis [7, 8]. Besides MG, a patient presenting with ptosis and diplopia may have isolated disease of CN III or a cranial polyneuropathy. Patients with ptosis from chronic progressive external ophthalmoplegia (CPEO) are generally spared of diplopia due to relatively symmetric weakness of the extraocular muscles, but this sparing is not universal. Dysthyroid orbitopathy can produce diplopia and eyelid *retraction*; however, a dysthroid patient with unilateral eyelid retraction may instead believe that he or she has contralateral ptosis, especially if reflex blepharospasm (in response to lid retraction-induced exposure keratopathy) is also present. The potential for confusion is also high in those patients who have both MG and auto-immune thyroid disease; either half of such comorbidity might remain initially undiagnosed.

Finally, patients with congenital phorias who are experiencing typical age-related reduction of fusional vergence amplitudes may report diplopia when tired. When such a decompensating congenital phoria, with consequent intermittent diplopia, occurs in a patient with incidental, non-myasthenic ptosis, the combination of ptosis and intermittent diplopia can temporarily suggest MG and obscure the correct underlying diagnoses. Despite "Occham's razor," then, for any individual patient it must be considered that the signs and symptoms of a rare disease like myasthenia may instead be due to the presence of two unrelated, common disorders.

Similarly, patients with partial, non-myasthenic ptosis may report some degree of palpebral fissure narrowing with fatigue. Recruitment of the frontalis muscle to raise the ptotic eyelid often occurs without conscious volition on the part of the patient. As the day progresses, this compensatory brow elevation may fatigue due to decreasing effort, allowing the eyebrow, and therefore the eyelid, to slowly droop, simulating the "diurnal variation" seen in true myasthenics. However, such a mechanism is very unlikely to produce the complete ptosis sometimes experienced by myasthenics in which, after prolonged use of the eyes, one or both eyelids *shut completely and will not open again* unless the upper eyelid is elevated digitally, or the patient rests with his eyes closed for a number of minutes. A confusingly similar history, involving intermittent complete closure of both eyes, may also be encountered in patients with benign essential blepharospasm.

When MG is suspected, sensorimotor testing with quantitative measurement of any ocular misalignment in different directions of gaze, with remeasurement for stability after several minutes, can be diagnostic. For example, esotropia in primary gaze that changes to an exotropia upon repeated measurement allows few other diagnoses besides MG. The extended "gaze-holding" required for such quantitative measurement also often serves as a test of eyelid fatigability; more usually, such fatigability is evaluated by having the patient maintain sustained upgaze for at least 60 s, while observing the patient for any drop in upper eyelid height that is *unaccompanied by lowering of gaze*. The eyelids may be further tested, especially after such attempts at fatiguing, by having the patient quickly shift gaze from downward to a primary-gaze target: an initial, momentary over-shoot of the lids, so that the supra-limbal sclera becomes visible for perhaps one-half to 1 s before being covered again as the lid fatigues, is very characteristic of myasthenia; this sign is termed the *Cogan lid twitch*, after its describer, David GlendenningC ogan [9].

The physical finding of orbicularis weakness, so that forced eyelid closure is either incomplete or weak (i.e., the lids are easily distracted by the examiner's fingers) is a frequent finding in patients with ocular symptoms from MG. Additionally, proximal muscle fatigability may also be tested, even in the ophthalmology office. A patient who is unable to keep the arms extended forward at shoulder level, or who is at first able to rise from the exam chair but can no longer do so after several repetitions, would be considered to have a positive exam. And, of course, if the patient walks into the office with a soft neck collar because of an as-yet-unexplained inability to maintain neck posture, MG is already suggested.

A myasthenia office test that takes advantage of the myasthenia's characteristic improvement with rest is the *rest test*. The patient is examined with attempt to fatigue the extraocular and eyelid muscles into maximum strabismus and/or ptosis. The patient is then placed into a reclined position in a dark, quiet room for perhaps 30 min, encouraged to sleep, and instructed to keep the eyes closed. After the prescribed time, the patient is awakened and, after the request to open the eyes is given, the examiner quickly measures any remaining ptosis or strabismus to check for improvement. Significant improvement after rest suggests MG. If prolonged measurement leads to return of the previous motility deficit, or a different deficit, that observation is confirmatory. Alternatively, an ice-pack, applied to both closed eyes during the time that the patient is reclined, is added to the rest test (the *ice test*); the addition of ice may improve the sensitivity of the test [10]. The increased muscle response in myasthenics after local cooling is mediated by an electromyographically demonstrated improvementinne uromusculartra nsmission [11].

Diagnosis:T esting

When MG is suspected or diagnosed after completion of appropriate history and examination, several options are available for confirmation of the diagnosis. The most dramatic test is the improvement of an easily visible paresis (for example, at least 2 mm of relative ptosis) in response to intravenously administered *edrophonium chloride ("Tensilon test")*. Edrophonium is a short-acting acetylcholine potentiator, blocking the action of acetylcholinesterase (AChE) so that ACh released at the synapse has a longer opportunity to bind with a receptor. The complete reversal of a previously obvious ptosis, strabismus, or neck flexion upon administration of edrophonium provides convincing proof of MG, and is one of the small thrills of medical diagnosis. The return of the paresis (after 1–3 min, typically) is confirmatory.

Unfortunately, the IV edrophonium test has drawbacks. It is difficult to perform in a busy out-patient office. As the medication potentiates ACh throughout the body, several side effects can be anticipated: salivation, lacrimation, increased gastro-intestinal motility with accompanying discomfort or nausea, and diffuse muscular fasciculations, often most visible in the orbicularis. Cardiac effects, including bradycardia, hypotension, and light-headedness or syncope may be encountered. Because of these potential problems, it is recommended that atropine be available for immediate IV administration whenever edrophonium is administered, and some testers give atropine prophylactically to block these muscarinic effects.

The risk for dangerous cardiac arrhythmia after edrophonium in patients with normal heart conduction seems to be quite low [12]; therefore, the physician planning to do an edrophonium test may decide to review a pre-procedure electrocardiogram (if a recent one has not been performed) in order to stratify the risk to each individual patient. Such precaution can prevent, for example, a suspected MG patient – who instead has the Kearns–Sayre variant of CPEO and pre-existing, undiagnosed atrioventricular (AV) cardiac conduction block – from receiving edrophonium, which could further inhibit AV conduction [13]. In addition, having a cardiopulmonary resuscitation cart with appropriately trained personnel available may be a consideration for some offices if edrophonium testing is to be offered.

The *pyridostigmine test* is an "oral form" of the edrophonium test; pyridostigmine is a *per ora* AChE-inhibitor. A 60-mg test dose can be given to the patient, who then remains in the clinic for intermittent observation so that monitoring of blood pressure and heart rate may be performed; 1 h later, if ptosis has not changed and the patient has suffered no side-effect symptoms or significant change in vital signs, an additional 60 mg is given (the average daily total dosage for myasthenics treated with pyridostigmine is 600 mg). As with edrophonium, if dosage sufficient to produce side-effects has not produced improvement of ptosis, the test is negative. The pyridostigmine test probably has a higher false-negative rate than the edrophonium test, but it serves the double-duty of determining whether or not the drug will be a safe, effective, tolerated therapy for the patient. The same cautions discussed above regarding edrophonium testing also apply to pyridostigmine.

Another standard diagnostic tool for MG is serum assay for myasthenia-specific auto-antibodies. Research has revealed a host of auto-antibodies in this disease, many of which are likely pathogenic to some extent. Current clinical testing, however, revolves around three main antibody types. *Anti-AChR antibodies* were the first auto-antibodies described in MG. Binding, blocking, and modulating antibody types are usually assayed, with binding antibodies being the most prevalent in patients with MG. Still, such antibodies will be undetectable in perhaps one-sixth of patients with generalized MG, and as many as half of those with ocular MG may be likewise" sero-negative" [14–16].

Anti-striated muscle (also: anti-skeletal muscle, ASM) antibodies are strongly correlated in myasthenics with the presence of thymoma, with a sensitivity of over 80% for myasthenics with thymoma; by contrast, sero-negative, non-thymoma myasthenics are rarely positive for ASM antibodies, and ASM-positivity in the absence of anti-AChR antibodies is not specific for MG. Therefore, this test may be more helpful in diagnosing thymoma than in diagnosing sero-negative patientsw ithM G [17, 18].

The *anti-muscle-specific kinase (anti-MuSK) antibody* may be present in up to 60% of patients with sero-negative MG [19]. Because MG in sero-negative patients is not caused by AChR antibodies, diagnostic tests that focus on that receptor (e.g., edrophonium test) will generally not be as helpful; therefore, the anti-MuSK antibody assay may be an exceedingly important test in the 50% of patients with ocular MG who are "sero-negative" [20, 21]. Nevertheless, many seronegative ocular MG patients are also anti-MuSKn egative [22].

Given the availability of serum auto-antibody testing for the diagnosis of MG, many practitioners will defer AChE-inhibitor (i.e., edrophonium or pyridostigmine) testing until these blood tests have been performed. If the titers are positive, the diagnosis is confirmed, and edrophonium trial is not needed; however, a "negative" antibody result does not rule out MG.

Electrophysiological testing will provide additional diagnostic options for some patients. In patients with generalized MG, conventional-needle electromyographic (EMG) testing with repetitive nerve stimulation can reveal the characteristic finding of MG: fatiguing response over time with recovery after rest or administration of edrophonium. In patients with ocular MG, single-fiber EMG recording may be required to uncover the diagnostic findings: large jitter (variability of the relative latency between two muscle fibers innervated by a common neuron) and blocking (non-response of one fiber) [23]. In ocular MG patients who are sero-negative, anti-MuSK-negative, and equivocal or negative on edrophonium testing, single-fiber EMG of a clinically weak muscle may provide the only available confirming evidence for MG.

All patients receiving the diagnosis of MG should be screened for the presence of thymoma. The diagnostic test of choice is a thoracic computed tomography (CT) scan [24]. The use of a non-contrast CT avoids the risk of possible immediate-onset, prolonged, life-threatening dyspnea (*myasthenic crisis*) in response to iodinated contrast agents [25, 26]. In addition, it is common for patients with new-onset ptosis (especially if coupled with binocular diplopia) to undergo MRI of the brain and orbits with and without contrast to look for other etiologies; MRI is particularly important if the patient's findings are unilateral, progressive, or nonfluctuating, but is often performed even when myasthenia is strongly suspected.

MedicalT herapy

Therapy of a patient with generalized MG will usually come under the direction of a neurologist. Standard therapy includes systemic immunosuppression (most commonly, with prednisone) [27]; in cases with bulbar or respiratory involvement, high-dose intravenous corticosteroids and immediate plasmapheresis under the direction of a hematologist are typically required; intravenous immunoglobulin (IVIg) infusion can be useful as well [28]. Rarely, a previously stable myasthenic will suddenly develop myasthenic crisis; such rapid decompensation can occur spontaneously, or be triggered by illness, certain medications,ors tress [29].

Occasionally, the treatment of ocular MG will be managed by the ophthalmologist. Pyridostigmine therapy may be tried, with a low initial dosage (60 mg p.o. three times a day) that is slowly titrated upward until satisfactory therapeutic effects (or unacceptable side-effects) are produced. The initial dose of pyridostigmine may be best administered in the supervised setting of the eye clinic or office, in the form of a "pyridostigmine test" (see above). Patients' acceptance of pyridostigmine therapy is typically limited by gastro-intestinal complaints, including cramping pain and loose stools; supplemental fiber-based stool bulking agents may be of benefit, and the use of a transdermal scopolamine patch (of the type usually used for motion sickness) may further reduce undesirable muscarinic symptoms. If an acceptable therapeutic dosage is reached, repeat electrocardiogram may be considered to rule out new, drug-induced atrioventricular block.

It is currently recommended that patients with ocular MG be started on prednisone. The regimen is typically one of an initial high dosage (40–80 mg p.o. daily), with taper after improvement of symptoms; most patients will require long-term low-dose (2.5–10 mg, daily or every other day) therapy to control symptoms [30]. Prednisone therapy is expected to result in a higher rate of diplopia and ptosis control than pyridostigmine, and to both delay and reduce the incidence of conversion of patients from ocular MG to generalized MG [31]. Given the numerous known side-effects of prednisone, care must be taken to minimize those problems, including steps to lessen bone-density loss (vitamin D and calcium supplements), to avoid peptic ulcers (antacids and anti-H_2 blocker therapy), and to monitor for diabetes mellitus and hypertension. It is recommended that the patient's primary care doctor be closely involved to help with medical oversight and prevention of adverse effects from systemic immunomodulatory therapy. Systemic corticosteroids may initially result in transient worsening of muscle weakness, particularly during the first few days of treatment; this risk is most worrisome for patients with generalized myasthenia already involving the respiratory and/or pharyngeal muscles.

In many patients – especially children, adolescents, and diabetics – the risks associated with corticosteroid treatment will prompt the selection of an alternative, non-steroidal immunosuppressive agent. Such agents may be used as adjuvant therapy with corticosteroids to minimize steroid dosage, either when treatment is started or when tapering the steroid dose, or even as initial monotherapy, avoiding corticosteroids altogether. Further, they may also be resorted to when steroid treatment has been ineffective. The most familiar agent is azathioprine [32], a purine analog that has long been used for immunosuppression in organ-transplant patients and those with severe auto-immune disease. It is considered a "first-line" agent and the most frequently used immunosuppressant (after prednisone) in MG.

After azathioprine, alternative therapies suffer from either unproven efficacy (especially for newer, "promising" drugs) or increased toxicity (for older, proven medications). They are therefore at this time usually reserved for cases poorly responsive to corticosteroid and azathioprine, or in special circumstances where those agents should not be used. Practitioners considering treatment options for their myasthenic patients should keep in mind that there are very few prospective, randomized-control studies showing efficacy of the immunosuppressants used in myasthenia [33].

Plasmapheresis and IVIg – mentioned earlier in the treatment of myasthenic crisis – may also be preferred treatments in children with generalized myasthenia, in order to minimize both steroid complications and long-term cancer risk from cytotoxic agents [34]. Rituximab, a monoclonal antibody directed against CD20-expressing B-cells, has been reported effective when used for some patients with refractory MG [35]. Mycophenolate mofetil (a purine-synthesis inhibitor) seems neither to add efficacy nor to speed taper for MG patients using concurrent corticosteroids; [36, 37] however, it may be useful as a chronic suppressant for ocular MG [38], and is a consideration for patients who develop or are at risk for azathioprine toxicity, especially patients with thiopurine *S*-methyltrans-/ferase deficiency [39]. It has, however, been associated with the development of progressive multifocal leukoencephalopathy [40].

Tacrolimus is a macrolide calcineurin inhibitor that functions as a T-cell suppressant, and is usually employed for transplant-recipient immunosuppression; it may be useful in the long-term suppression of myasthenic symptoms, though its precise mode of action in MG is not clear [41]. Cyclosporine A is also a calcineurin inhibitor effective against T-cells, and has been used for MG refractory to first-line agents [42]. Cyclophosphamide is a powerful alkylating cytotoxin, often employed as a myelo-ablative in hematopoietic stem cell ("bone marrow") transplantation; the risks for toxicity with cyclophosphamide are substantial. Nevertheless, it has been used in lower, sub-ablative dosages for refractoryM G [43].

SurgicalT herapy

Patients with MG on occasion require surgical care. MG patients with thymoma will usually undergo thymectomy; in fact, consideration toward thymectomy is sometimes weighed even in MG patients with a CT-normal thymus, particularly with generalized myasthenia. Minimally invasive, video-assisted thorascopic thymectomy is one of the several possible surgical approaches [44].

Besides thoracic surgery, specific oculoplastic or strabismus-correction procedures are in some instances recommended for patients with myasthenia, despite the variability of the disease. Some myasthenic patients may have ptosis and/or strabismus due to another, unrelated condition. The clinician is frequently alerted to this condition on follow-up examinations by finding that the patient has evolved a persistent, nonvariable ptosis or strabismus, or that the patient's variability oscillates around this constant. An edrophonium test may be used to confirm the non-myasthenic nature of the repeatable deficit. Timely recognition of "fixed" ptosis or strabismus in a patient with known MG may prevent the decision to use higher dosages of medication, or more aggressive therapies, to treat what seems to be "refractory" MG.

When such non-myasthenic ptosis (or strabismus) is discovered in a patient with MG, additional diagnostic tests may be indicated to determine the etiology. Medical therapy for the stable portion of the ptosis and prismatic glasses for diplopia can be offered. Given the variable nature of MG symptoms, surgical correction is generally and understandably deemed unwise. However, in some cases, it may be appropriate to offer surgical correction of ptosis or strabismus to eliminate the fixed portion of the deficit, if this is reasonably expected to result in reduction of symptoms. Successful ptosis surgery has been reported in myasthenic patients with stable ptosis that failed to respond to medical therapy for MG [45]. Nevertheless, myasthenics with immunologically active disease and fluctuating ptosis are more likely to experience an unsatisfactory outcome (especially under-correction or recurrent ptosis)follo wingptos iss urgery.

References

1. Juel VC, Massey JM. Myasthenia gravis. Orphanet J Rare Dis. 2007;2:44. http://www.ojrd.com/content/2/1/44
2. von Noorden GK, Campos EC. Binocular vision and ocular motility. 6th ed. St. Louis, MO: Mosby; 2002. p. 102. http://telemedicine.orbis.org/bins/content_page.asp?cid=1-2193
3. Tindall RS. Humoral immunity in myasthenia gravis: clinical correlations of anti-receptor antibody avidity and titer. Ann N Y Acad Sci. 1981;377:316–31.
4. Kupersmith MJ, Latkany R, Homel P. Development of generalized disease at 2 years in patients with ocular myasthenia gravis. Arch Neurol. 2003;60(2):243–8.
5. Ortiz S, Borchert M. Long-term outcomes of pediatric ocular myasthenia gravis. Ophthalmology. 2008;115(7):1245–8.
6. Weinberg DA, Lesser RL, Vollmer TL. Ocular myasthenia: a protean disorder. Surv Ophthalmol. 1994;39(3):169–210.
7. Lepore FE, Sanborn GE, Slevin JT. Pupillary dysfunction in myasthenia gravis. Ann Neurol. 1979; 6(1):29–33.
8. Glass JP, Halpern J, Grossman RG. Uncovering ocular pseudomyasthenia. Ann Ophthalmol. 1993;25(11): 418–21.
9. Cogan DG. Myasthenia gravis: a review of the disease and a description of lid twitch as a characteristic sign. Arch Ophthalmol. 1965;74:217–21.
10. Kubis KC, Danesh-Meyer HV, Savino PJ, Sergott RC. The ice test versus the rest test in myasthenia gravis. Ophthalmology. 2000;107(11):1995–8.
11. Borenstein S, Desmedt JE. Local cooling in myasthenia. Improvement of neuromuscular failure. Arch Neurol.1975;32(3):152–7.
12. Mitrani RD, Kloosterman EM, Huikuri H, Dylewski J, Atapattu S, Interian Jr A, et al. Muscarinic receptor stimulation with edrophonium hydrochloride does not elevate ventricular fibrillation thresholds in humans. J Cardiovasc Electrophysiol. 1999;10(6): 809–16.
13. Arsura EL, Brunner NG, Namba T, Grob D. Adverse cardiovascular effects of anticholinesterase medications. Am J Med Sci. 1987;293(1):18–23.
14. Hsu SY, Tsai RK, Wang HZ, Su MY. A comparative study of ocular and generalized myasthenia gravis. Kaohsiung J Med Sci. 2002;18(2):62–9.
15. Soliven BC, Lange DJ, Penn AS, Younger D, Jaretzki III A, Lovelace RE, et al. Seronegative myasthenia gravis. Neurology. 1988;38(4):514–7.
16. Limburg PC, The TH, Hummel-Tappel E, Oosterhuis HJ. Anti-acetylcholine receptor antibodies in myasthenia gravis. Part 1. Relation to clinical parameters in 250 patients. J Neurol Sci. 1983;58(3):357–70.
17. Lanska DJ. Diagnosis of thymoma in myasthenics using anti-striated muscle antibodies: predictive value and gain in diagnostic certainty. Neurology. 1991;41(4):520–4.
18. Kuks JB, Limburg PC, Horst G, Oosterhuis HJ. Antibodies to skeletal muscle in myasthenia gravis. Part 2. Prevalence in non-thymoma patients. J Neurol Sci.1993; 120(1):78–81.
19. Sanders DB, El-Salem K, Massey JM, McConville J, Vincent A. Clinical aspects of MuSK antibody positive seronegative MG. Neurology. 2003;60(12): 1978–80.
20. Caress JB, Hunt CH, Batish SD. Anti-MuSK myasthenia gravis presenting with purely ocular findings. Arch Neurol. 2005;62(6):1002–3.
21. Hanisch F, Hain B, Zierz S. [Ocular involvement in MuSK antibody-positive myasthenia gravis]. Klin Monatsbl Augenheilkd. 2006;223(1):81–3.
22. Luchanok U, Kaminski HJ. Ocular myasthenia: diagnostic and treatment recommendations and the evidence base. Curr Opin Neurol. 2008;21(1):8–15.
23. Schwartz MS, Stålberg E. Myasthenic syndrome studied with single fiber electromyography. Arch Neurol.1975; 32(12):815–7.
24. Batra P, Herrmann Jr C, Mulder D. Mediastinal imaging in myasthenia gravis: correlation of chest radiography, CT, MR, and surgical findings. Am J Roentgenol. 1987;148(3):515–9.
25. Chagnac Y, Hadani M, Goldhammer Y. Myasthenic crisis after intravenous administration of iodinated contrast agent. Neurology. 1985;35:1219–20.
26. Ferrer X, Ellie E, Deleplanque B, Lagueny A, Julien J. [Myasthenic crisis after intravenous injection of iodine contrast product.]. Presse Méd. 1992;21:1127–8.
27. Tackenberg B, Hemmer B, Oertel WH, Sommer N. Immunosuppressive treatment of ocular myasthenia gravis. BioDrugs. 2001;15(6):369–78.
28. Díaz-Manera J, Rojas-García R, Illa I. Treatment strategies for myasthenia gravis. Expert Opin Pharmacother.2009; 10(8):1329–42.
29. Chaudhuri A, Behan PO. Myasthenic crisis. QJM. 2009;102(2):97–107.
30. Kupersmith MJ, Ying G. Ocular motor dysfunction and ptosis in ocular myasthenia gravis: effects of treatment. Br J Ophthalmol. 2005;89(10):1330–4.
31. Kupersmith MJ. Ocular myasthenia gravis: treatment successes and failures in patients with long-term follow-up. J Neurol. 2009;256(8):1314–20.

32. Juel VC, Massey JM. Autoimmune myasthenia gravis: recommendations for treatment and immunologic modulation. Curr Treat Options Neurol. 2005; 7(1):3–14.
33. Hart IK, Sharshar T, Sathasivam S. Immunosuppressant drugs for myasthenia gravis. J Neurol Neurosurg Psychiatry.2009; 80(1):5–6.
34. Chiang LM, Darras BT, Kang PB. Juvenile myasthenia gravis. Muscle Nerve. 2009;39(4):423–31.
35. Zebardast N, Patwa HS, Novella SP, Goldstein JM. Rituximab in the management of refractory myasthenia gravis. Muscle Nerve. 2010;41(3):375–8.
36. Sanders DB, Hart IK, Mantegazza R, Shukla SS, Siddiqi ZA, De Baets MH, et al. An international, phase III, randomized trial of mycophenolate mofetil in myasthenia gravis. Neurology. 2008;71(6):400–6.
37. Muscle Study Group. A trial of mycophenolate mofetil with prednisone as initial immunotherapy in myasthenia gravis. Neurology. 2008;71(6):394–9.
38. Chan JW. Mycophenolate mofetil for ocular myasthenia. J Neurol. 2008;255(4):510–3.
39. Gold R, Schneider-Gold C. Current and future standards in treatment of myasthenia gravis. Neurotherapeutics.2008; 5(4):535–41.
40. US Food and Drug Administration. Communication about an ongoing safety review of CellCept (mycophenolate mofetil) and Myfortic (mycophenolic acid). April 10, 2008. http://www.fda.gov/Drugs/DrugSafety/PostmarketDrugSafetyInformationforPatientsandProviders/DrugSafetyInformationforHeathcareProfessionals/ucm072438.htm
41. Ponseti JM, Gamez J, Azem J, López-Cano M, Vilallonga R, Armengol M. Tacrolimus for myasthenia gravis: a clinical study of 212 patients. Ann N Y Acad Sci.2008; 1132:254–63.
42. Lavrnic D, Vujic A, Rakocevic-Stojanovic V, Stevic Z, Basta I, Pavlovic S, et al. Cyclosporine in the treatment of myasthenia gravis. Acta Neurol Scand. 2005;111(4):247–52.
43. Drachman DB, Adams RN, Hu R, Jones RJ, Brodsky RA. Rebooting the immune system with high-dose cyclophosphamide for treatment of refractory myasthenia gravis. Ann N Y Acad Sci. 2008;1132:305–14.
44. Meyer DM, Herbert MA, Sobhani NC, Tavakolian P, Duncan A, Bruns M, et al. Comparative clinical outcomes of thymectomy for myasthenia gravis performed by extended transsternal and minimally invasive approaches. Ann Thorac Surg. 2009;87(2):385–90.
45. Bradley EA, Bartley GB, Chapman KL, Waller RR. Surgical correction of blepharoptosis in patients with myasthenia gravis. Ophthal Plast Reconstr Surg. 2001;17:103–10.

Chapter 12
Neurogenic Blepharoptosis

Jonathan W. Kim

Abstract Neurogenic blepharoptosis is an important entity to recognize since there are specific considerations in its evaluation and treatment. Most cases are caused by lesions of the oculomotor nerve or a disruption of the oculosympathetic pathway. Neurogenic ptosis can be distinguished from involutional blepharoptosis by the associated findings of pupillary and/or ocular motility abnormalities. The etiology and localization of the lesion is determined by a careful review of the history, associated signs and symptoms, and appropriate neuroimaging studies. The initial treatment approach is aimed at correcting the underlying pathologic process. For patients who require surgical repair of the ptosis, frontalis sling is the only viable option for patients with oculomotor nerve palsy, while both levator resection and Müllerectomy are effective procedures for patients with Horner syndrome.

Introduction

The vast majority of blepharoptosis cases encountered in clinical practice are due to involutional or myopathic etiologies. Neurogenic blepharoptosis is relatively rare but an important entity to recognize since there are specific considerations in its evaluation and treatment. Most cases of neuropathic ptosis encountered in clinical practice are caused by lesions of the oculomotor nerve or a disruption of the oculosympathetic pathway (i.e., Horner syndrome). These entities can be distinguished in almost all cases by the associated ocular findings of pupillary and/or ocular motility abnormalities. Rarely, cortical pathology may cause neurogenic blepharoptosis due to a disruption of the cortico-bulbar pathways. There are also unusual brainstem syndromes causing a supranuclear inhibition of levator tonus or a disruption of levator muscle initiation (e.g., apraxia of eyelid opening). Finally, eyelid synkinesis following facial nerve paresis or congenital "miswiring" conditions, such as the Marcus Gunn jaw-winking phenomenon may be broadly defined as neurogenic ptosis. The clinical history, accompanying neurologic signs, and a careful ophthalmologic examination are all critical in making the correct diagnosis. Neurogenic ptosis should not be missed by the clinician since the treatment is usually aimed at correcting the underlying pathologic process causing the neurologic injury.

Cortical and Supranuclear Blepharoptosis

Although rare, both unilateral and bilateral cortical lesions may cause neurogenic blepharoptosis [1–3]. The cortical damage may be located in

J.W. Kim (✉)
Department of Ophthalmology, Stanford Medical Center, 900 Blake Wilbur Drive, W3001, Stanford, CA, 94304, USA
e-mail: J Kim6@stanford.edu

A.J. Cohen and D.A. Weinberg (eds.), *Evaluation and Management of Blepharoptosis*,
DOI 10.1007/978-0-387-92855-5_12, © Springer Science+Business Media, LLC 2011

various regions of the cerebral hemispheres such as the temporal lobe, temporo-occipital regions, the angular gyrus, or frontal lobes. The precise anatomic pathways responsible for "cerebral" or cortical ptosis have not been defined, but the blepharoptosis in these cases may be related to a disruption of the cortico-bulbar fibers that connect to the third nerve nucleus in the midbrain. Cortical blepharoptosis is most commonly unilateral and contralateral to the lesion in the brain, although bilateral cortical ptosis has also been reported with extensive nondominant hemispheric lesions [1]. There may be other signs of cortical dysfunction such as gaze deviation, ocular motor apraxia, and facial nerve weakness, with the latter masking the blepharoptosis due to the presence of concomitant eyelid retraction. Given its rarity, cortical or cerebral blepharoptosis is a diagnosis of exclusion; an abnormality should be present in neuroimaging studies, and clinical signs of other conditions, such as myasthenia gravis, oculomotor palsy, or external ophthalmoplegia, should be absent. Treatment is mainly supportive since cortical ptosis is usually transient, lasting weeks to months before resolving [1, 2].

The extrapyramidal system may affect the eyelid position by modifying the normal supranuclear control of the blink reflex or contributing to apraxia of eyelid opening (AEO). Patients with AEO demonstrate an inability to initiate eyelid opening, despite the presence of normal levator excursion. AEO is thought to be related to an interruption of the supranuclear signal which initiates levator action, or due to a lack of coordinated inhibition of the antagonistic orbicularis contraction during eyelid opening [4]. Patients display symmetric, bilateral ptosis, and marked frontalis contraction during voluntary attempts to open the eyelids [5]. AEO may be seen in otherwise healthy patients or in association with CVA, progressive supranuclear palsy (PSP), Wilson's disease, Parkinson's disease, and benign essential blepharospasm [4–6]. Treatment of AEO is initially aimed at the underlying etiology, but if that strategy fails the blepharospasm component can be treated with low dose botulinum toxin injections (into the pretarsal orbicularis). Recalcitrant cases of AEO may respond to bilateral frontalis sling ptosis repair.

Third Nerve (Oculomotor) Palsy

Diagnosis

Third nerve palsy is a common cause of neurogenic ptosis. The diagnosis of a third nerve palsy as the cause of an acquired blepharoptosis should not be missed since the ptosis is always accompanied by other ophthalmic findings, such as extraocular muscle paresis and pupillary mydriasis. The blepharoptosis is usually profound with markedly diminished levator excursion (<10 mm) (Fig. 12.1a). There is typically a large-angle exotropia and hypotropia; the eye on the involved side is deviated "down and out" from residual tone in the fourth cranial nerve (superior oblique muscle) and sixth cranial nerve (lateral rectus muscle). Clinically, patients with even a subtle third nerve palsy demonstrate an incomitant, vertical strabismus, which may not be noted by the patient due to the presence of the ptosis. Therefore, clinicians should have a low suspicion for evaluating ptosis patients for subclinical strabismus with alternate cover testing or the single Maddox rod in all cardinal positions of gaze. Rarely, a patient with an orbital process demonstrates a superior division third nerve palsy, involving the superior rectus and levator muscles and sparing the pupil (Fig. 12.2a, b). These patients typically present with a progressive blepharoptosis and a hypotropia on the involved side which increases in upgaze. A useful method for assessing ptosis patients for subtle superior rectus weakness is the single Maddox rod. If there is no vertical separation of the two images in a binocular patient in upgaze, oculomotor nerve palsy is not the cause of the blepharoptosis or there is concurrent pathology on the contralaterals ide.

The pupil in a third nerve palsy patient is typically mid-dilated (Fig. 12.1b) (never >7–8 mm) causing an anisocoria more noticeable in a brightly-lit room (Fig. 12.1c). The pupillary dilation results from dysfunction of the parasympathetic fibers which originate in the Edinger–Westphal subnucleus of the oculomotor nuclear complex. These preganglionic fibers

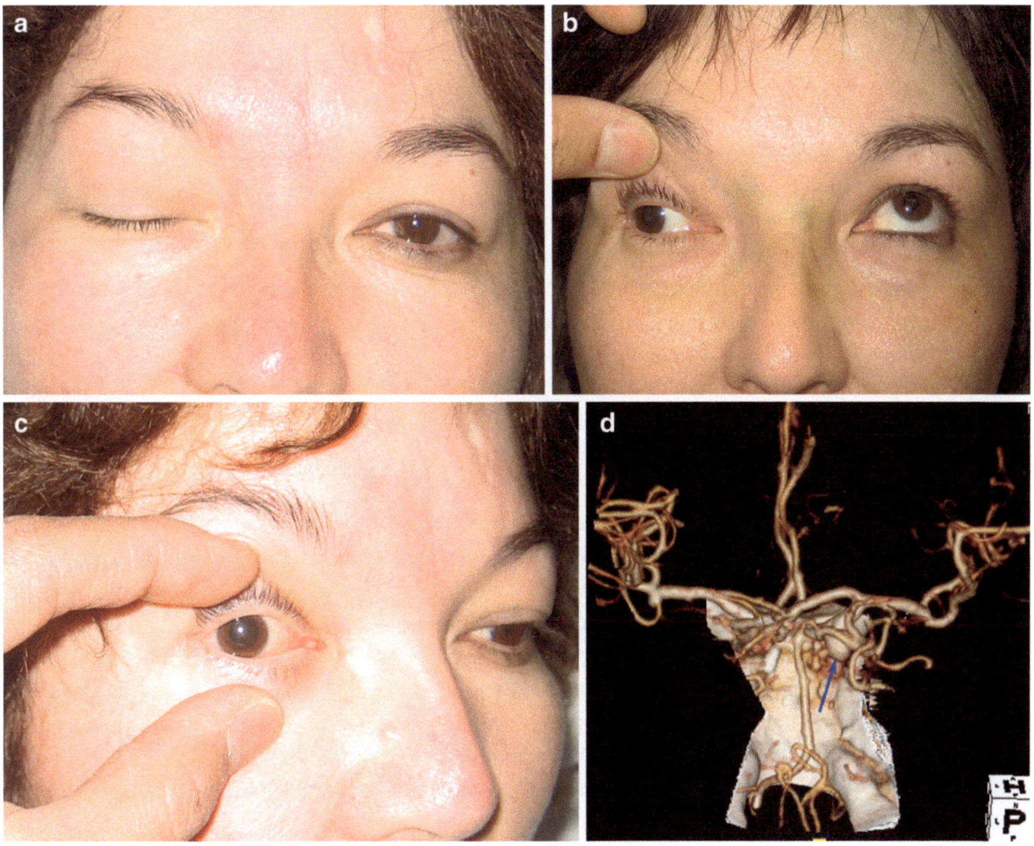

Fig. 12.1 Fifty-four-year-old woman with an acute right third nerve palsy causing profound blepharoptosis (**a**), strabismus (**b**), and mid-dilated pupil (**c**). Three-dimensional reformation of computed tomography angiogram showing a right posterior communicating artery aneurysm (**d**, *arrow*)

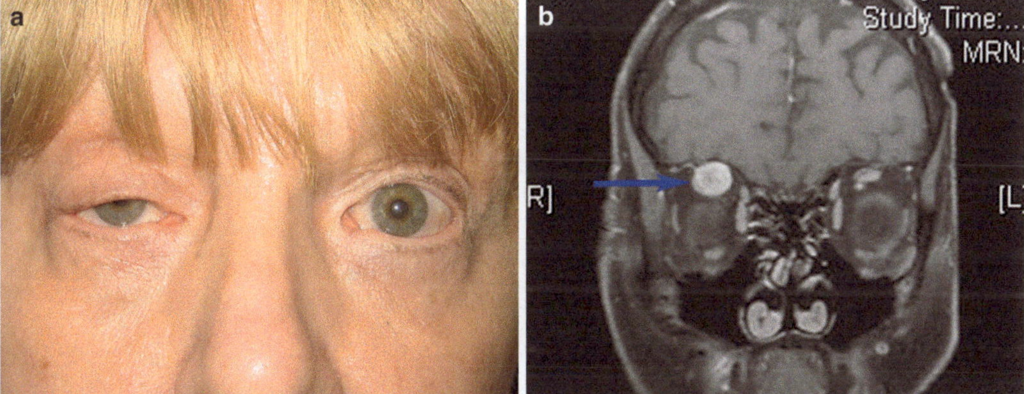

Fig. 12.2 Seventy-two-year-old woman who presented with a superior division third nerve palsy causing right upper lid ptosis and superior rectus weakness without anisocoria (**a**). Coronal magnetic resonance imaging study demonstrating a mass lesion in the superior orbit (**b**). Orbital biopsy demonstrated an undifferentiated adenocarcinoma, and the patient was found to have widespread metastatic disease from an unidentified primary malignancy

travel with the third nerve fascicle and peripheral nerve before joining the branch to the inferior oblique muscle in the orbit and synapsing at the ciliary ganglion. As a rule, pupillary dilation is always present in a third nerve palsy except in the following scenarios: discrete nuclear lesions (sparing the Edinger–Westphal subnucleus), ischemic third nerve palsies involving the subarachnoid segment, superior division third nerve palsies in the orbit, and cavernous sinus lesions which produce a concurrent Horner syndrome. One of the more difficult settings to diagnose a third nerve palsy is following severe orbital trauma. The presentation of traumatic third nerve palsy may be identical to a patient with a traumatic mydriasis, traumatic ptosis, and extraocular motility limitation due to an orbital fracture. Pharmacologic testing is not effective in reducing the etiology of the mydriasis in this setting since both conditions respond to 1% pilocarpine. A careful clinical examination may reveal the diffuse, saccadic slowing of a third nerve palsy and the relative preservation of abduction. Blunt trauma to the levator muscle should resolve spontaneously by 3 months (rarely by 6 months), whereas traumatic third nerve palsy typically demonstrates incomplete recovery and evidence of aberrant regeneration (Fig. 12.3). Adie's tonic pupil should not be confused with a pupil-involving third nerve palsy given the absence of ptosis and strabismus with the former condition. In difficult cases, pharmacologic testing with dilute pilocarpine (0.1%) can be used to demonstrate the denervation supersensitivity of Adie's tonicpupil.

Localization of a Third Nerve Palsy

The third nerve may be affected anywhere along its pathway from the oculomotor nucleus within the midbrain to its distal branches innervating the levator superioris muscle within the orbit (Fig. 12.4). Localization of the lesion responsible for a third nerve palsy is based on both the neuroimaging findings and the clinical symptoms and signs. Blepharoptosis arising from a nuclear midbrain lesion is typically bilateral, symmetric, and associated with other signs of dorsal mesencephalic dysfunction. Both levator muscles are controlled by a single midline subnucleus located at the caudal end of the oculomotor nerve complex; therefore, a nuclear lesion almost always produce bilateral ptosis. Rarely, a discrete nuclear lesion involving the caudal region of the oculomotor complex may produce an isolated midbrain ptosis without other third nerve signs. More commonly, a nuclear lesion is present with bilateral oculomotor abnormalities since the superior rectus muscle has contralateral nuclear innervation. Fascicular lesions of the

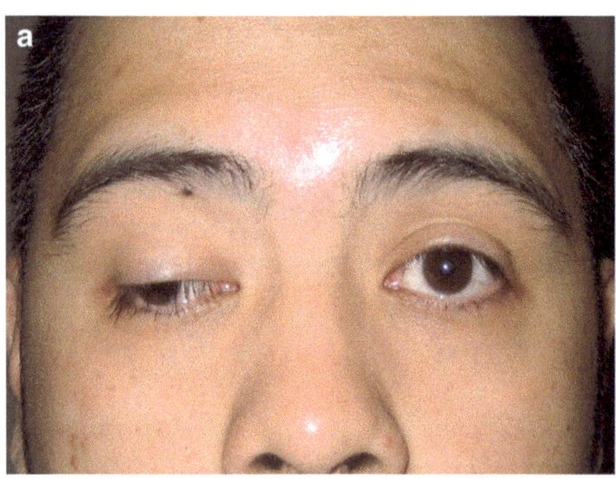

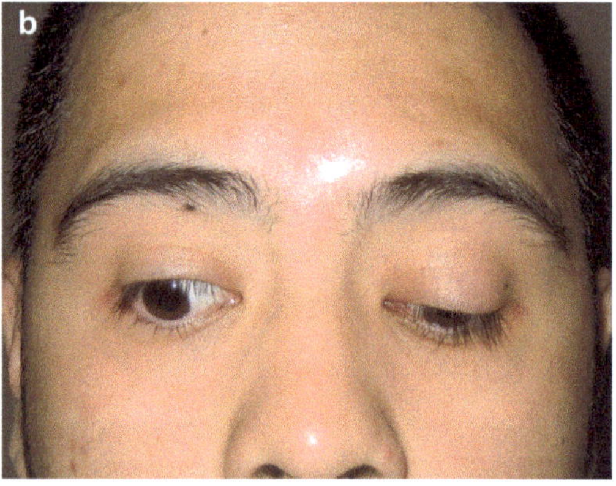

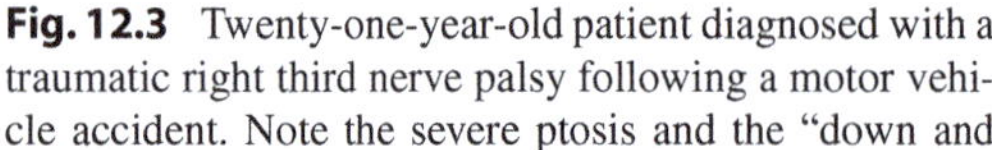

Fig. 12.3 Twenty-one-year-old patient diagnosed with a traumatic right third nerve palsy following a motor vehicle accident. Note the severe ptosis and the "down and out" position of the right eye (**a**). In downgaze, the patient demonstrates aberrant regeneration causing upper lid retraction (**b**)

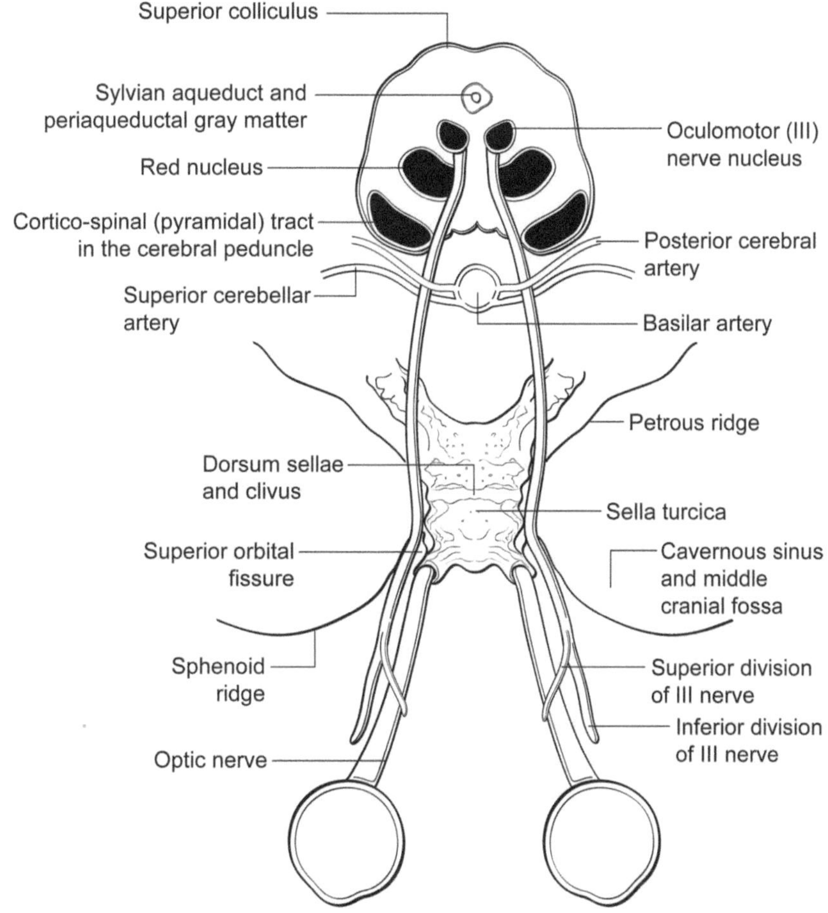

Fig. 12.4 Anatomicpa thwayof t het hird(oculomotor)ne rve

oculomotor nerve within the brainstem are present with partial or complete signs of unilateral oculomotor nerve dysfunction, often in association with a contralateral hemiplegia, rubral tremor, or cerebellar ataxia. Benedikt syndrome of the upper midbrain causes ipsilateral third cranial nerve palsy, contralateral flapping hand tremor (rubral tremor from red nucleus involvement), and ataxia. Weber syndrome results from a slightly more ventral lesion with the involvement of the cerebral peduncle giving rise to contralateral hemiplegia or hemiparesis along with ipsilateral third cranial nerve palsy.

Blepharoptosis that accompanies a lesion of the subarachnoid segment is typically profound and invariably accompanied by ophthalmoplegia. In this location, the fibers to the levator muscle travel in proximity with the neurons innervating the extraocular muscles. However, pupillary involvement with lesions involving the subarachnoid portion of the third nerve can vary depending on the etiology. The pupillary fibers from the Edinger–Westphal nucleus are located superficially in the superomedial aspect of the nerve and an intrinsic ischemic insult (e.g., diabetic third nerve palsy) commonly spares the pupil. Conversely, an extrinsic, compressive third nerve injury from a posterior communicating artery aneurysm almost always causes pupillary dilation. Involvement of the third nerve within the cavernous sinus should not occur in isolation since the sixth, fourth, and fifth cranial nerves travel together before entering the superior orbital fissure. The sixth nerve is particularly vulnerable to compression within the cavernous sinus, and an ipsilateral abduction deficit, however minor, can be very helpful in localizing a third nerve palsy. Coexisting fourth nerve palsy can be difficult to detect in the presence of a complete third nerve paresis, but intorsion can be assessed on attempted downgaze by observing an ocular landmark, such as the conjunctival vessels at the limbus. Lesions at the orbital apex typically cause orbital signs, such as proptosis, conjunctival chemosis, and an optic neuropathy.

Common Etiologies for Third Nerve Palsy

Diagnostic considerations for acquired third nerve palsy vary to a great extent on the anatomic location of the injury (see Table 12.1) [7]. Nuclear or brainstem causes for third nerve palsy include neoplasm (e.g., glioma), stroke (e.g., basilar artery occlusion), inflammation (e.g., abscess), infiltration, and extrinsic compression. The fascicular portion of the third nerve is most commonly affected by vascular processes causing midbrain infarction. Multiple sclerosis is a rare cause of third nerve palsy and when it occurs, the lesion must involve the white matter of the third nerve fascicle before it leaves the brainstem. The most common lesion to affect the third nerve in its subarachnoid segment is a posterior communicating artery aneurysm (Fig. 12.1d). In addition to the acute ocular findings, there may be signs of subarachnoid hemorrhage, including sudden severe headache, stiff neck, and photophobia. Other causes of third nerve palsy in this location include basal infiltration by metastatic tumors, meningeal infection (bacterial, fungal, viral), and granulomatous inflammation, such as sarcoidosis or tuberculosis. Within the cavernous sinus, the third nerve is susceptible to compression from a variety of pathologic processes, including aneurysms, meningiomas, metastatic tumors, lymphomas, carotid-cavernous fistulas, and lateral extension of pituitary adenomas (e.g., apoplexy). Nonspecific, granulomatous inflammation within the cavernous sinus causing painful ophthalmoplegia has been termed Tolosa–Hunt syndrome; this is a rare condition that is considered a diagnosis of exclusion when all neoplastic and structural lesions have been ruled out. Ophthalmoplegic migraine is a nonstructural cause of episodic third nerve palsy starting in childhood, with recurring bouts of ipsilateral headache and third nerve palsy that can last several weeks per episode.

Treatmento fB lepharoptosis in Third Nerve Palsy

For patients diagnosed with oculomotor palsy, treatment of the blepharoptosis is aimed at the primary lesion causing the neurogenic injury. For example, aneurysms of the posterior communicating artery are treated with either interventional neuroradiology techniques or an open surgical approach, i.e., craniotomy. Surgical options include gluing, coiling, or wrapping of the berry aneurysm to relieve the pressure on the third nerve and prevent future bleeding episodes.

Table12.1 Common etiologies for third nerve palsy

Location			
Midbrain	Subarachnoid	Cavernouss inus	Orbit
Ischemia/stroke	Aneurysm	Meningioma	Perineurali nvasion
Neoplasm(glioma)	Meningitis	Aneurysm	Lymphoma
Infiltration	Carcinomatosis	Metastatict umor	Cavernoushe mangioma
Abscess	Granulomatous inflammation	Carotid-cavernousfi stula	Orbital pseudotumor (idiopathic orbital inflammation)
Multiples clerosis	Schwannoma	Tolosa–Hunts yndrome	

In general, clipping is considered the most effective method for relieving the clinical symptoms of third nerve palsy since it removes the mass effect of the aneurysm on the nerve fibers. Ischemic injuries of the third nerve are managed conservatively as the majority of patients spontaneously improve without treatment over 6–16 weeks. These patients should have a comprehensive medical evaluation and systemic issues, such as diabetes or hypertension addressed appropriately by their internist. Metastatic tumors may benefit from radiotherapy and/or chemotherapy, although recovery of third nerve function is variable even with dramatic regression of the lesions following successful treatment. In general, surgical removal of neoplastic lesions causing third nerve palsy rarely leads to complete recovery of its function and this should be kept in mind when considering treatment options.

When a patient demonstrates partial or no recovery of the blepharoptosis 6–12 months following the onset of a third nerve palsy, surgical repair of the ptosis may be considered. Since the levator muscle has a neurogenic injury, performing traditional aponeurosis advancement or resection is NOT an effective strategy. Shortening the paretic levator muscle does not improve the blepharoptosis without creating significant lagophthalmos. Since these patients often have an absent Bell's phenomenon due to concurrent superior rectus weakness, postoperative lagophthalmos may lead to severe exposure keratopathy. Therefore, frontalis sling is the only viable surgical option for blepharoptosis in patients with oculomotor nerve palsy [8]. Materials chosen for the frontalis sling depend on the patient's age and the surgeon's preference, but a silicone rod (Seiff frontalis suspension set, made by BD Visitec, 1 Becton Drive, Franklin Lakes, NJ 07417) works well in the vast majority of patients. Rarely, a patient with partial third nerve palsy may demonstrate levator function greater than 8 mm and levator resection may be considered. It should be emphasized that the surgical results following levator surgery in third nerve palsy cases are extremely disappointing. For patients with minimal levator function and evidence of aberrant regeneration, consideration may be given to disinsert the levator muscle completely, in order to prevent synkinetic movements of the upper eyelid, at the same time that the frontalis sling is placed. Finally, strabismus surgery should always precede ptosis repair in these cases since any adjustment of the vertical extraocular muscles may alter the eyelid fissure.

HornerSyndr ome

Diagnosis

Horner syndrome results from a disruption of the sympathetic innervation to the eye and face, causing the classic triad of blepharoptosis, pupillary miosis, and anhidrosis. The blepharoptosis results from the denervation of Müller's muscle in the upper eyelid, resulting in a lid drop of approximately 2 mm (Figs. 12.4 and 12.5). The eyelid fissure is further decreased by the "upside down ptosis" of the lower lid, caused by an atonic inferior tarsal muscle. The combination of the upper lid drooping and lower lid elevation contributes to a sunken or enophthalmic appearance on the affected side. Miosis results from weakness of the pupillary dilator muscle, leading to an anisocoria which is accentuated with dim illumination. In normal room lighting, the anisocoria may be 1.0 mm or less; therefore even subtle miosis on the same side as the ptosis may be significant. Since miosis always accompanies Horner syndrome, the diagnosis can be essentially eliminated if there is no anisocoria or the pupil on the ptotic side is larger. Dilation lag of the pupil may be noted when the room lights are turned down, although this is not considered a reliable finding in Horner syndrome. Ipsilateral anhidrosis results from an interruption of the sudomotor fibers of the sympathetic pathway. Anhidrosis affects the ipsilateral side of the body with central, first-order neuron lesions and the ipsilateral face with second-order neuron lesions. Anhidrosis is absent or is limited to the ipsilateral eyebrow with third order lesions since the sudomotor fibers travel with the external carotid

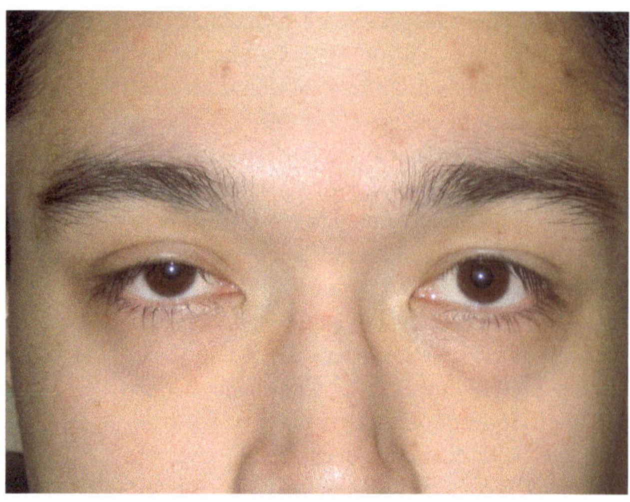

Fig. 12.5 Classic findings of Horner syndrome: right upper lid ptosis, pupillary miosis, and "upside down ptosis" of right lower lid

Table 12.2 Clinical findings in Horner syndrome

Ptosis (2 mm)
Miosis
Anhidrosis/lack of flushing
Lower lid elevation
Increased accommodation
Heterochromia (congenital)
Lower intraocular pressure (transient)
Injected conjunctival vessels
Apparent enophthalmos

artery. As a clinical sign, anhidrosis is difficult to assess on examination but patients may occasionally describe a lack of sweating on one side of the face after exercise. Iris heterochromia is seen in congenital Horner syndrome or when the condition is acquired less than 2 years of age. The clinical signs of Horner syndrome are summarized in Table 12.2.

Pharmacologic Evaluation

Since physiologic anisocoria is present in 20% of the population, and asymmetric levator dehiscence ptosis is common, numerous patients with "pseudo-Horner syndrome" are encountered in clinical practice. If there is clinical suspicion for Horner syndrome based on the findings of ipsilateral ptosis and pupillary miosis, pharmacologic testing should be performed to confirm the diagnosis before considering radiographic studies. Clinical testing with 4 or 10% cocaine has been the standard for many years to diagnose Horner syndrome [9]. Cocaine inhibits the reuptake of norepinephrine from the synaptic cleft, dilating the normal pupil with intact sympathetic innervation. In an eye with Horner syndrome, pupillary dilation is limited due to the absence, or reduced quantity, of endogenous norepinephrine in the synapse. The maximum pupillary response with cocaine testing is seen 40–60 min after the instillation of two drops into both eyes. In a patient with Horner syndrome, the difference in pupil size should increase after the instillation of cocaine drops, and anisocoria greater than 0.8 mm is considered a positive test. However, it should be noted that for the results to be valid, the smaller Horner pupil should dilate less than 2 mm and the normal pupil should dilate more than 2 mm.

Recently, clinicians have been using apraclonidine drops to diagnose Horner syndrome because of the difficulty in obtaining and maintaining cocaine solution in the office setting [10–12]. Apraclonidine (0.5 or 1%) is now considered a practical and reliable alternative to cocaine for the routine testing of Horner syndrome. Apraclonidine is an ocular hypotensive agent and a weak, direct-acting alpha-1 and alpha-2 receptor agonist. Apraclonidine has little or no effect on a normal pupil, but patients with Horner syndrome develop denervation

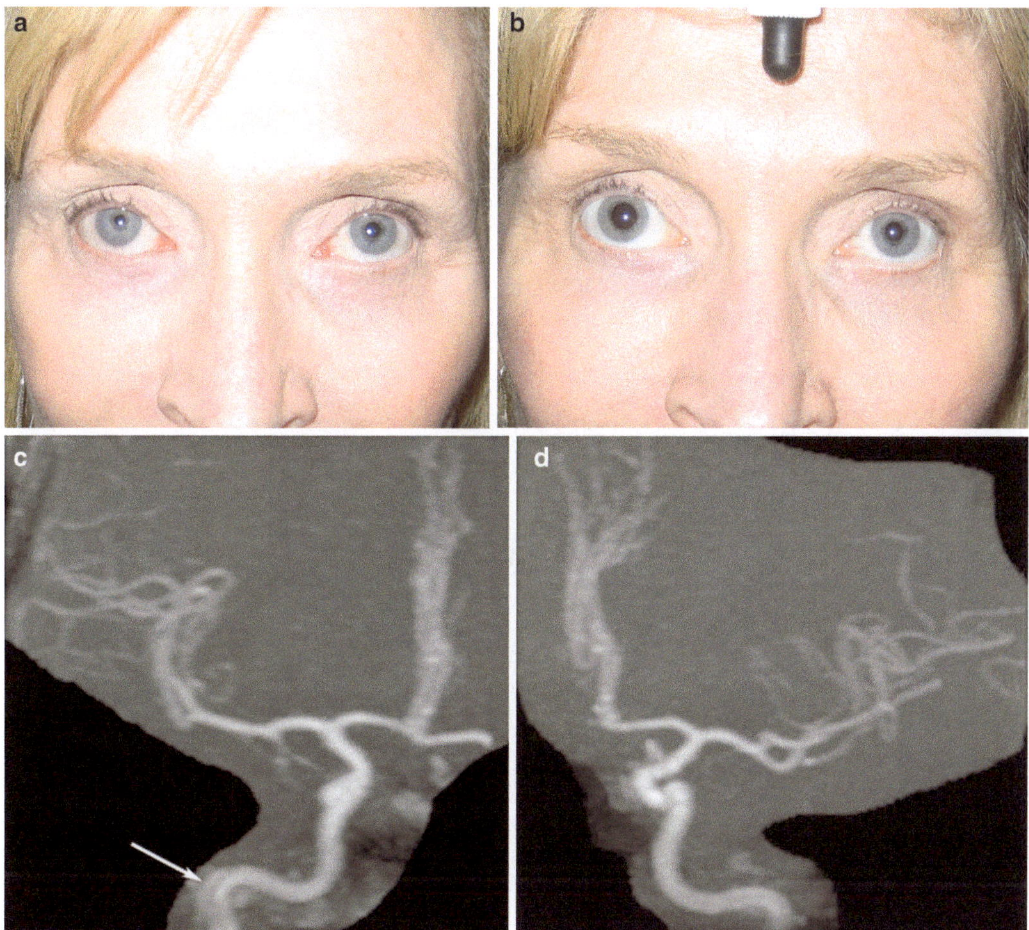

Fig. 12.6 Fifty-nine-year-old woman referred for evaluation of anisocoria. Note the subtle right upper lid ptosis and miotic right pupil (**a**); reversal of anisocoria following 0.5% apraclonidine (**b**). Computed tomography angiogram demonstrating dissection of the right internal carotid artery (**c**, *arrow*) and normal left internal carotid artery (**d**)

supersensitivity of the iris dilator muscle. The Horner pupil dilates in response to apraclonidine due to the upregulation of alpha-1 receptors, resulting in a reversal of the anisocoria after bilateral instillation of apraclonidine (Fig. 12.6a, b). False negative results may occur in acute cases as it takes a few weeks for the upregulation of these receptors to occur. After confirming the diagnosis of Horner syndrome with either cocaine or apraclonidine, hydroxyamphetamine 1% drops may be used to localize the lesion [13]. Hydroxyamphetamine stimulates the release of norepinephrine from postganglionic nerve terminals, dilating the pupil in patients with an intact third-order neuron to an equal or greater extent than the normal side. However, patients with postganglionic or third-order neuron lesions do not respond to hydroxyamphetamine testing [14]. Finally, it should be noted that pharmacologic testing for Horner syndrome should always be performed a minimum of 24 h after the instillation of any topical ophthalmic medications.

Localization of Horner Syndrome

A lesion at any point along the anatomic pathway of the sympathetic system may result in Horner syndrome (Fig. 12.7). First-order (central) Horner syndrome affects the sympathetic pathway that extends from the posterolateral hypothalamus,

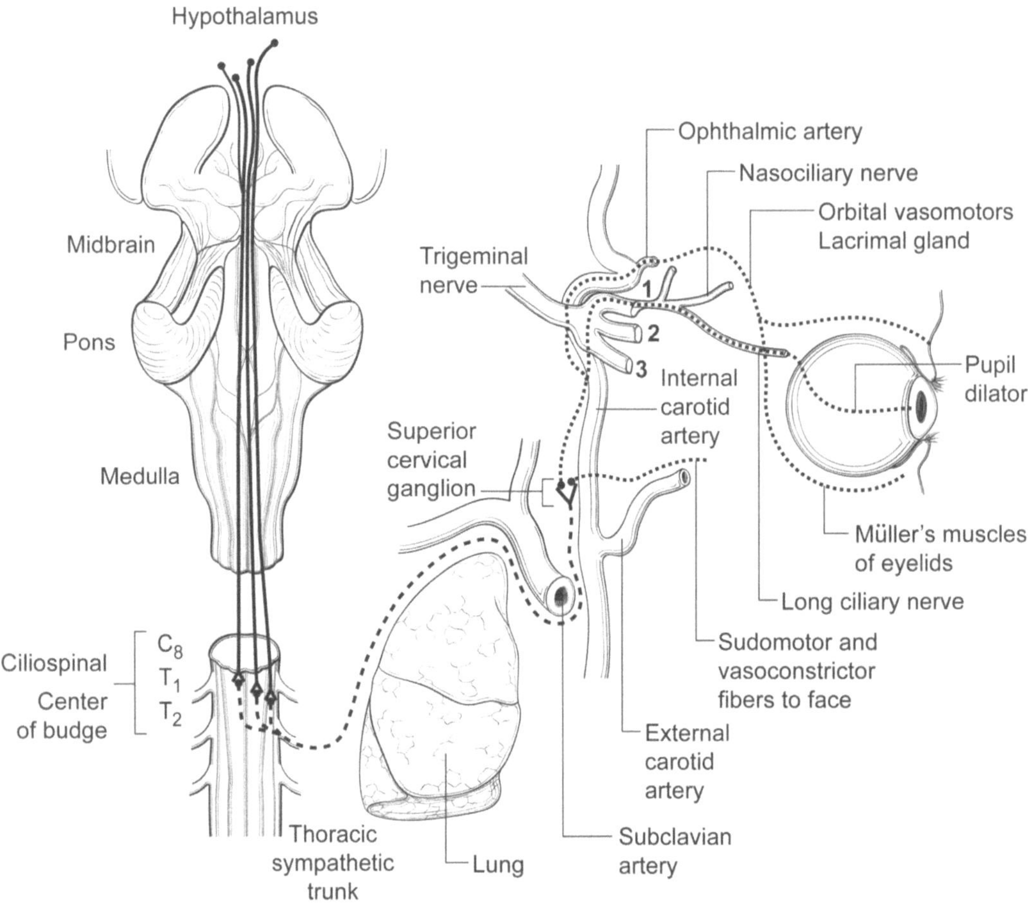

Fig. 12.7 Diagram of oculosympathetic pathway

midbrain and pons, to the intermediolateral gray column of the spinal cord at the level of C8-T2 (ciliospinal center of Budge). Second-order Horner syndrome involves the preganglionic fibers that exit the spinal cord at the level of T1 and extend through the cervical sympathetic chain, over the pulmonary apex and the subclavian artery, to synapse at the superior cervical ganglion at the level of the bifurcation at the common carotid artery. Third-order postganglionic fibers exit the superior cervical ganglion and ascend along the internal carotid artery to enter the cavernous sinus. From the cavernous sinus, fibers travel with the abducens nerve and enter the orbit through the superior orbital fissure to innervate the eyelid muscles, lacrimal gland, and pupillary dilator muscle. With a thorough knowledge of the anatomy of the sympathetic pathway, an astute clinician can often localize a Horner syndrome by identifying the accompanying clinical signs and symptoms.

In clinical practice, first-order neuron lesions are rare or perhaps overlooked due to the presence of obvious brainstem signs and symptoms, such as hemisensory loss, dysarthria, dysphagia, ataxia, vertigo, and nystagmus. It would be extremely unusual for a patient to develop first-order Horner syndrome as the presenting sign of a brainstem lesion. On the other hand, isolated second-order Horner syndrome cases are commonly encountered in clinical practice, and there is typically a history of neck, chest, or spinal cord trauma (Table 12.3). Iatrogenic causes of Horner syndrome are a common source for referrals in tertiary medical centers, particularly following thoracic or neck surgery,

Table12 .3 Commone tiologiesf orH orners yndrome

Location			
First-order	Second-order	Third-order	Children
Tumor (brainstem glioma)	Pancoast lung tumor	Internal carotid artery dissection	Birtht rauma
Ischemia/stroke	Neck or chest trauma	Raeder syndrome/cluster headaches	Neuroblastoma
Basal skull tumor	Aortic artery dissection	Carotid-cavernous fistula	Brainstemv ascular malformation
Meningitis	Centralv enous catheterization	Cavernous sinus mass/ tumor	
Vertebral artery dissection	Surgical trauma (thyroidectomy)		
Syringomyelia	Mediastinalt umor		
Arnold–Chiarim alformation	Neuroblastoma		

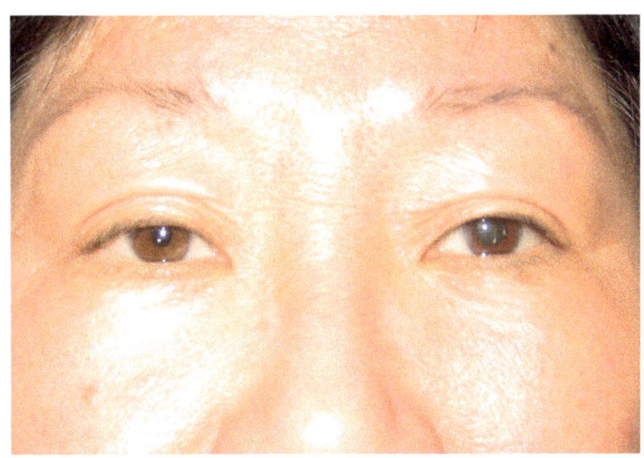

Fig.12.8 Fifty-five-year-old woman diagnosed with right-sided Horner syndrome following thyroidectomy

chest tube insertion, or central venous catheter placement (Fig. 12.8). A classic but rare entity causing second-order Horner syndrome is the Pancoast tumor, a squamous cell or adenocarcinoma which invades the upper chest wall and apical pleura-pulmonary groove. Patients suspected to have an apical lung tumor should be asked about their previous tobacco history, shoulder or arm pain, an unusual cough or recent hemoptysis, the presence of hand atrophy, and facial anhidrosis. The third-order, or postganglionic, Horner syndrome is caused by a pathologic process distal to the carotid bifurcation. The most urgent condition causing a third-order Horner syndrome is a carotid artery dissection, which typically involves the internal carotid artery as it extends upward from the carotid bifurcation to enter the cavernous sinus [15]. In this location, the postganglionic sympathetic fibers destined for the eye travel with the extracranial and intracranial segments of the internal carotid artery, and an arterial dissection can cause an isolated Horner syndrome without other neurologic signs (Fig. 12.1c). More distal sympathetic lesions in the cavernous sinus and orbital apex are likely to be accompanied by diplopia due to a concomitant sixth, fourth, or third cranial nerve palsy.

RadiographicEval uation

After the diagnosis is confirmed with pharmacologic testing, the next step is the radiographic evaluation to determine the etiology of the Horner syndrome. There are many presumed cases of Horner syndrome that have a negative radiographic workup. These patients tend to do well clinically, and it may be that the pharmacologic testing was erroneous or the patient suffered an undocumented traumatic injury. Patients with a postoperative, isolated Horner syndrome following recent neck or chest surgery do not require further evaluation for an etiology. However, any patient with a newly diagnosed, unexplained Horner syndrome should undergo immediate neuroimaging. As previously mentioned, the most urgent condition to rule out in an adult patient with an acquired Horner syndrome is a carotid dissection, which can lead to an ipsilateral hemispheric stroke if left untreated. In certain cases, neuroimaging is ordered even before pharmacologic testing is performed, particularly when a patient presents to the Emergency Department with acute ptosis, miosis, and severe neck pain. In most centers, MRI (and MRA) of the head and neck is preferred over computed tomography angiography (CTA) since the former also rules out infiltrative lesions in the cavernous sinus and orbital apex. If a vascular abnormality is identified on MRA, a CTA or formal angiogram may be performed to confirm the diagnosis. Patients with carotid dissection are typically treated with anticoagulation. If neuroimaging is negative, consideration can be given to performing a chest CT to rule out a lesion in the thorax (e.g., lung apex lesion). If both the MRI and chest CT are unrevealing, the patient can be monitored clinically, with consideration of other studies, such as a PET scan or lumbar puncture if the clinical findingsprogre ss.

Horner Syndrome in Children

Horner syndrome in children may be developmental, related to birth trauma, or caused by an acquired neoplasm [16]. Typically, the clinical finding which initiates the evaluation for Horner syndrome in a child is unilateral blepharoptosis, since subtle miosis is easily overlooked by the parents and even the pediatrician. Before undertaking a workup for possible Horner syndrome, it is important to date and document the presence of blepharoptosis in photographs, since the parents may have missed the presence of mild ptosis at birth. Congenital Horner syndrome cases or those arising before the age of 2 years may also demonstrate iris heterochromia. The iris on the affected side is paler in these children due to the impaired development of iris melanophores. Infants with preganglionic Horner syndrome may be noted to have a hemifacial flush, with the affected side of the face demonstrating pallor due to impaired facial vasodilation; this may be seen after atropine drops or when the infant nurses or cries. Pharmacologic testing for Horner syndrome in children is similar to adults except that it may be prudent to use 4% cocaine rather than the 10% solution to decrease systemic levels of the drug in infants. In children less than 6 months of age, apraclonidine is contraindicated because of sporadic reports of lethargy, bradycardia, and respiratory depression in infants, evenw iththe lo wer 0.5%c oncentration [17].

When considering the diagnostic workup for children with documented Horner syndrome, it is critical to distinguish between the congenital and acquired forms [18]. The definition of congenital Horner syndrome denotes infants diagnosed in the first month of life. Birth trauma is probably the most common etiology for Horner syndrome diagnosed at this age, most commonly due to an injury of the sympathetic plexus along its course in the neck or near the thoracic outlet. In some cases, upper extremity weakness may be present due to concomitant damage to the ipsilateral brachial plexus. The most feared clinical entity when a young child presents with an acquired Horner syndrome is neuroblastoma, typically from a thoracic primary extending into the cervical area [19]. Since neuroblastoma developing in utero or in the first 4 weeks of life would be rare, infants with Horner syndrome diagnosed at this early age typically do not require further workup, particularly if there is a history of birth trauma. The diagnostic evaluation for possible childhood neuroblastoma is handled by a pediatric neuro-oncologist, but the referring physician may be asked to order some of the preliminary tests. Urine tests for

Table12.4 Surgicalopt ionsf orne urogenicpt osis

Procedure		
Frontaliss ling	Levatora dvancement/resection	Müllerectomy
Third nerve palsy	Horner syndrome	Horner syndrome
Apraxia of eyelid opening	Negative response to phenylephrine	Positive response to phenylephrine
	Ptosis >2 mm	Ptosis <2 mm
	Dermatochalasis	
	Previous levator surgery	

vanillylmandelic acid (VMA) and homovanillic acid (HVA) (24-h collection) are obtained to look for elevated catecholamine levels [20]. A serologic laboratory panel is rarely diagnostic but can be used to guide further testing (liver function tests, CBC, LDH, ferritin levels). Chest and abdominal imaging with CT scans is the mainstay for evaluating the thoracic and retroperitoneal cavities. MRI is recommended for evaluating the head, neck, and paraspinal regions. Finally, a methyliodobenzyguanadine (MIBG) scan is a specific method for documenting skull and skeletal metastases in neuroblastoma since this agent accumulates in catecholaminergic cells.

Treatment

As with other causes of neurogenic ptosis, the strategy for treating Horner syndrome is aimed at correcting the underlying etiology. However, even with successful treatment of the primary disease, it is not uncommon for the blepharoptosis to persist, particularly for patients with longstanding Horner syndrome. Since levator excursion is normal in Horner syndrome, the blepharoptosis can be treated with either an anterior approach (i.e., levator surgery) or posterior approach (i.e., Müllerectomy) ptosis repair. Determining a patient's candidacy for posterior approach ptosis repair is based on the patient's response to topical phenylephrine; if eyelid elevation is adequate following the instillation of 2.5% phenylephrine, Müllerectomy can be recommended. The prognostic effect of topical phenylephrine in Horner syndrome patients cannot be adequately explained on an anatomic basis. The clinical response of Müller's muscle to phenylephrine suggests that the muscle fibers can be pharmacologically activated by its adrenergic receptors. However, the surgical success of Müllerectomy in Horner syndrome patients is somewhat surprising since the denervated muscle is atonic. Glatt and Putterman postulated that the mechanism of action of Müllerectomy in these cases is independent of its effect on Müller's muscle, and likely related to a shortening or augmentation of the levator aponeurosis [21]. In any case, the surgical approach for correcting eyelid ptosis in a Horner syndrome patient is based on the response to topical phenylephrine and other preoperative surgical factors(s eeT able 12.4).

References

1. Caplan LR. Cerebral ptosis. J Neurol Neurosurg Psychiatry.1974; 34:1–7.
2. Averbuch-Heller L, Leigh RJ, Mermelstein V, Zagalsky L, Streifler JY. Ptosis in patients with hemispheric strokes. Neurology. 2002;58:620–4.
3. Krohel GB, Griffin JF. Cortical blepharoptosis. Am J Ophthalmol.1978; 85:632–4.
4. Boghen D. Apraxia of eyelid opening: a review. Neurology.1997; 48:1491–4.
5. Lepore FE, Duvoisin RC. "Apraxia" of eyelid opening: an involuntary levator inhibition. Neurology. 1985;35:423–7.
6. Jordan DR, Anderson Rl, Digre K. Apraxia of lid opening in blepharospasm. Ophthalmic Surg. 1990;21:331–4.
7. Richards BW, Jones FR, Younge BR. Causes and prognosis in 4278 cases of paralysis of the oculomotor, trochlear, and abducens cranial nerves. Am J Ophthalmol.1992; 113:489–96.
8. Carter SR, Meecham WJ, Seiff SR. Silicone frontalis slings for the correction of blepharoptosis:

indications and efficacy. Ophthalmology. 1996; 103(4):623–30.
9. Kardon RH, Denison CE, Brown CK, Thompson HS. Critical evaluation of the cocaine test in the diagnosis of Horner's syndrome. Arch Ophthalmol. 1990;108: 384–7.
10. Koc F, Kavuncu S, Kansu T, Acaroglu G, Firat E. The sensitivity and specificity of 0.5% apraclonidine in the diagnosis of oculosympathetic paresis. Br J Ophthalmol.2005; 89(11):1442–4.
11. Brown SM, Aouchiche R, Freedman KA. The utility of 0.5% apraclonidine in the diagnosis of horner syndrome. Arch Ophthalmol. 2003;121(8):1201–3.
12. Morales J, Brown SM, Abdul-Rahim AS, Crosson CE. Ocular effects of apraclonidine in Horner syndrome. Arch Ophthalmol. 2000;118:951–4.
13. Cremer SA, Thompson HS, Digre KB, Kardon RH. Hydroxyamphetamine mydriasis in Horner's syndrome. Am J Ophthalmol. 1990;110:71–6.
14. Maloney WF, Younge BR, Moyer NK. Evaluation of the causes and accuracy of pharmacologic location of Horner's syndrome. Am J Ophthalmol. 1980;90: 394–402.
15. Kline LB, Vitek JJ, Raymon BC. Painful Horner's syndrome due to spontaneous carotid artery dissection. Ophthalmology. 1987;94:226–30.
16. Jeffery AR, Ellis FJ, Repka MX, Buncic JR. Pediatric Horner syndrome. J AAPOS. 1998;2:159–67.
17. Watts P, Satterfirld D, Lim MK. Adverse effects of apraclonidine used in the diagnosis of Horner syndrome in infants. J AAPOS. 2007;11(3):282–3.
18. George ND, Gonzalez G, Hoyt CS. Does Horner's syndrome in infancy require investigation? Br J Ophthalmol.1998; 82:51–4.
19. Musarella MA, Chan HS, DeBoer G, Gallie BL. Ocular involvement in neuroblastoma: prognostic implications. Ophthalmology. 1984;91:936–40.
20. Mahoney NR, Liu GT, Menacker SJ, Wilson MC, Hogarty MD, Maris JM. Pediatric Horner syndrome: etiologies and roles of imaging and urine studies to detect neuroblastoma and other responsible mass lesions. Am J Ophthalmol. 2006;142:651–9.
21. Glatt HJ, Putterman AM, Fett DR. Müller's muscle-conjunctival resection procedure in the treatment of ptosis in Horner's syndrome. Ophthalmic Surg. 1990;21(2):93–6.

Chapter 13
Traumatic Blepharoptosis

Nariman S. Boyle and Eli L. Chang

Abstract The objective of this chapter is to review the various etiologies and management of traumatic blepharoptosis. Iatrogenic causes constitute the most common category of factors in traumatic ptosis. This includes ptosis postintraocular surgery and posteyelid and adnexal procedures. Contact lens wear, various systemic interventions, and birth trauma are other iatrogenic causes reported in the literature in association with upper lid blepharoptosis. Lacerations and blunt traumatic injuries to the upper eyelid are frequently associated with various degrees of blepharoptosis. Neurogenic ptosis secondary to head trauma can occur secondary to third nerve injury, superior orbital fissure syndrome, or traumatic facial nerve palsy. The prognosis and management of traumatic ptosis depends on the underlying mechanism of injury.

Introduction

Traumatic blepharoptosis is an abnormally low upper eyelid following trauma. There are a multitude of mechanisms resulting in traumatic blepharoptosis. Ptosis can be mild, moderate, or severe depending on the complexity of injury to the eyelid structures, including the levator muscle and aponeurosis. Nearly half of the traumatic cases are iatrogenic in nature with inadvertent injury to the levator muscle or aponeurosis [1]. Iatrogenic causes are numerous and are secondary to a large repertoire of surgical and nonsurgical interventions.

Etiology and Mechanisms of Traumatic Ptosis

Iatrogenic Causes of Ptosis

Ptosis Postintraocular Surgery

One of the most common causes of blepharoptosis is the iatrogenic category, which encompasses a broad range of etiologies and mechanisms. Ptosis postintraocular surgery is commonly observed. The incidence of ptosis after cataract surgery has been quoted to be approximately 5–7% [2, 3]. By comparison, glaucoma filtering surgery and other types of complicated intraocular surgeries have a slightly higher incidence of ptosis when compared to simple cataract extraction. Although the mechanism of ptosis postintraocular surgery is uncertain, there are numerous articles pointing to the use of a speculum during ocular surgery [4]. The exact mechanism is unknown, but it is thought to be secondary to levator aponeurosis dehiscence. Bridle suture and anesthesia myotoxicity have also been implicated in postcataract ptosis [5]. The type of local

E.L. Chang (✉)
Doheney Eye Institute, University of Southern California, Los Angeles, CA, USA
e-mail: echang@doheny.org

A.J. Cohen and D.A. Weinberg (eds.), *Evaluation and Management of Blepharoptosis*,
DOI 10.1007/978-0-387-92855-5_13, © Springer Science+Business Media, LLC 2011

anesthesia used in cataract surgery does not seem to affect the incidence of postoperative ptosis [2]. A randomized, double-masked study of 317 patients revealed the incidence of ptosis at 90 days to be 5.5% in patients who received retrobulbar anesthesia and 5.8% in the peribulbar anesthesiagroup [2].

Ptosis Posteyelid and Adnexal Procedures

Ptosis may occur as a complication of a wide range of eyelid and adnexal procedures, through various mechanisms. Ptosis as a consequence of blepharoplasty can be transient secondary to postoperative eyelid edema or hematoma. Inadvertent levator dehiscence during resection of a wide strip of pretarsal orbicularis may result in permanent ptosis with a high lid crease [6, 7]. Direct repair of the ptosis secondary to an aponeurotic defect in the immediate postoperative period is instrumental in correcting ptosis afterble pharoplasty [7].

Resection of conjunctival or eyelid tumors with violation of the levator complex or Müller muscle may cause ptosis. Excision of conjunctival tumors with or without cryotherapy may result in scarring or symblepharon between the bulbar conjunctiva and the posterior surface of eyelid. This may lead to ptosis secondary to mechanical limitation of the eyelid excursion. In these cases, release of the symblepharon and grafting the defect with mucous membrane or amniotic membrane may improve the ptosis and prevent recurrence of the symblepharon. Use of antimetabolites, such as mitomycin C, is useful in patients who are predisposed to exuberant scar formation [8, 9]. Young patients who sustain a chemical burn are a good example in this category.

Excision of eyelid tumors resulting in large full thickness lid defect necessitates reconstruction. The lid may be tight for many weeks. Lid elevation may be mechanically restricted by a horizontally tight eyelid, a vertical traction band, a swollen eyelid, or a bulky scar or skin graft. Limited lid elevation secondary to a horizontally tight eyelid gradually resolves with time. On the other hand, vertical traction bands, bulky scars, and skin grafts may necessitate surgical revision to resolve the mechanical restriction and improve lid elevation.

Ptosis is commonly observed in patients with an anophthalmic socket [10, 11]. It can be true ptosis or pseudoptosis. True ptosis can be due to levator muscle damage during enucleation, scarring of the levator secondary to socket surgery or preexisting involutional ptosis. Pseudoptosis, on the other hand, is due to the loss of volume in the anophthalmic socket or inadequate prosthesis size. It is also due to the abnormal mechanical forces in the anophthalmic socket with loss of support of Whitnall's ligament and straightening of the course of the levator [10]. Inferior migration of the orbital implant is another mechanism for pseudoptosis (Fig. 13.1). This can be verified in clinic by applying digital pressure on the implant to push it superiorly and noticing the improvement of the ptosis. Enucleation technique may contribute to the development of ptosis. Imbrication of the rectus muscles after enucleation over spherical implants may lead to upper lid ptosis in addition to implant migration [12]. The imbricated muscles over a spherical implant may slip off the implant, usually inferonasally, resulting in migration of the implant to the supero-temporal tenon space in the orbit. As a result, the superior fornix and upper lid are pulled forward and downward which may explain theptos is [12].

Vertical rectus muscle surgery is known to affect upper and lower lid position [13]. Recession of the superior or inferior rectus leads to widening of the palpebral fissure. On the other hand, resection or advancement of the vertical rectus muscles may lead to narrowing of the palpebral fissure. Resection of the superior rectus is less likely to result in upper eyelid blepharoptosis if careful dissection is performed [13]. It is advised that all intermuscular septum and fascial connections to be dissected about 12–15 mm posterior to the muscle insertion to separate the superior rectus from levator and Müller muscles.

Botulinum toxin has a broad array of cosmetic and functional applications. While it has

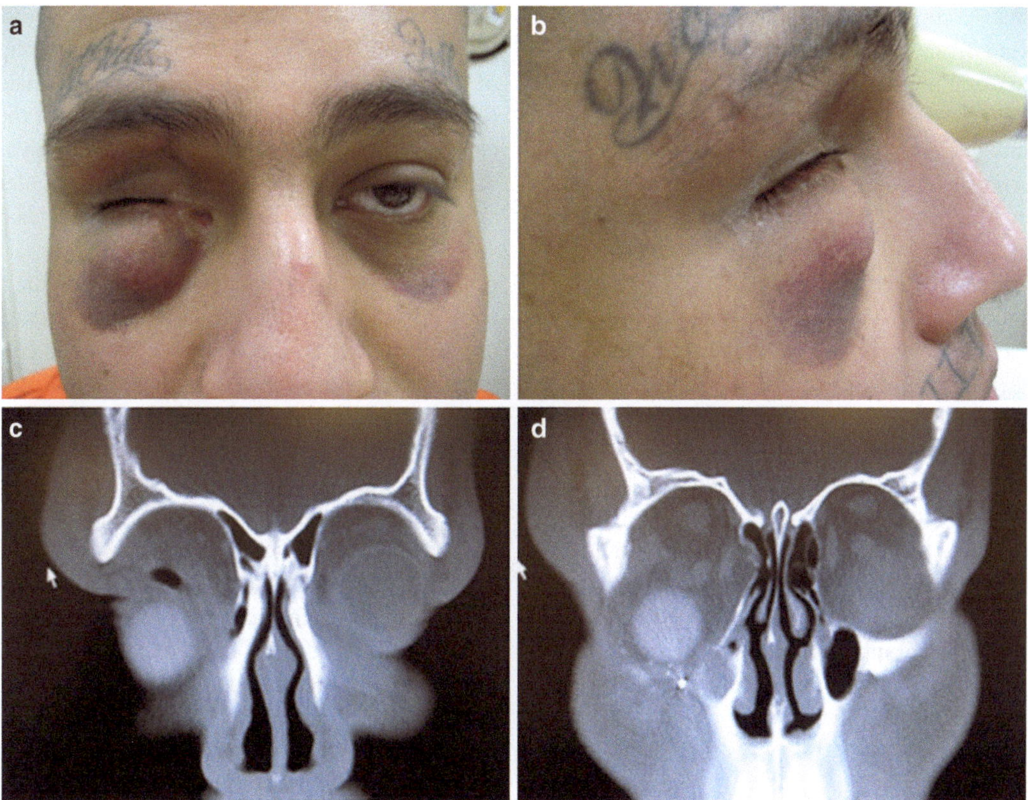

Fig.13.1 An inferiorly displaced orbital implant into the lower eyelid at the inferior orbital rim secondary to blunt trauma with a fist

been safely and effectively used, adverse reactions are possible. Transient upper lid blepharoptosis is the most common example. Ptosis results from inadvertent injection or diffusion of the botulinum toxin behind the orbital septum, affecting the levator muscle function [14]. The effect typically lasts about 3 months. A careful history, inquiring about any recent botulinum toxin injections around the eyes, may spare these patients unnecessarys urgery.

ContactL ensW ear

Usage of contact lenses, particularly rigid gas permeable and hard is another cause of iatrogenic ptosis. Several reports suggest the association of acquired nonsenile ptosis with prolonged use of contact lenses [15, 16]. In one series, contact lens use was identified in 47% of patients with acquired ptosis in the young to middle aged group [15]. It is often progressive and bilateral in 58% of cases and unilateral in the remaining 42% [15]. Levator aponeurosis dehiscence and thinning was found in the majority of those patients who underwent surgery [15, 16]. Another histopathology study showed fibrosis of Müller muscle and levator aponeurosis in patients with blepharoptosis and a history of prolonged hard contact lens use [17]. In comparison, patients with involutional ptosis were found to have mild Müller muscle fibrosis and substantial fatty degeneration of the levator muscle.

The mechanism of ptosis in contact lens wearer is attributed to recurrent traction on the levator aponeurosis during contact lens removal with lateral pulling of the lids. Another unusual and rare mechanism for ptosis associated with contact lens wear is intrapalpebral migration of the contact lens by eroding into the tissue. It is a rare complication. Clinical presentation may vary from simple upper eyelid ptosis to more unusual findings, such as a conjunctival mass in the superior fornix, a movable hard mass simulating a neoplasm, or an orbital mass [18–23]. Another manifestation of contact lens migration can be pseudochalazion, where the contact lens is embedded in the tarsal conjunctiva [24]. Patients often have unilateral ptosis and may recall losing a contact lens on the same side. Double lid eversion may reveal the retained contact lens. Imaging may be required in cases where there is an encysted mass.

A more common complication of contact lens use is giant papillary conjunctivitis (GPC). Papillary changes in the tarsal palpebral conjunctiva can occur as part of an immunoglobulin E (IgE)-mediated hypersensitivity reaction. Patients with GPC may present with ptosis attributed to local inflammation and edema. The ptosis is usually reversible once contact lens use is discontinueda ndthe G PCis tre ated [19].

Ptosis Following Systemic Interventions

Horner syndrome has been well described as a complication in thoracic and neck surgery [25, 26]. It has been reported following coronary bypass surgery with a frequency ranging from 1.3 to 7.7% [27, 28]. It tends to be isolated and unrelated to a C8-T1 plexopathy. In a study of 248 patients, hypertensive and diabetic patients had a higher incidence of Horner syndrome than normotensive patients (10.6 vs. 2.9%); there was no correlation with the cardiopulmonary bypass time. Horner syndrome persisted in 4% of patient at 6 months after surgery [27]. Another study revealed Horner syndrome in 1.3% of patient undergoing a variety of thoracic procedures, including thoracotomy, chest tube insertion, and thoracic trauma [25]. Transient Horner syndrome has been reported in patients with tension pneumothorax. Chest tube insertion relieved the tension pneumothorax and reversed the ptosis and miosis on the same side [29]. On the other hand, chest tube insertion itself can precipitate a transient or permanent Horner syndrome [30, 31] due to damaged preganglionic sympathetic fibers. In one case, CT scan showed that the tip of the chest tube was resting against the stellate (cervicothoracic) ganglion. Repositioning of the chest tube led to resolution of the Horner syndrome [31]. Thoracoscopy and internal jugular venous cannulation have also been associated with Horner syndrome [26, 32, 33]. Surgical procedures involving the neck, including radical neck dissection for tumors, parathyroid surgery, thyroidectomy, carotid endarterectomy, and cervical spine fusion, may cause Horner syndrome secondary to sympathetic denervation from damaget ot hec ervicothoracicg anglion [26, 34].

Another iatrogenic cause of Horner syndrome is epidural anesthesia [35], which may or may not display associated cranial nerve palsies. Horner syndrome has been described following lumbar epidural analgesia for labor with low concentration (0.04%) bupivacaine [35, 36]. Therefore, if patients become symptomatic following epidural infusion, a diagnostic work up may be unnecessary. Transient Horner syndrome has also been reported in a patient who underwent thoracic epidural analgesia for multiple rib fractures [37].

BirthT rauma

Birth trauma secondary to forceps delivery, vacuum extraction, fetal rotation, and shoulder dystocia may result in ptosis manifesting at birth [38]. Ptosis can be secondary to a stretched or dehiscent levator aponeurosis [39]. Horner syndrome is another potential cause of ptosis in newborns (Fig. 13.2). A study conducted to define the etiologies of Horner syndrome in the pediatric age revealed a history of birth trauma in 53% of patients [38]. Ptosis due to congenital Horner syndrome may be differentiated from garden-variety congenital ptosis based on history of birth trauma, as well as the absence of anisocoria and the presence of lid lag in downgaze in congenital ptosis. Children with congenital Horner syndrome and a history of a forceful delivery may not require the extensive work up otherwise mandated in the absence of a history of birth trauma [38].

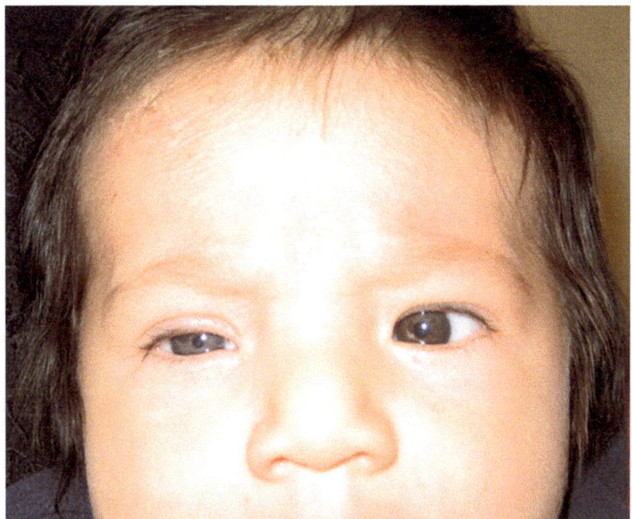

Fig.13.2 CongenitalH orners yndromes econdaryt obi rtht rauma

BluntT rauma

Blunt trauma can result in ptosis secondary to edema or stretching or dehiscence of the levator aponeurosis. Ptosis secondary to blunt trauma is usually transient, with full recovery of levator function in most cases. Patients who constantly rub their eyelids are predisposed to blepharoptosis. It is thought to be the result of repetitive microtrauma to the levator aponeurosis [40].

LaceratingT rauma

Traumatic lacerations of the upper eyelid involving the levator aponeurosis and/or muscle result in various degrees of ptosis (Fig. 13.3). Small lacerations, when properly repaired, with repositioning of prolapsed preaponeurotic fat, usually do well. On the other hand, eyelid avulsion is a more challenging scenario with a higher incidence of permanent ptosis. Exploration of the laceration, identification, and reapproximation of the levator muscle can improve outcomes of thesee xtensivei njuries [41].

Traumatic Ptosis Secondary to Restrictive Scarring

Sharp injuries to the upper eyelid, whether traumatic or iatrogenic following surgical procedures, may result in restrictive eyelid scarring. It may be due to improper repair of the wound with poor attention to the anatomical layers. Adhesions between the levator muscle and the skin or between the eyelid and the orbital rim may create a tethering effect and restrict the levator muscle motility and eyelide xcursion(Figs . 13.4a nd 13.5).

Traumatic Ptosis Following Facial Fractures

Facial fractures involving the inferior or medial orbital wall or the zygomatico-maxillary complex (ZMC) may result in enophthalmos (Figs. 13.5 and 13.6), with potential esthetic and functional consequences. The functional deficits that accompany enophthalmos include gaze-evoked diplopia, eyelid malposition, and exposure keratitis [42]. A sunken globe may affect the support of Whitnall's ligament, thereby altering eyelid mechanics [10]. Enophthalmos also

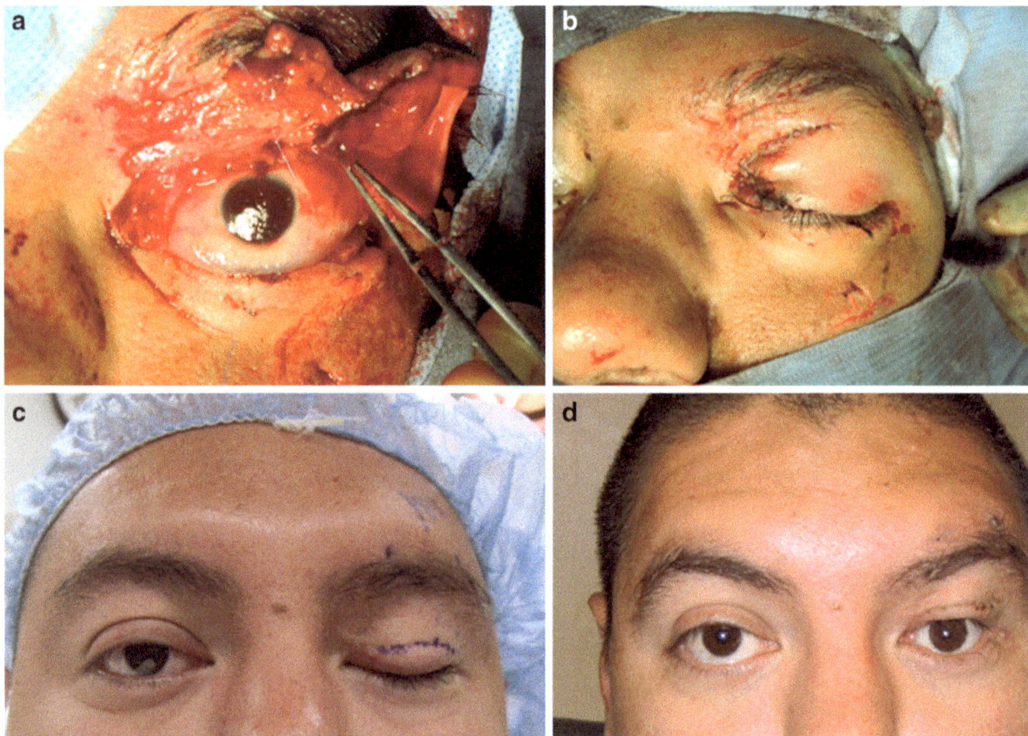

Fig. 13.3 (**a**) Complete avulsion of the left upper eyelid following severe motor vehicle accident. (**b**) The eyelid was explored, and levator was reapproximated with 6-0 vicryl suture. He also had a ruptured globe that was repaired initially. He underwent subsequent enucleation and prosthesis fitting. (**c**) Six months following the injury, patient had persistent complete ptosis and underwent a frontalis sling procedure. (**d**) Two weeks status postfrontalis sling procedure

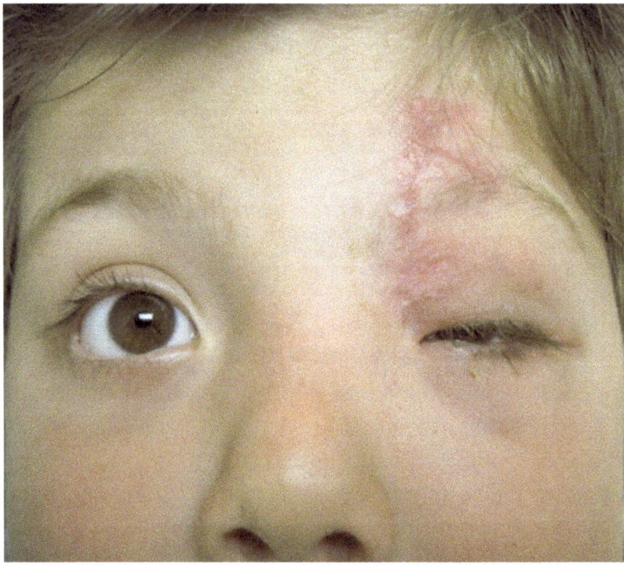

Fig.13.4 A 4-year-old boy with history of penetrating injury to the medial canthus by a wooden stick. Restrictive scarring of the medial aspect of upper eyelid and brow contributing to right upper eyelid blepharoptosis

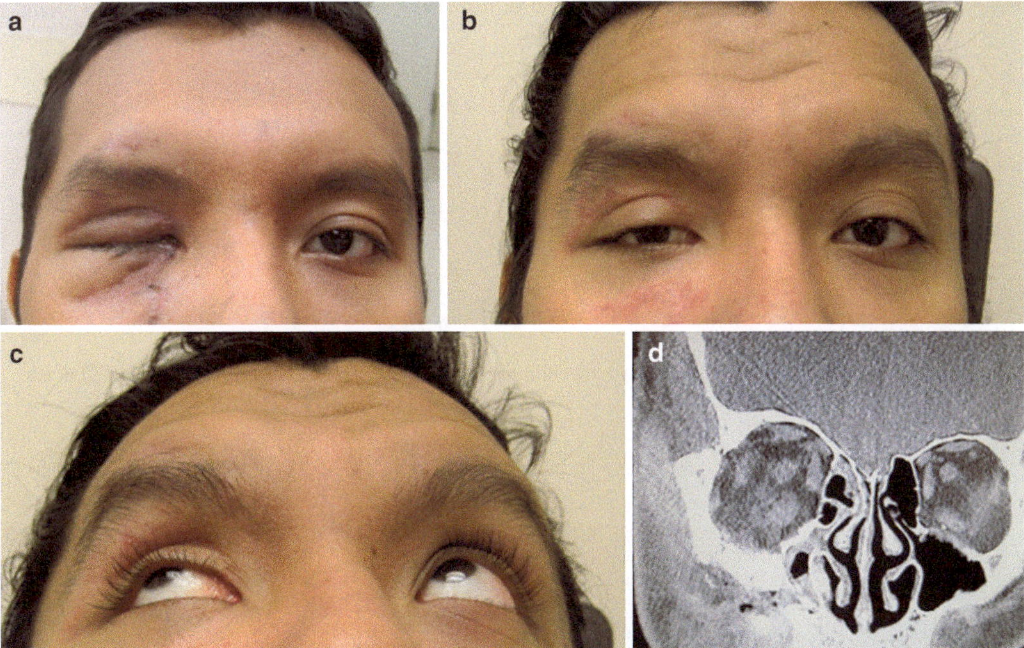

Fig. 13.5 (**a**) Right enophthalmos and ZMC fracture secondary to motor vehicle accident. The right upper eyelid is bound down to the superior orbital rim. The right upper eyelid laceration was used for surgical access to repair the fractures by nonophthalmology service leading to this complication. (**b**) Six month post-trauma, there is persistent enophthalmos and ptosis. The restrictive component has improved in part. (**c**) Coronal view of CT scan revealing a persistent ZMC malalignment

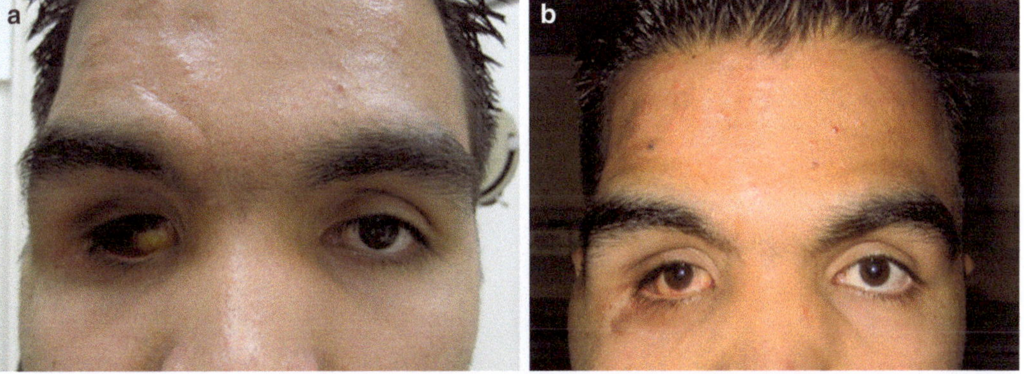

Fig.13.6 (**a**) Severe enophthalmos after a motor vehicle accident with multiple skull and facial bones fractures. (**b**) The ptosis improved markedly after the treatment of enophthalmos

induces narrowing of the palpebral fissure and hence upper lid pseudoptosis (Fig. 13.7). The levator muscle function is usually normal. Correction of the enophthalmos may alleviate the ptosis (Figs. 13.8 and 13.9). Ptosis, commonly transient, may accompany orbital roof ("blow-in") fractures due to bone fragments that impinge upon the levator-superior rectus muscle complex. Ptosis repair may be necessary if it does not resolve spontaneously over time [43–45].

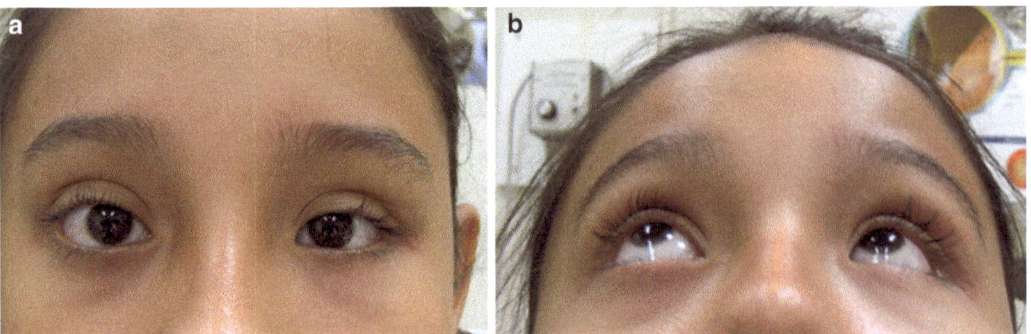

Fig.13.7 (**a**, **b**) Left enophthalmos following blowout floor fracture. There is mild pseudoptosis of the left upper eyelidw ithnor male yelidc rease

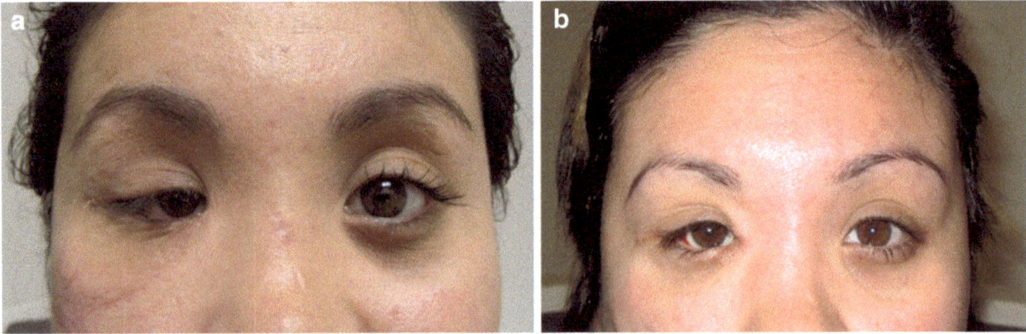

Fig. 13.8 A 25-year-old female post Le Fort II fractures secondary to motor vehicle accident. (**a**) She has right upper lid ptosis and residual enophthalmos. (**b**) The right upper eyelid blepharoptosis improved after the correction of enophthalmos. She underwent Y-to-V medial canthoplastya ndr etrobulbarf ati njection

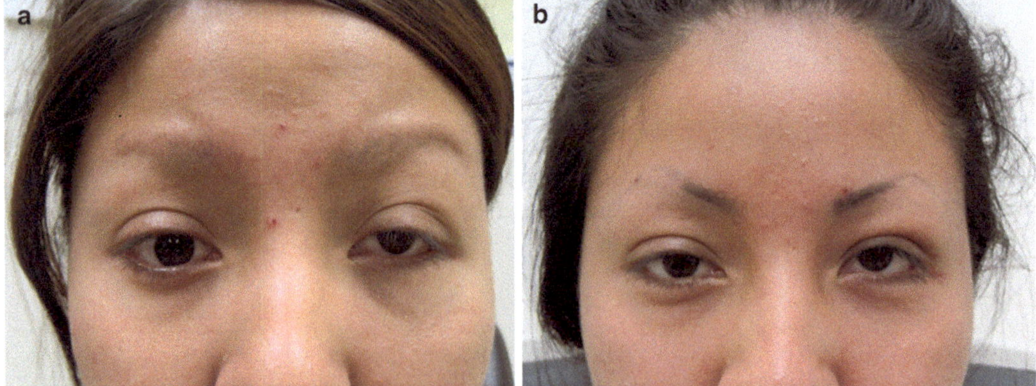

Fig. 13.9 (**a**) Left enophthalmos following blowout fracture of the orbital floor. (**b**) The residual ptosis, after the correction of the enophthalmos with a high-density porous polyethylene implant, was addressed with external levator resection and eyelid crease formation

Neurogenic Ptosis Secondary to Trauma

Traumatic Superior Orbital Fissure Syndrome

Superior orbital fissure syndrome (SOFS) can develop secondary to tumors, inflammation, infection, and trauma (Fig. 13.10), which may impact cranial nerves III, IV, V (ophthalmic division of the trigeminal nerve), and VI. The manifestations are external ophthalmoplegia, corneal anesthesia, proptosis, and ptosis. Traumatic SOFS may occur secondary to Le Fort II and III fractures, zygomatic fractures, and frontobasal skull fracture [46]. The common pathway of injury in all of these types of fractures is disruption of the bony margins of the SOF and the concomitant compression of the nerves secondary to bony fragments and/or edema. In most cases of linear fractures along the SOF and/or optic canal, spontaneous recovery with resolution of the SOFS syndrome is expected [47]. On the other hand, surgical intervention with decompression of the orbital apex is recommended in cases of fractures with signs of progressive, or persistent, ophthalmoplegia and optic neuropathy [48]. In these cases, CT scan usually reveals narrowing of the SOF or optic canal with displaced bony fragments [49, 50].

Blepharoptosis Secondary to Traumatic Third Nerve Palsy

Head trauma can result in injury to the oculomotor nerve either directly or secondary to uncal herniation with compression of the nerve [51].

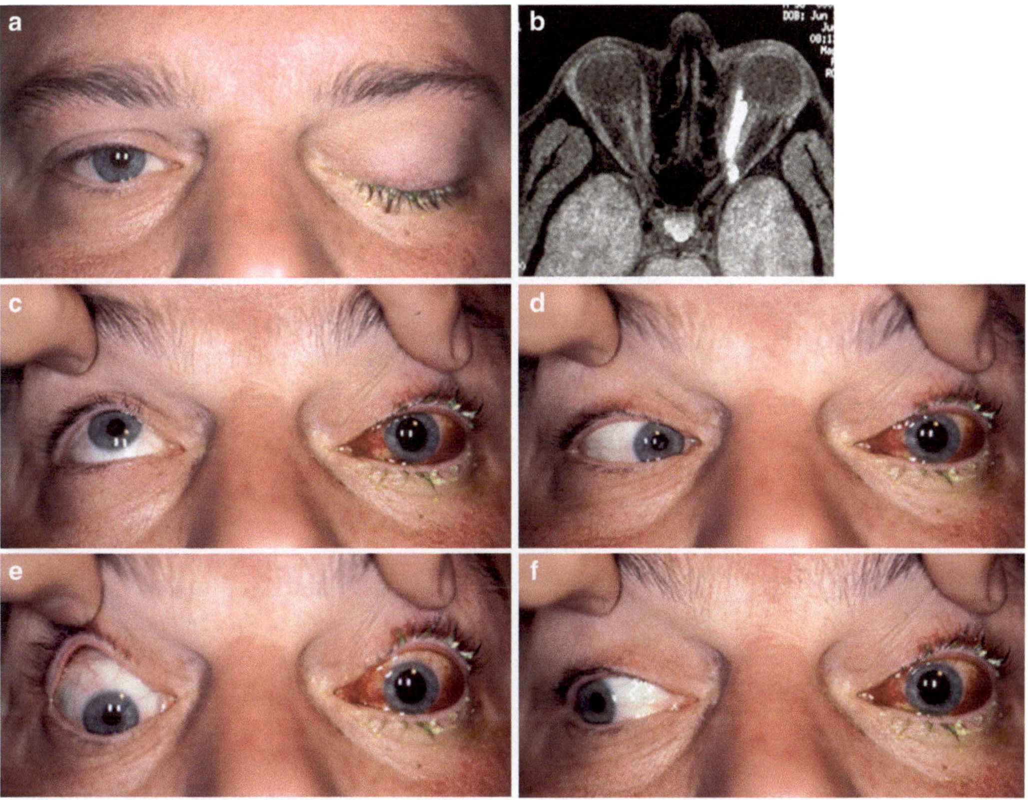

Fig. 13.10 A gentleman with complete left upper eyelid ptosis (**a**) who was impaled with baling wire that penetrated his medial left orbit, reaching the superior orbital fissure, as noted on MRI (**b**). Note complete loss of supraduction (**c**), abduction (**d**), infraduction (**e**), and adduction (**f**), along with a dilated, nonreactive pupil, in the left eye, consistent with a complete left internal and external ophthalmoplegia. The SOFS largely resolved spontaneously over time, with some residual deficits (courtesyof D avidA .W einberg,M D)

A blunt frontal head blow, usually due to a motor vehicle accident, is the most common scenario. Most patients have associated skull fractures with neurologic and ophthalmologic manifestations. Blepharoptosis is often complete, with limitation of adduction, depression, and elevation of the eye. Recovery of the levator muscle function occurs in most cases over a 1-year period [52]. Abberrant regeneration occurs in half of the cases and is seen as early as 9 months following the injury [52]. Surgical correction of blepharoptosis following direct injury to the third nerve should be delayed for 1 year, with the exception of young children, who are at risk for amblyopia. In these children, frontalis sling is usually the procedure of choice due to poor levator function. External levator resection is another option if the levator function is more than 5 mm.

Isolated Neurogenic Ptosis

Isolated neurogenic ptosis, with transient loss of levator function after forceful anterior displacement of the upper eyelid, has been reported [53]. The injury is due to a finger placed under the upper eyelid, typically in an altercation or sports-related injury. There is complete loss of levator function with minimal eyelid edema and preserved superior rectus muscle function. The site of injury is presumed to be the oculomotor nerve branch to the levator palpebrae muscle near its insertion. The blepharoptosis is transient with complete resolution within 2 weeks [53]. In contrast, levator aponeurosis dehiscence, which commonly occurs in blunt trauma, is not transient and is associated with relatively preserved levatorfunc tion.

Traumatic "Ptosis" Secondary to Facial Synkinesis

Traumatic facial nerve palsy may result in aberrant regeneration. Renervation of the lower face is misdirected to the upper eyelid, resulting in partial closure of the upper eyelid with lower face movements. The levator muscle innervation is intact; however, there is increased tone in the orbicularis oculi muscle that mimics blepharoptosis [40], and you probably also see "reverse ptosis" of the lower eyelid, as well, due to the orbicularismus clec ontraction.

Managemento fT raumatic Blepharoptosis

Management of traumatic ptosis depends on the underlying etiology. Injuries such as blunt trauma, contact lens wear, and intraocular surgery, leading to a stretched levator aponeurosis, are treated surgically, usually with external levator resection. Müllerectomy is an option in mild cases that have a positive response to the phenylephrine test. Patients with Horner syndrome, regardless of the etiology, are good candidates forM üllerectomy [54].

Complex lacerations of the upper eyelid have a better chance of recovery of levator function when repaired primarily [40]. Exploration of the laceration and identification of the levator muscle is essential. The lost levator muscle can be traced by pulling the conjunctiva forward or by identifying Whitnall's ligament leading to the levator muscle. Reapproximation of the levator muscle or aponeurosis can then be performed. If the patient is under local anesthesia, grasping the tissue suspected to be the levator and asking the patient to close and open their eyes, or look up, may help to confirm that the tissue in question contains, or is attached to, the levator muscle before surgical reapproximation. Delayed repair of the ptosis can be challenging because of cicatricial changes, with loss of natural tissue planes [55]. Within 3 weeks of the injury, scars are still soft and the wound can be pulled apart easily for surgical exploration. After 3 weeks, it is preferable to wait for the scar to remodel, which can takeupto6months [40].

Neurogenic, traumatic ptosis is dependent on the recovery of the third nerve palsy. Spontaneous recovery is the usual scenario, occurring over several months to a year. Therefore, these patients should be observed [52]. Surgical management of the residual ptosis depends on the levator function. Patients with poor levator function are candidates for a frontalis sling procedure. External levator function is an option in those with levator function greater than 4 mm.

Synkinetic ptosis secondary to traumatic facial nerve palsy has no surgical treatment, unlike cases of Marcus Gunn jaw winking ptosis. In the latter case, disinserting the levator and applying a sling offers a reasonable cosmetic result [56]. With the increased orbicularis oculi tone in synkinetic ptosis following facial nerve palsy, botulinum toxin injection to the orbicularis oculi is an option to consider in these patients. Surgical denervation of the orbicularis oculi muscle leaves patient with severe paralytic lagophthalmos, and renervation usually occurs over time. The use of botulinum toxin injections has been reported in a family with familial Bell's palsy and synkinesis of the eyelid with the orbicularis oris [57]. In addition, the utility of botulinum toxin in synkinetic ptosis could be extrapolated from its reported efficacy in cases of hyperlacrimation secondary to "crocodile tears," or gustatory hyperlacrimation, following facialne rvepa lsy [58].

References

1. Crawford JS. Ptosis as a result of trauma. Can J Ophthalmol.1974 ;9:244–8.
2. Fiebel RM, Custer PL, Gordon MO. Post cataract ptosis: a randomized, double-masked comparison of peribulbar and retrobulbar anesthesia. Ophthalmology. 1993;100(5):660–5.
3. Hosal BM, Tekeli O, Gursel E. Eyelid malposition after cataract surgery. Eur J Ophthalmol. 1998;8(1):12–5.
4. Paris GL, Quickert MH. Disinsertion of the aponeurosis of the levator palpebrae superioris muscle after cataract extraction. Am J Ophthalmol. 1976;81:337–40.
5. Bernardino CR, Rubin PA. Ptosis after cataract surgery. Semin Ophthalmol. 2002;17(3–4):144–8.
6. Wolfort FG, Poblete JV. Ptosis after blepharoplasty. Ann Plast Surg. 1995;34(3):264–6.
7. Bosniak SL. Complications: diagnosis and treatment. Cosmetic blepharoplasty. New York: Raven; 1990. p. 101–2.
8. Henderson HW, Collin JR. Mucous membrane grafting. Dev Ophthalmol. 2008;41:230–42.
9. Espana EM, Prabhasawat P, Grueterich M, Solomon A, Tseng SC. Amniotic membrane transplantation for reconstruction after excision of large ocular surface neoplasias. Br J Ophthalmol. 2002;86(6):640–5.
10. Heinz GW, Nunery WR. Anophthalmic socket evaluation and management. Oculoplastic Surgery. 3rd ed. New York: Raven; 1995. p. 609–36.
11. Christmas NJ, Van Quill K, Murray TG, Gordon CD, Garonzik S, Tse D, et al. Evaluation of efficacy and complications: primary orbital implants after enucleation. Arch Ophthalmol. 2000;118(4):503–6.
12. Allen L. The argument against imbricating the rectus muscles over spherical orbital implants after enucleation. Ophthalmology. 1983;90(9):1116–20.
13. Kushner BJ. A surgical procedure to minimize lower eyelid retraction with inferior rectus recession. Arch Ophthalmol.1992; 110:1011–4.
14. Carruthers JA, Lowe NJ, Menter MA, Gibson J, Nordquist M, Mordaunt J, et al. A multicenter, double-blind, randomized, placebo-controlled study of the efficacy and safety of botulinum toxin type A in the treatment of glabellar lines. J Am Acad Dermatol. 2002;46(6):840–9.
15. Kersten RC, de Conciliis C, Kulwin DR. Acquired ptosis in the young and middle-aged adult population. Ophthalmology. 1995;102(6):924–8.
16. Thean JH, McNab AA. Blepharoptosis in RGP and PMMA lens wearers. Clin Exp Optom. 2004;87(1): 11–4.
17. Watanabe A, Araki B, Noso K, Kakizaki H, Kinoshita S. Histopathology of blepharoptosis induced by prolonged hard contact lens wear. Am J Ophthalmol. 2006;141(6):1092–6.
18. Tossounis CM, Saleh GM, McLean CJ. The long and winding road: contact lens-induced ptosis. Ophthal Plast reconstr Surg. 2007;23(4):324–5.
19. Patel NP, Savino PJ, Wenber DA. Unilateral eyelid ptosis and a red eye. Surv Ophthalmol. 1998;43(2): 182–7.
20. Jones D, Livesey S, Wilkins P. Hard contact lens migration into the upper lid: an unexpected lid lump. Br J Ophthalmol. 1987;71(5):368–70.
21. Zola E, van der Muelen IJ, Lapid-Gortzak R, van Vliet JM, Nieuwendaal CP. A conjunctival mass in the deep superior fornix after a long retained hard contact lens in a patient with keloids. Cornea. 2008;27(10):1204–6.
22. Friedberg ML, Abedi S. Encysted hard contact lens appearing as an orbital mass. Ophthal Plast Reconstr Surg.1989; 5(4):291–3.
23. Beyer-Machule CK, Shapiro A. Eyelid penetration of a hard contact lens, simulating a neoplasm. Ophthalmic Surg. 1986;17(2):101–2.
24. Sebag J, Albert DM. Pseudochalazion of the upper lid due to hard contact lens embedding- case reports and literature review. Ophthalmic Surg. 1982;13(8): 634–6.

25. Kaya SO, Liman ST, Bir LS, Yuncu G, Erbay HR, Unsal S. Horner syndrome as a complication in the thoracic surgical practice. Eur J Cardiothorac Surg. 2003;24(6):1025–8.
26. Allen AY, Meyer DR. Neck procedures resulting in Horner syndrome. Ophthal Plast Reconstr Surg. 2009;25(1):16–8.
27. Barbut D, Gold JP, Heinemann MH, Hinton RB, Trifiletti RR. Horner syndrome after coronary artery bypass surgery. Neurology. 1996;46(1):181–4.
28. Shaw PJ, Bated D, Cartlidge NE, Heaviside D, French JM, Julian DG, et al. Neuro-ophthalmological complications of coronary artery bypass graft surgery. Acta Neurol Scand. 1987;76(1):1–7.
29. Cook T, Kietzman L, Leibold R. Pneumo-ptosis in the emergency department. Am J Emerg Med. 1992;10(5):431–4.
30. Fleishman JA, Bullock JD, Rosset JS, Beck RW. Iatrogenic Horner syndrome secondary to chest tube thoracostomy. J Clin Neuroophthalmol. 1983;3(3): 205–10.
31. Levy M, Newman-Toker D. Reversible chest tube Horner syndrome. J Neuroophthalmol. 2008;28(3):212–3.
32. Guye E, Lardy H, Piolat C, Bawab F, Becmeur F, Dyon JF, et al. Thoracoscopy and solid tumors in children: a multicenter study. J Laparoendosc Adv Surg Tech A. 2007;17(6):825–9.
33. Ford S, Lauder G. Case report of Horner syndrome complicating internal jugular venous cannulation in a child. Paediatr Anaesth. 2007;17(4):396–8.
34. Solomon P, Irish J, Gullane P. Horner's syndrome following a thyroidectomy. J Otolaryngol. 1993;22(6): 454–6.
35. Chandrasekhar S, Peterfreund RA. Horner syndrome following very low concentration bupivacaine infusion for labor epidural analgesia. J Clin Anesth. 2003;15(3):217–9.
36. Narouze SN, Basali A, Mandel M, Tetzlaff JE. Horner syndrome and trigeminal nerve palsy after lumbar epidural analgesia for labor and delivery. J Clin Anesth.2002;14(7) :532–4.
37. Menendez C, MacMillan DT, Britt LD. Transient Horner syndrome in a trauma patient with thoracic epidural analgesia: a case report. Am Surg. 2000;66(8):756–8.
38. Jeffery AR, Ellis FJ, Repka MX, Buncic JR. Pediatric Horner syndrome. J AAPOS. 1998;2(3):159–67.
39. Putnam JR, Nunery WR, Tanenbaum M, McCord AD. Blepharoptosis. Oculoplastic surgery. 3rd ed. New York: Raven; 1995. p. 175–6.
40. Silkiss RZ, Baylis HI. Management of traumatic ptosis. Adv Ophthalmic Plast Reconstr Surg. 1988;7:149–55.
41. Berke RN. Surgical treatment of traumatic blepharoptosis. Am J Ophthalmol. 1971;72:691–8.
42. Rubin PA, Rumelt S. Functional indications for enophthalmos repair. Ophthal Plast Reconstr Surg. 1999;15(4):284–92.
43. Fulcher TP, Sullivan TJ. Orbital roof fractures: management of ophthalmic complications. Ophthal Plast Reconstr Surg. 2003;19:359–63.
44. Sullivan WG. Displaced orbital roof fractures: presentation and treatment. Plast Reconstr Surg. 1991;87:657–61.
45. Karesh JW, Kelman SE, Chirico PA, Mirvis SE. Orbital roof "blow-in" fractures. Ophthal Plast Reconstr Surg. 1991;7:77–83.
46. Bun RJ, Vissinik A, Bos RM. Traumatic superior orbital fissure syndrome: report of two cases. J Oral Maxillofac Surg. 1996;54:758–61.
47. Postma MP, Seldomridge GW, Vines FS. Superior orbital fissure syndrome and bilateral internal carotid pseudoaneurysms. J Oral Maxillofac Surg. 1990;48(5):503–8.
48. Murakami I. Decompression of the superior orbital fissure. Am J Ophthalmol. 1965;59:803–8.
49. Unger JM, Gentry LR, Grossman JE. Sphenoid fractures: prevalence, sites and significance. Radiology. 1990;175(1):175–80.
50. Zachariades N. The superior orbital fissure syndrome. Oral Surg. 1982;53(3):237–40.
51. Memon MY, Paine KW. Direct injury of the oculomotor nerve in craniocerebral trauma. J Neurosurg. 1971;35(4):461–4.
52. Krohel GB. Blepharoptosis after traumatic ptosis. Am J Ophthalmol. 1979;88(3):598–601.
53. McCulley TJ, Kersten RC, Yip CC, Kulwin DR. Isolated unilateral neurogenic blepharoptosis secondary to eyelid trauma. Am J Ophthalmol. 2002;134(4): 626–7.
54. Glatt HJ, Putterman AM, Fett DR. Müller's muscle-conjunctiva resection procedure in the treatment of ptosis in Horner syndrome. Ophthalmic Surg. 1990;21:93–6.
55. Smith B, Obear MF. Traumatic blepharoptosis. Surg Clin North Am. 1967;47:515–20.
56. Bowyer JD, Sullivan TJ. Management of Marcus Gunn jaw winking synkinesis. Ophthal Plast Reconstr Surg.2004; 20(2):92–8.
57. Zaidi FH, Gregory-Evans K, Acheson JF, Ferguson V. Familial Bell's palsy in females: a phenotype with a predilection for eyelids and lacrimal gland. Orbit. 2005;24(2):121–4.
58. Keegan DJ, Geerling G, Lee JP, Blake G, Collin JR, Plant GT. Botulinum toxin treatment for hyperlacrimation secondary to aberrant regenerated seventh nerve palsy or salivary gland transplantation. Br J Ophthalmol.2002; 86(1):43–6.

Chapter 14
Anophthalmic Ptosis

Ann P. Murchison and Jurij R. Bilyk

Abstract Anophthalmic ptosis should never be considered as an entity in isolation, and in this regard it is unlike other forms of acquired ptosis. Surgical anophthalmia changes the relationship between the eyelids and the orbital contents. Furthermore, changes within the orbital soft tissue may secondarily manifest as ptosis. Conversely, lower lid laxity associated with anophthalmia may result in a downward displacement of the ocular prosthesis, resulting in masking of underlying ptosis. In all likelihood, the majority of anophthalmic ptosis is the result of multiple factors and must always be evaluated in relation to associated orbital and periocular soft tissues. Effective management of the ptotic lid in anophthalmia can be difficult and must take into account these orbital and periocular factors as well as prosthesis fitting.

Anophthalmic ptosis should never be considered as an entity in isolation, and in this regard it is unlike other forms of acquired ptosis. Surgical anophthalmia changes the relationship between the eyelids and the orbital contents. Furthermore, changes within the orbital soft tissue may secondarily manifest as ptosis. Conversely, lower lid laxity associated with anophthalmia may result in a downward displacement of the ocular prosthesis, resulting in masking of underlying ptosis. In all likelihood, the majority of anophthalmic ptosis is the result of multiple factors and must always be evaluated in relation to associated orbital and periocular soft tissues. Effective management of the ptotic lid in anophthalmia can be difficult and must take into account these orbital and periocular factors as well as prosthesis fitting.

Etiology

In most cases, anophthalmic ptosis occurs secondary to changes in deeper orbital soft tissue. In 1982, Tyers and Collin described a "postenucleation socket syndrome" manifesting as enophthalmos, ptosis with deepening of the superior sulcus, and laxity of the lower eyelid (Fig. 14.1) [1, 2].

The exact mechanism that leads to this constellation of findings remained obscure until Smit et al. provided CT data on the anophthalmic socket in two studies [3, 4]. By comparing parasagittal views of anophthalmic socket, either with or without an orbital implant, to the normal contralateral orbit in a series of 20 patients, the authors concluded that a rotation of orbital soft tissue occurs. Put simply, there is a migration of superior soft tissue posteriorly, and posterior soft tissue inferiorly (Fig. 14.2a). This results in a net rotation of orbital soft tissue inferiorly with a concomitant loss superiorly. Second, enucleation without orbital implant placement results in an anterior displacement of Tenon's capsule with a

J.R. Bilyk (✉)
Department of Ophthalmology, Jefferson University Hospitals and Thomas Jefferson University Medical College, Philadelphia, PA, USA
e-mail: jrbilyk@aol.com

A.J. Cohen and D.A. Weinberg (eds.), *Evaluation and Management of Blepharoptosis*,
DOI 10.1007/978-0-387-92855-5_14, © Springer Science+Business Media, LLC 2011

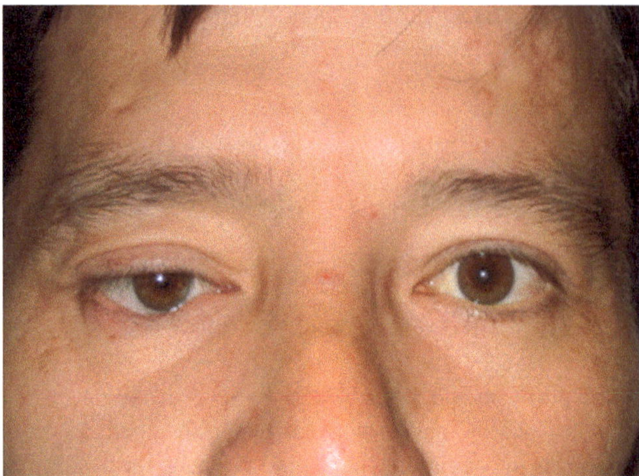

Fig. 14.1 Right anophthalmic ptosis secondary to postenucleation socket syndrome. Note the right enophthalmos and lower lid laxity, leading to prosthesis dystopia. The orbital volume deficit and lower lid laxity must be addressed prior to attempted ptosis repair

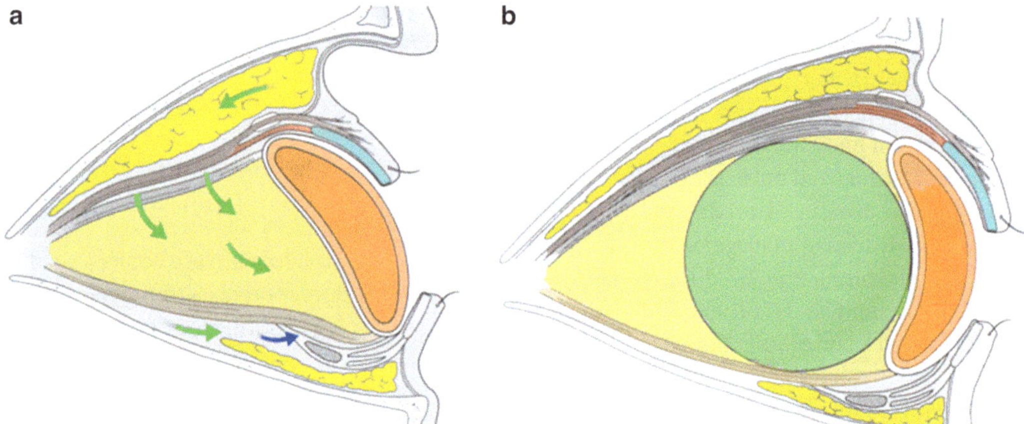

Fig. 14.2 (**a**) In an anophthalmic socket, absence of an orbital implant can result in a rotation of the intraconal orbital fat (*light yellow*) inferiorly. The levator (*dark gray*) is also displaced away from the orbital roof while the inferior rectus (*light brown*) migrates superiorly (*blue arrow*), shallowing the inferior fornix. The result of this soft tissue movement is a posterior tilting of the superior edge of the prosthesis (*orange*), posterior slippage of the orbital septum and preaponeurotic fat (*bright yellow*), poor support for the levator (*dark gray*), and Müller muscle (*maroon*) complex, manifesting clinically as ptosis with a deep superior sulcus. A similar mechanism occurs with an undersized orbital sphere (modified from [2]). (**b**) Placement of an appropriately sized orbital sphere (*green*) helps to maintain the orbital soft tissue relationships in a more normal configuration. Compare the anatomy in this figure with Fig. 14.2a (modified from [2])

simultaneous anterior migration of intraconal fat. Finally, the authors found evidence of a superior migration of the inferior rectus muscle from an unclear mechanism. Whether this inferior rectus muscle movement occurs because of the absence of the globe and further facilitates orbital soft tissue rotation inferiorly, or is a result of that rotation, remains unclear. More recent MRI studies of extraocular muscle positions in anophthalmic sockets show the path and volume of the muscles is not significantly changed, though the length appears decreased [5].

Smit et al. [3, 4] also reported that the levator–superior rectus complex was displaced inferiorly (away from the orbital roof), confirming earlier findings by Vistnes [6] and Soll [7]. This levator sag is postulated to result in a relative lengthening of the muscle, resulting in ptosis. However, CT studies of Smit et al. also noted that this perceived lengthening may be counterbalanced by retraction of the levator muscle. Tyers and Collin provide a different theory for anophthalmic ptosis: rotation of the intraconal soft tissue causes shallowing of the inferior fornix and a posterior tilting of the ocular prosthesis, with a resultant loss of support for the "fulcrum" of the levator muscle, which manifests clinically as ptosis.

In addition to volume loss and soft tissue rotation, other mechanisms for anophthalmic ptosis may also be present [8]. Iatrogenic injury to the levator muscle or to the superior division of the oculomotor nerve may occur during enucleation. Overzealous manipulation of orbital soft tissue or excessive bleeding may disrupt the normal orbital fascial matrix or cause fibrosis. Postoperatively, progressive orbital soft tissue contracture may lead to worsening enophthalmos and resultant ptosis. Of note, despite previous hypotheses that orbital fat atrophy plays a significant role in postenucleation socket syndrome [1], this has not been borne out in CT studies [3, 4]. However, undersizing of the orbital implant does play a role in enophthalmos and in all likelihood facilitates the previously described orbital soft tissue rotation. A volume loss of 6–7 cc was noted in the anophthalmic side by Smit et al., but the authors did not specifically study implant size in their series [3, 4].

Direct imbrication of the levator muscle, either during extraocular muscle fixation to the implant or during closure of Tenon's capsule, may injure or restrict the levator mechanism. A poorly fitted ocular prosthesis may either change the function of the levator mechanism or directly injure it. Chronic papillary conjunctivitis secondary to the prosthesis may result in chronic eyelid edema and eventual stretching of soft tissues. Excessive manipulation of the prosthesis could also result in eyelid laxity and ptosis.

Of note, the same mechanisms that result in anophthalmic ptosis may simultaneously act to mask its presence. Kaltreider et al. noted that ectropion and lower lid laxity often resulted in a downward displacement of the ocular prosthesis, resulting in a relative elevation of the upper lid [8]. Manual tightening of the lower eyelid with temporary repositioning of the prosthesis would unmask the ptosis.

Forniceal shortening or more severe contraction of the socket ("malignant socket contracture") [9] may also occur and lead to eyelid malposition and difficulty in retaining a prosthesis. This challenging presentation often requires a staged approach; as with all anopthalmic ptosis, patients with any orbital volume insufficiency should have this addressed before final evaluation and possible ptosis repair.

Evaluation

Anopthalmic patients presenting with eyelid abnormalities require a full examination of the orbit, upper and lower eyelids (including fornices), and the ocular prosthesis. Evaluation of the ptosis alone is inadequate and frequently leads to unsatisfactory results. With the prosthesis in place, the patient should first be evaluated for any significant enophthalmos. If this is present, there is little to be gained from ptosis repair; the enophthalmic socket should be reconstructed first. The superior sulcus should be examined for deepening and symmetry when compared to the opposite side. The presence of a significant conjunctival papillary reaction should be recorded. The size of the prosthesis and the amount of superior prosthetic buildup should also be evaluated. In general, a large prosthesis typically connotes an orbital soft tissue volume deficit and results in a higher incidence of lower lid laxity, both of which may need to be addressed before ptosis repair.

The upper eyelid position should be noted and levator function evaluated. Significant rotation of the prosthesis may occur after initial fitting. This may result in a migration of the pupil in relation to the contralateral side and ptosis evaluation may become inaccurate. When evaluating the upper eyelid, it is important to assure that the lower eyelid is in correct position. If laxity is present, the lower lid should be manually tightened by gently pulling it toward the lateral canthus. This may result in significant upward movement of the prosthesis and a relative worsening of the ptosis.

The movement of the prosthesis should be evaluated as compared to the contralateral eye. Poor movement can be due to fornix abnormalities, enophthalmos or poor prosthesis fit. The prosthetic should then be removed and evaluated for size and integrity. The socket should be evaluated for inflammation, excessive mucous, giant papillary conjunctivitis under the upper eyelid, and pyogenic granulomas. The forniceal depth should be noted, specifically noting if the superior fornix is excessively deep or if the fornices are not well defined. The tissue over the implant should be examined for thinning, fistula, or exposure. Lastly, palpation of the socket can determine the presence or absence of an implant and the position of the implant within the orbit.

In all monocular patients, the remaining eye must also be evaluated in a serial fashion, with the frequency determined by the patient's age, history, and health of the eye. The patient should always be reminded about monocular precautions and the use of polycarbonate safety glasses, and this conversation should be documented in the medical record.

Solutions

The solutions to anophthalmic ptosis vary in invasiveness. Care should first be taken to rule out ptosis which is secondary to orbital volume deficiency or lower eyelid laxity; these issues should be addressed before addressing the ptosis (Fig. 14.2b).

One minimally invasive option is a ptosis crutch on the patient's glasses. The crutch must be fit individually and for patients unable or unwilling to have surgery, it can clear the ptosis from the patient's "visual axis." Proper prosthesis fitting, sometimes with a "sulcus crutch" or built-up superior ledge may help raise the upper lid. In cases with minimal ptosis, this may be a good option, although motility is generally reduced. With greater ptosis, care must be taken not to create a large, heavy prosthetic to avoid subsequent problems.

There are several surgical techniques to address residual ptosis after orbital volume and lower eyelid laxity have been addressed. Levator surgery, including external levator resection, or posterior procedures work well in patients with good levator function. However, the latter must be performed with care to avoid shortening the superior fornix. If there is complete ptosis with little to no levator function, a frontalis sling may correct the ptosis. In such cases, patients must be counseled that a conventional unilateral frontalis sling may fail to correct the ptosis to any significant degree because there is no visual advantage to frontalis contracture in a nonseeing (or prosthetic) eye. In cases of poor levator function, a maximal levator resection or a tethering of the upper eyelid via a frontalis sling may be options, but the patient must be warned about the need for possible postoperative lubrication of the prosthesis and the potential cosmetic outcome of a static lid and decreased prosthetic motility. Details on each of the surgical techniques may be found in subsequent chapters.

Conclusion

Upper eyelid ptosis in the anophthalmic socket typically has multiple etiologies and the evaluation and management can be complex. While true, isolated ptosis may occur, upper eyelid dystopia due to poor support from the prosthesis, decreased orbital volume from an undersized implant, orbital soft tissue rotation, abnormal implant location, and lower eyelid malposition are usually present in various degrees. A systematic approach taking into account orbital, periocular, and prosthetic dynamics should be used in the evaluation and treatment of the anophthalmic patientpre sentingw itha pparentptos is.

References

1. Tyers AG, Collin JRO. Orbital implants and post enucleation socket syndrome. Trans Ophthalmol Soc UK.1982;102:90–2.
2. Collin JRO. Enucleation, evisceration and socket surgery. In: Collin JRO, editor. A manual of systematic eyelid surgery. 3rd ed. London: Elsevier; 2006. p. 208–23.
3. Smit TJ, Koornneef L, Zonneveld FW, Groet E, Otto AJ. Computed tomography in the assessment of the postenucleation socket syndrome. Ophthalmology. 1990;97(10):1347–51.
4. Smit TJ, Koornneef L, Zonneveld FW, Groet E, Otto AJ. Primary and secondary implants in the anopthalmic orbit. Preoperative and postoperative computed tomographic appearance. Ophthalmology. 1991; 98(1):106–10.
5. Detorakis ET, Engstrom RE, Straatsma BR, Demer JL. Functional anatomy of the anopthalmic socket: insights from magnetic resonance imaging. Invest Ophthalmol Vis Sci. 2003;44(10): 4307–13.
6. Vistnes LM. Mechanism of upper lid ptosis in the anophthalmic orbit. Plast Reconstr Surg. 1976;58: 539–45.
7. Soll DB. Evolution and current concepts in the surgical treatment of the anophthalmic orbit. Ophthal Plast Reconstr Surg. 1986;2:163–71.
8. Kaltreider SA, Sheilds MD, Hippeard SC, Patrie J. Anophthalmic ptosis: investigation of the mechanisms and statistical analysis. Ophthal Plast Reconstr Surg.2003; 19(6):421–8.
9. Mustardé JC. Repair and reconstruction in the orbital region. 2nd ed. Edinburgh: Churchill Livingstone; 1980.p.222.

Chapter15
LashPt osis

Renzo A. Zaldívar, Michael S. Lee, and Andrew R. Harrison

Abstract Eyelash ptosis can occur as a congenital or acquired condition. Careful clinical assessment will help distinguish between the two and assist in surgical planning. The appropriate surgical procedure, based on the diagnosis, is likely to result in an excellent long-term outcome.

Introduction

Lash ptosis (LP), or eyelash ptosis, occurs when the lashes of the upper eyelid begin pointing in a more horizontal to inferior orientation (Fig. 15.1) [1, 2]. Lash ptosis can be congenital or acquired; however, most cases are in association with acquired blepharoptosis and therefore often overlooked. Other conditions that may be associated with lash ptosis include floppy eyelid syndrome (FES), congenital lamellar ichthyosis, longstanding ocular leprosy, bilateral acoustic neuroma, thyroid eye disease, and latanoprost-induced LP [2–8].

Pathophysiology

Lash ptosis has been found in association with several conditions. Review of these cases offers clues to the etiology of LP. Hypotheses are largely based on anatomical changes within the upper eyelid [1]. The eyelid margin is separated by the gray line into the anterior (skin and muscle) and posterior (tarsus and conjunctiva) lamellae. The eyelash bulbs of the upper eyelid lie in a space between the Riolan muscle and the pretarsal orbicularis oculi. The eyelash follicles may extend posteriorly to embed in the tarsus. The eyelashes emerge through this space and exit through the eyelid margin. The eyelashes project downward initially, then curve superiorly and anteriorly, projecting away from the globe (Fig. 15.2a,b).

Conditions such as FES where there is an abnormality in the elastin of the tarsus and pretarsal orbicularis may explain the presence of lash ptosis in these cases [9]. Eyelid laxity diminishes the support needed for the lash to maintain the appropriate vector, leading to lash ptosis [10]. Mulhern et al. [6] studied patients with facial palsy and found that 42% had LP as a long-term consequence. Loss of tone of the pretarsal orbicularis and Riolan muscles may compromise support to these muscle fibers and eyelash follicles. Excess skin laxity, as in dermatochalasis, could also alter the underlying eyelid muscle tension. Lash ptosis in association with trichomegaly secondary to usage of a prostaglandin analog, such as latanoprost, may be due to the weight of the relatively large lashes overwhelming the support structures that maintain proper follicle projection [3]. Changes to the tarsus may alter the direction of eyelashes because the hair follicles embed posteriorly within the tarsus. Terminal fibers of the levator aponeurosis weave

A.R.H arrison (✉)
Departmentof O phthalmology,
UniversityofM innesota, Minneapolis, MN USA
e-mail:ha rri060@umn.edu

A.J. Cohen and D.A. Weinberg (eds.), *Evaluation and Management of Blepharoptosis*,
DOI 10.1007/978-0-387-92855-5_15, © Springer Science+Business Media, LLC 2011

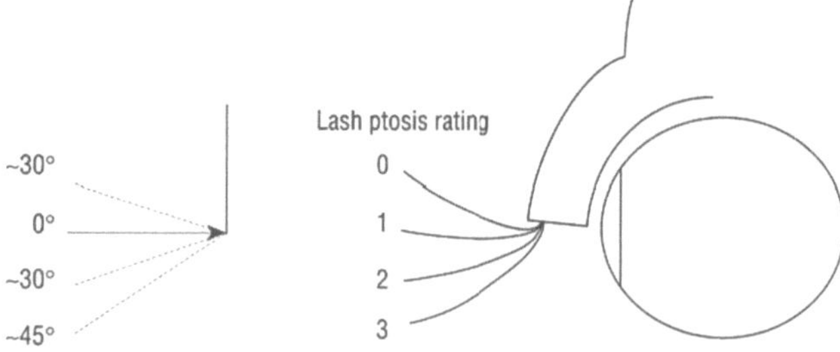

Fig. 15.1 Diagram illustrating eyelash ptosis rating scale

through the orbicularis oculi to insert into the subcutaneous tissue and skin. Disruption of these fibers by congenital ptosis leads to a poor eyelid crease and lack of eyelash support [9]. The close proximity of the aponeurosis and orbicularis suggests that loss of these aponeurotic fibers may alter the eyelid anatomy and mechanically cause laxity of the overlying eyelid skin and muscle, producing LP. Lash ptosis in congenital and acquired blepharoptosis may stem from a laxity of anterior lamellar structures and an underlying connective tissue deformation.

Clinical Evaluation

As previously described with eyelid ptosis, lash ptosis evaluation should begin with a complete history. Careful assessment will help determine if it is congenital vs. acquired, in addition to possible comorbid conditions, as seen in FES and sleep apnea. The physical exam should include a complete oculofacial exam as well as a complete eye exam. Slit lamp exam is critical as it may reveal pseudolash ptosis secondary to cicatricial entropion. This should be assessed by eversion of the upper lid and examination of the tarsus and conjunctiva. Management will differ greatly if lash ptosis is due to cicatricial entropion (see below). When evaluating the eyelash orientation, you should ensure that the patient is in primary gaze with the chin parallel to the ground. In addition, it is important to examine the patient from both frontal and lateral perspectives.

Documentation of eyebrow position and the relationship to and contribution from possible eyelid ptosis should be noted. Careful assessment of the degree of levator dehiscence via measurement of the lid crease is important, as this is likely the most common cause of LP. A simple, semiquantitative grading scale to categorize LP by severity has been developed by Malik et al. In their study, each eyelid was assessed using a 4-point rating scale: 0 indicates no LP; 1, minimal; 2, moderate; and 3, severe [11]. A lash ptosis rating (LPR) of 0 represented the natural position of eyelashes relative to the eyelid margin (0° to ≥30° *above* the horizontal). Eyelashes oriented nearly parallel to the horizontal meridian relative to the eyelid margin (0–30° *below* the horizontal) are rated as having an LPR of 1. A LPR of 2 characterizes eyelashes with an orientation that is 31–45° below the horizontal meridian. Eyelashes oriented at more than 45° below the horizontal meridian characterize an LPR of 3. They found that patients with congenital ptosis had a mean LPR of 2.1 and it was 1.3 for those with acquired blepharoptosis. Finally, it is important to document the degree of lash ptosis in each eyelid as it may differ, and you should adjust your surgical technique accordingly.

Surgical Management

Management depends on the severity of the lash ptosis, and surgical technique is modified in cases with associated blepharoptosis, both acquired and congenital. The following scenarios illustrate surgical interventions based on clinical findings.

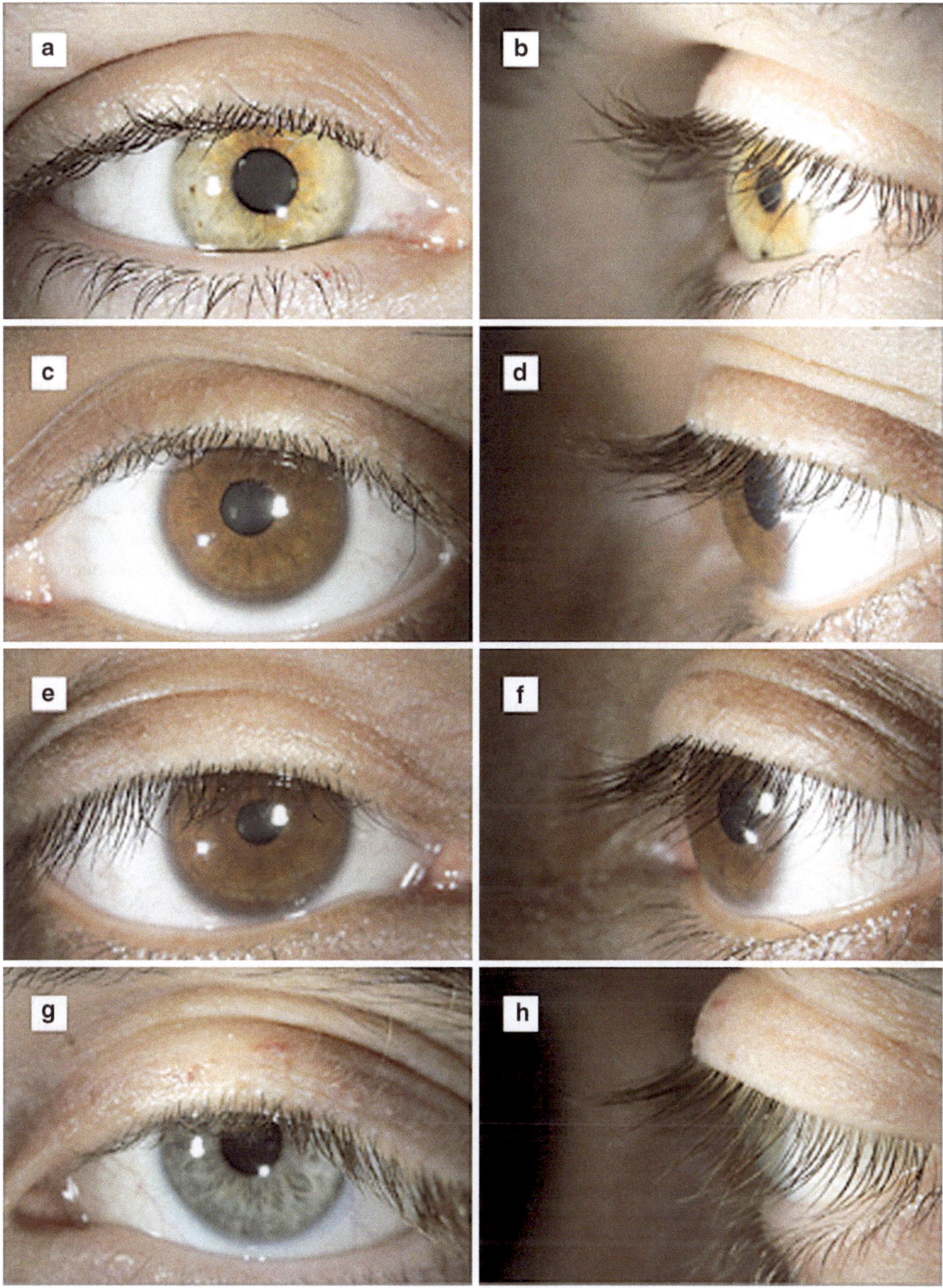

Fig. 15.2 Clinical photographs illustrating variations in the degree of lash ptosis from frontal and lateral perspectives. (**a, b**) No lash ptosis (lash ptosis rating, LPR, 0). (**c, d**) Minimal lash ptosis (LPR, 1). (**e, f**) Moderate ptosis (LPR, 2). (**g, h**) Significant lash ptosis (LPR, 3)

Minimal Lash Ptosis

The lash ptosis is addressed after the excess skin is removed (to address concurrent dermatochalasis), and the levator is advanced in cases of blepharoptosis. Interrupted bites of 6–0 chromic sutures are used to attach skin to the deep levator aponeurosis just above the superior tarsal border. It is important to note that as the sutures are tightened, often the subsequent sutures are more difficult to place; therefore, we often preplace the sutures prior to tying them down to ensure that each one is appropriately placed. The number of sutures placed depends on the size of the incision; however, we typically place five to six sutures in each eyelid. The preplaced sutures are then tied down and any remaining skin gaps are closed with 6–0 fast-absorbing gut suture. The careful attention to closure, by ensuring the incorporation of the levator aponeurosis, accomplishes two goals. First, it reforms the lid crease, and second, it causes enough of a vertical traction on the anterior lamella to improve the angle of the eyelash orientation. We aim for slight overcorrection, as the lashes are expected to drop slightly in the postoperative period.

Moderate to Severe Lash Ptosis

These cases can be challenging to correct and therefore require a more powerful procedure to improve the vertical vector forces on the lash base. Again, in cases of either acquired or congenital blepharoptosis, we prefer to address this first. Once we have the lid height in the desired position and just prior to closure, we address the lashes. For moderate cases, we like to use a polygalactin double-armed 5–0 or 6–0 horizontal mattress suture through the upper third of the tarsus and exit just above the lash base. These sutures are placed along the same level of the tarsus across the eyelid and exit in the same position immediately above the lash base to ensure symmetric elevation across the lashes. Once tied down, the closure of the skin is completed with a running 6–0 fast-absorbing gut suture.

For more severe cases of lash ptosis, we employ a similar technique as described above with a couple of modifications. Instead of using a dissolvable suture, we like to use a permanent suture, such as silk and remove it around postoperative week 6 to minimize the chance of postoperative descent. In addition, we reinforce the vertical traction by closing the skin similar to that described for minimal lash ptosis.

In patients with FES, the lash ptosis is corrected with a horizontal tightening procedure. The authors' preference is to use a full-thickness pentagonal wedge resection at the junction of the lateral ¼ and medial ¾ of the eyelid. The eyelid is closed using standard marginal and layered closure techniques. In our experience, rarely will floppy eyelid patients need additional rotational suture techniques as described above. Lash ptosis secondary to cicatricial entropion needs to be corrected by treatment of the underlying etiology having caused, or causing, the cicatricial changes. Once the cicatrix has stabilized, or if protection of the ocular surface warrants sooner intervention, surgery can be undertaken. The approach depends on the severity of the cicatrix, but usually requires incisional relaxation of the cicatrix and placement of a spacer graft. If the anterior lamellar anatomy has not been chronically disrupted, the lash ptosis may resolve; however, residual lash ptosis may need to be addressed secondarily using one of the above procedures.

In all of our techniques we aim for mild to moderate overcorrection, as the lash angle is expected to drop slightly in the postoperative period.

Conclusion

Lash ptosis is associated with various conditions, and the etiology of the lash ptosis may be secondary to the underlying condition, i.e., congenital or acquired blepharoptosis, FES, etc. Preoperatively, it is important to document the severity of the lash ptosis and grade it accordingly in order to determine the best surgical technique to employ.

The combined approach of addressing the underlying condition along with the severity of the lash ptosis will lead to an improved outcome and the greater likelihood of a satisfied patient.

References

1. Langford JD, Linberg JV. A new physical finding in floppy eyelid syndrome. Ophthalmology. 1998; 105(1):165–9.
2. Guimarães FC, Cruz AV. Eyelid changes in long-standing leprosy. Ophthal Plast Reconstr Surg. 1998;14(4):239–43.
3. Casson RJ, Selva D. Lash ptosis caused by latanoprost. Am J Ophthalmol. 2005;139(5):932–3.
4. McNab AA. Floppy eyelid syndrome. Ophthalmology. 1998;105(11):1977–8.
5. Singh AJ, Atkinson PL. Ocular manifestations of congenital lamellar ichthyosis. Eur J Ophthalmol. 2005;15(1):118–22.
6. Mulhern MG, Aduriz-Lorenzo PM, Rawluk D, Viani L, Eustace P, Logan P. Ocular complications of acoustic neuroma surgery. Br J Ophthalmol. 1999;83(12): 1389–92.
7. McNab AA. Floppy eyelid syndrome and obstructive sleep apnea. Ophthal Plast Reconstr Surg. 1997;13(2): 98–114.
8. Culbertson WW, Ostler HB. The floppy eyelid syndrome. Am J Ophthalmol. 1981;92(4):568–75.
9. Netland PA, Sugrue SP, Albert DM, Shore JW. Histopathologic features of the floppy eyelid syndrome: involvement of tarsal elastin. Ophthalmology. 1994;101(1):174–81.
10. Dutton JJ. Surgical management of floppy eyelid syndrome. Am J Ophthalmol. 1985;99(5):557–60.
11. Malik KJ, Lee MS, Park DJJ, Harrison AR. Lash ptosis in congenital and acquired blepharoptosis. Arch Ophthalmol.2007; 125(12):1613–5.

PartI V
Treatment

Chapter16
TheN onsurgicalT reatmento fPt osis

Ippolit C. A. Matjucha

Abstract The surgical treatment of blepharoptosis is in most cases dependably effective and safe; by comparison, nonsurgical treatment generally provides less satisfactory results and can be difficult for the patient to tolerate. Therefore, relatively few patients will prefer medical treatment for symptomatic, chronic ptosis, except as a temporizing measure before a definitive procedure. The possible mechanisms for lifting the eyelid nonsurgically are external mechanical devices (skin-taping, adhesives, or spectacle-based lid crutches) to retract the upper lid, topical eye drops to stimulate Müller's muscle, and injectable botulinum toxin to weaken orbicularis tone.

Introduction

Given the availability and effectiveness of the surgical treatments for blepharoptosis discussed elsewhere in this volume, the use of medical therapies for this problem is perhaps becoming eclipsed. Nevertheless, some patients with chronic ptosis may prefer nonsurgical treatment; and even those patients choosing surgery may require interim therapy while their procedure is being planned and scheduled. Therefore, a review of available nonsurgical treatments for ptosis is presented, along with guidelines for patient selection for such therapy, keeping in mind that medical therapy is often not well tolerated over time.

The most common nonsurgical treatment is the mechanical lifting of the upper lid by tape, skin adhesives, and lid crutches. Pharmacological options for improving ptosis include topical ocular adrenergic agents and botulinum toxin. In the specific case of ptosis from myasthenia gravis, control of ptosis is best achieved by appropriate therapy for that disease (see Chapter 11: "MyastheniaG ravis").

PatientSel ection:Et iological Disease

Successful medical treatment for ptosis starts with proper patient selection, and patients with ptosis as part of Horner syndrome may be particularly appropriate for consideration of medical therapy. As discussed in more detail below, patients with mild ptosis due to sympathetic denervation of Müller's muscle in the upper (and lower) eyelid have at their disposal a readily available, effective topical medication, apraclonidine 0.5%, to improve their ptosis with few potential side effects; therefore, patients with symptomatic ptosis from Horner syndrome, as well as those with temporary ptosis as a side effect of botulinum toxin injections, are considered good candidates for medical treatment as an initial step.

In some patients with other disease states, ptosis of the upper eyelid may be accompanied by weakness of eyelid closure. In these cases,

I.C.A.M atjucha (✉)
Neuro-opthalmologist,C omprehensiveS urgical Ophthalmologist,Pri vatePr actice, Sudbury, MA, USA
e-mail:ic matjucha@verizon.net

A.J. Cohen and D.A. Weinberg (eds.), *Evaluation and Management of Blepharoptosis*,
DOI 10.1007/978-0-387-92855-5_16, © Springer Science+Business Media, LLC 2011

surgical elevation of the ptotic eyelid may promote exposure keratoconjunctivitis, even with a frontalis sling procedure that allows patient-adjustable eyelid opening. By contrast, the temporary and easily reversible eyelid elevation provided by nonsurgical methods may be a safer alternative for these patients and should be carefully considered. Examples of disease where ptosis is combined with orbicularis weakness include myasthenia gravis (MG), myotonic dystrophy, and chronic progressive external ophthalmoplegia (CPEO). Combined cranial nerve (CN) III and VII palsies are rarely seen together due to a single lesion in nondevastated patients, given the anatomical distance between the nuclei of CN III and VII in the brainstem and throughout their courses. However, such combined palsies can be seen as part of cranial polyneuropathy presentation of infectious or noninfectious etiology [1–3].

In Bell's palsy, the palpebral fissure will usually widen, as the weakened orbicularis allows the upper eyelid to rise and the lower eyelid to fall; occasionally, however, the frontalis weakness in Bell's palsy produces sufficient brow ptosis to cause a secondary, mechanical blepharoptosis. Similarly, patients with Möbius syndrome (congenital CN VI and VII weakness) or myotonic dystrophy can present with facial weakness and ptosis [4]. Orbicularis oculi weakness can increase the risk of postoperative keratopathy, so surgical correction of ptosis in this setting must be weighed carefully, and in some patients avoided.

Just as patients with CN VII weakness are at special risk for ocular exposure problems after surgical correction of ptosis, so too are patients with coexisting ptosis and corneal hypesthesia. Combined CN III and V disease (due to compression or inflammation at the orbital apex, superior orbital fissure, or cavernous sinus) occurs with reasonable clinical frequency. Also, corneal hypesthesia can represent an independent finding (as a complication, for instance, of recurrent herpetic corneal infections or trigeminal ablative procedures for ameliorating *tic douloureux*) in a patient with any etiology of ptosis. Because of the higher risk of corneal complications after surgical ptosis treatment when the cornea is hypesthetic, such patients may prefer only medical methods to reduce their blepharoptosis.

Patients whose underlying disease produces ptosis that is unpredictably variable (e.g., MG), temporary (e.g., ischemic CN III palsy), or addressable via means other than eyelid surgery (e.g., prednisone treatment for MG or Tolosa–Hunt syndrome) will also usually choose medical treatment of ptosis. And, of course, patients who have external or internal ophthalmoplegia in addition to ptosis may choose to leave the ptosis completely untreated – or treated medically from time to time – to minimize symptomatic diplopia or photophobia, respectively

PatientSel ection:Ot her Considerations

Patients who are considered quite fragile medically, whether from advanced age or disease, may choose to avoid the relatively low surgical risk associated with a ptosis repair procedure, and may therefore choose medical treatment alone. A few patients will not be able to tolerate the surgery without general anesthesia, which presents additional risks to some patients, especially those with advanced cardiac or pulmonary disease. Also, some patients will refuse surgical treatments for other reasons.

Some patients will be limited to medical treatment because they represent "bad surgical risks." Besides the very ill, such patients might include those with poor nutrition, those receiving chemotherapy, and those who have received radiation therapy in the surgical field, so that the risk of slow, incomplete healing (with complicating infection) is considerable. Others may be unable to follow postoperative directions dependably and simultaneously lack the reliable social support needed to help them perform those tasks; available social and medical services, such as a temporary visiting nurse, can sometimes remove such roadblocks to surgery.

While surgical risks may be unacceptable for certain patients, it does not follow that medical therapies are entirely benign: any of the medical treatments for ptosis carry the risk of significant side effects, such as skin injury from repetitive taping and contact allergy from topical agents. Therefore, the clinician should also be aware that a patient who originally chooses a medical treatment option for chronic symptomatic ptosis may over time reconsider surgical options if no absolute contraindications exist.

MechanicalM easures

LidC rutches

A "lid crutch" (or "ptosis crutch") is an attachment to the rear of the spectacle frame meant to hold the eyelid in place by friction after it has been elevated and the crutch applied [5, 6]. It is typically a small arc (one point of frame attachment), bow, or double-loop [7] (with two points of attachment) extending from the rear surface of a spectacle frame and meant to elevate the lid by directly contacting it (see Fig. 16.1a, b). The crutch is typically made of a spring-metal wire (sometimes covered with plastic tubing for comfort), but examples in plastic can be encountered.

The spectacles can be placed on the face in a way to allow the wires first to contact the eyelid skin and then, as the spectacles are pushed up the nasal bridge toward its resting place, to elevate the lid. Most patients quickly learn to do this maneuver. Alternatively, the patient may manually lift the eyelid and then put the spectacles in place so that the wire holds the lid in place.

Because of their effectiveness and general lack of side effects, *ptosis crutches are often the preferred nonsurgical method of controlling chronic ptosis*; in contrast, patients with temporary ptosis often do not choose to invest in this relatively expensive approach. Finding an optician who can dependably craft spectacle frames with crutches and then adjust them correctly for the individual patient can be difficult; therefore, an ophthalmology or plastic surgery office that sees many patients with ptosis may well consider working with an optician to develop such a service for these patients wherever it does not alreadye xist [8].

Side effects from the use of lid crutches are expected to be few. Injury to the ocular surface by wire contact can be anticipated if the spectacles are put on hastily and without care, or perhaps if the spectacles are forcefully struck by accident. Although no such injuries have been reported, other spectacle-related injuries [9] seem to imply that such injury is possible. Contact allergy to the plastic tubing (if any) covering the wires can develop, and contact dermatitis from certain steel and titanium alloys has been reported [10, 11].

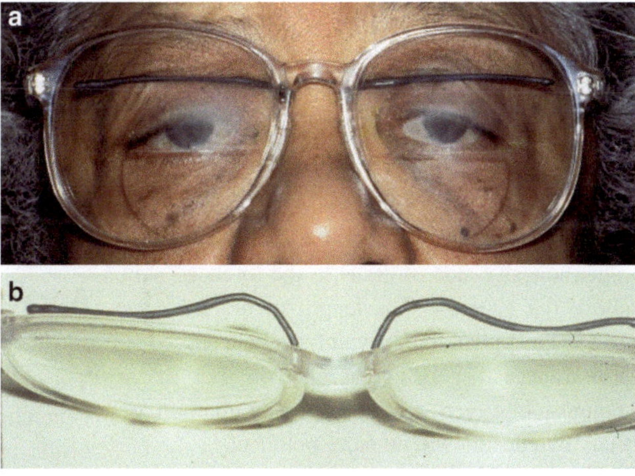

Fig.16.1 (**a**) Ptosis crutch mounted on spectacles (courtesy of Robert Lesser, MD). (**b**) Ptosis crutch elevating eyelids (courtesy of Robert Lesser,M D)

Eyelid Taping

Perhaps the simplest method of raising the eyelid (other than pulling it up with a finger) is by use of adhesive tape to the upper eyelid. Occasionally, patients with ptosis may have already begun to use this method on their own when first encountered in the ophthalmology or plastic surgery clinic.

As a chronic measure, taping has disadvantages. Patients can develop contact allergy to the adhesive, simple skin irritation, or traumatic injury to the epidermis from repeated tape removal [12]. Because tape loosens from the skin with prolonged wear, some patients may find it necessary to reapply tape several times a day, to substitute a tape with stronger adhesive, or to add an additional adhesive such as tincture of benzoin; these measures may further increase the risk of skin trauma and allergic reaction [13].

An ideal method of eyelid taping has not been proposed and is likely to vary with different individual patients. However, an effective taping method would mimic the surgical goals of the frontalis sling operation: connecting the tarsal-plate region of the upper eyelid to the frontalis region of the forehead while bypassing the uppermost eyelid skin and lower eyebrow. Such a method would allow variable opening of the eyelid based on raising the eyebrow, permitting the tape to glide over the eyebrow and its cilia with minimal inadvertent epilation.

A preprepared eyelid tape for such application may already be commercially available in the form of "knuckle" adhesive bandages typically used to cover finger knuckles; they are available in a selection of sizes. These H- or hourglass-shaped bandages would allow the patient to apply one long side of the adhesive "H" horizontally across the lid, then position the nonadhesive gauze in contact with the eyebrow, and finally apply the other adhesive side of the H to the forehead skin above the eyebrow. The length of the adhesive arm to be applied to the eyelid can be trimmed to size if necessary before application. For many patients, however, a simpler taping method of their own design will be more practical.

Glues

Medical cyanoacrylate-type glues are now commercially available, both in over-the-counter formulations for superficial wound dressing and as a skin adhesive for wound closure by medical professionals.

While incidents of accidental, temporary eyelid closure from skin-bonding using nonmedical household glues are well known, deliberate eyelid opening by use of strong glues has rarely been described [14]. In concept, especially in an older patient with redundant upper eyelid skin, such glue can be used to plicate the pretarsal eyelid skin and fix it superiorly to lid skin just below the eyebrow. For such use, bandage-level glues probably provide minimally sufficient adhesion; wound-closure glues are expensive and relatively difficult to access; and hardware-grade glues lack medical testing and can produce more heat while curing.

Precautions regarding this approach are numerous and include difficulty of accurate application by the patient, the slow spontaneous reversibility of the adhesion (whether the glue is well or inaccurately applied), possibility of allergic dermatitis, and the scarcity of published experience to use as a resource. Even if successful in an individual patient, the duration of action of eyelid skin gluing may be simultaneously "too long and too short:" it is harder to reverse (compared to taping) if eyelid closure is prevented, increasing the risk of exposure, and yet also would be expected to begin to lose effective adhesion within 24 h with bandage-level glue, and within 72 h even with the strongest skin-bonding agents.

Medical Measures: Topical Medication

Apraclonidine

Treatment of ptosis with topical medication is generally marked by lack of efficacy, with one bright exception: in cases of mild ptosis due to sympathetic denervation of Müller's muscle, the use of topical apraclonidine is dependably effective, often leading to complete resolution of ptosis [15].

Müller's muscle (or the superior tarsal muscle) is a sympathetically innervated smooth muscle located just above the superior tarsal border (in the upper eyelid), between the palpebral conjunctiva and the levator aponeurosis. When activated by the sympathetics, it elevates the upper lid by 1–2 mm; a similar muscle in the lower eyelid, the inferior tarsal muscle, acts to retract it slightly as well. Its subconjunctival position in the midportion of the lid makes Müller's muscle easy to expose to topical medication.

Apraclonidine (available as 0.5 or 1% ophthalmic solution) is an alpha-2 adrenergic agonist used to lower intraocular pressure. However, it is also a weak alpha-1 agonist. In Horner syndrome, sympathetic denervation results in an adrenergic supersensitivity, in which alpha-1 receptors do not appreciably increase in density (number per unit of cell membrane area), but become instead more efficient in stimulating muscle contraction [16]. This denervation supersensitivity allows even a weak alpha-1 agonist like apraclonidine to produce noticeable mydriasis and resolution of ptosis in Horner syndrome [17, 18].

Conversely, one should expect that in the absence of denervation hypersensitivity, apraclonidine would produce less eyelid retraction than stronger agonists such as phenylephrine and epinephrine. However, it has been suggested that apraclonidine 1% topical solution can be as effective as other topical adrenergic agents in raising the eyelid [19], and a 0.5% solution has been suggested as a reasonably effective treatment for temporary ptosis complicating botulinum toxin A injection to the *orbicularis oculi* or *corrugator supercilii* muscles [20]. Just as when used for glaucoma, apraclonidine has been given on a three times daily dosing schedule for management of botulinum toxin-induced ptosis. However, whether its duration of action as a lid retractor is equal to its duration as an ocular hypotensive agent (8 h for the 0.5% solution and 12 h for the 1% solution) has not been reported.

Intolerance of apraclonidine typically results from ocular irritation, including, in some patients, contact allergy manifesting as follicular conjunctivitis [21]. When allergy develops, there is little choice but to stop the medication; a related alpha-2 agonist, brimonidine, is more selective and does not have the same alpha-1 activity [22]; hence, it cannot substitute for apraclonidine as a treatment for ptosis. Another source of possible intolerance, especially in patients with Horner syndrome, is that apraclonidine is expected to produce not only elimination of ptosis but noticeable mydriasis as well. The photophobia and loss of focus that can accompany mydriasis may be unacceptable to some patients (see below).

Epinephrine,Di pivefrin and Phenylephrine

Epinephrine would be expected, by direct action on Müller's muscle, to elevate the eyelid perhaps 2 mm in most subjects, and to be most effective in patients with paresis of Müller's muscle due to Horner syndrome; however, it has been suggested that epinephrine lid effects are also obvious in selected cases of "senile" (levator aponeurotic) ptosis [23].

By the late 1970s, ophthalmologists had significant experience with the use of topical epinephrine (typically, 1% solution) as an ocular hypotensive agent for the treatment of glaucoma. Multiple side effects were encountered, such as systemic hypertension (perhaps dangerously so for any patient on a monoamine oxidase inhibitor), cystoid macular edema, ocular discomfort, and black "adrenochrome" deposits in the conjunctiva and cornea; while myocardial infarction or cardiac arrhythmia have occurred with injectable epinephrine, they have not been reported as a complication of topical ocular use.

These problems with topical epinephrine prompted the development of dipivefrin [24]. A more lipophilic form of epinephrine with greater ability to penetrate the cornea, dipivefrin could be used at 0.1% solution strength, resulting in a significantly lower incidence of side effects without loss of ocular efficacy. The development of more effective ocular hypotensives has resulted in both drugs falling into disuse; hence, ophthalmic epinephrine and dipivefrin are no longer commercially available in the US.

Phenylephrine (2.5 and 10% solutions) is the staple alpha-1-agonist mydriatic of ophthalmic diagnosis and is readily available. Little is known about the side effects of phenylephrine in long-term use, but given its chemical similarity to epinephrine and even higher solution concentration, problems similar to those encountered with chronic topical ophthalmic epinephrine use might be expected. Its action on ptosis would be expected to be similar to other adrenergic agents discussed, with eyelid elevation of up to 2 mm [25, 26]. While the 10% solution has a somewhat higher risk of adverse cardiovascular events than the 2.5%, the stronger solution is nevertheless frequently used in both diagnostic and surgical settings for patients with poor pupil dilation. Still, the potential risk and perhaps a shorter duration of action (3–6 h as a mydriatic) make this drug less appealing than apraclonidine for medical treatment of ptosis.

All strong alpha-1 adrenergic agents will share two visual side effects when applied to the eyes: photophobia from dilation of the pupil, and blurred vision from reduced depth-of-field focus, as the "pinhole" optical effect of a small pupil is lost. To reduce these problems (and to produce even greater reduction in eye pressure), topical epinephrine for the treatment of glaucoma was for a time produced as a combined preparation, mixed with the miotic pilocarpine. Such an approach has very little attractiveness if the goal is anything but lowered eye pressure: pilocarpine, for most patients, will have side effects that are even less tolerable than those of epinephrine. Also, one must consider that the simultaneous instillation of pilocarpine and phenylephrine has traditionally been considered the most efficient way, in those patients at risk, to induce acute angle-closure glaucoma [27].

Medical Measures: Botulinum Toxin

Both botulinum toxins A and B are available commercially, with toxin B generally reserved for the treatment of individuals who have become allergic to toxin A. Used for years as a standard treatment for benign essential blepharospasm, hemifacial spasm, and other dystonias, most practitioners are well acquainted with the ability of botulinum toxin to treat pseudoptosis associated with these conditions.

Regarding true ptosis, botulinum is perhaps more often thought of as a cause rather than as a treatment: inadvertent temporary paresis of the *levator palpebrae* muscle when treating the *orbicularis* and *corrugator* muscles is a well-known complication of botulinum toxin injection to the upper face (see above). Additionally, the levator muscle can be injected intentionally to cause temporary ptosis (a "chemical tarsorrhaphy") in the treatment of certain ocular surface diseases [28].

Toxin-mediated paresis of the orbicularis can in fact also serve to temporarily lessen true ptosis. Lid fissure height is determined by the balance between forces widening the fissure (muscle tone in the upper eyelid levator, lower eyelid retractor, and Müller's muscle; gravity on the lower eyelid; and degree of exophthalmos) and those narrowing the fissure (orbicularis tone, gravity on the upper eyelid, and degree of enophthalmos). When the orbicularis muscle tone is reduced by use of botulinum, the fissure will widen, but the effect may be small [29]. Successful temporary paralysis of the orbicularis, of course, carries the risk of symptomatic lagophthalmos.

There exists, as discussed above, the risk of worsening the ptosis by simultaneously weakening the levator when attempting to weaken the orbital or preseptal portion of the orbicularis and of weakening the frontalis or corrugator muscles enough to produce eyebrow ptosis with secondary mechanical eyelid ptosis. To minimize these risks, injection of botulinum toxin to improve ptosis should avoid the frontalis and corrugator muscles entirely; avoid the midline of the orbicularis muscle, as the levator lies beneath the muscle centrally; utilize as anterior (subdermal) an injection depth as is practical; and utilize small-volume aliquots of toxin, to minimize its migration away from the injection site. Also, as is standard with any botulinum injection protocol, a minimal number of injection sites should be placed at first, allowing for titration via additionalinje ctionla ter,ifre quired.

References

1. Mullaney PB, Nabi NU, Thorner P, Buncic R. Ophthalmic involvement as a presenting feature of nonorbital childhood parameningeal embryonal rhabdomyosarcoma. Ophthalmology. 2001;108(1): 179–82.
2. Mohan S, Ahmed SI, Alao OA, Schliep TC. A case of AIDS associated cryptococcal meningitis with multiple cranial nerve neuropathies. Clin Neurol Neurosurg. 2006;108(6):610–3.
3. Sood BR, Sharma B, Kumar S, Gupta D, Sharma A. Facial palsy as first presentation of acute myeloid leukemia. Am J Hematol. 2003;74(3):200–1.
4. Miller MT, Strömland K. The Möbius sequence: a relook. J AAPOS. 1999;3(4):199–208.
5. Lapid O, Lapid-Gortzak R, Barr J, Rosenberg L. Eyelid crutches for ptosis: a forgotten solution. Plast Reconstr Surg. 2000;106(5):1213–4.
6. Morrison J. Ptosis spectacles. Med Techn Bull. 1951;2(2):41–3.
7. Lundie RNG. The Lundie Loop. Myasthenia Gravis Association. https://www.mga-charity.org/web/guest/the-lundie-loop.
8. Walsh G, Rafferty PR, Lapin J. A simple new method for the construction of a ptosis crutch. Ophthalmic Physiol Opt. 2006;26(4):404–7.
9. Jain V, Natarajan S, Shome D, Gadgil D. Spectacle-induced ocular trauma: an unusual mechanism. Cornea.2007;26(1):109–10.
10. Suhonen R, Kanerva L. Allergic contact dermatitis caused by palladium on titanium spectacle frames. Contact Dermatitis. 2001;44(4):257–8.
11. Summer B, Fink U, Zeller R, Rueff F, Maier S, Roider G, et al. Patch test reactivity to a cobalt-chromium-molybdenum alloy and stainless steel in metal-allergic patients in correlation to the metal ion release. Contact Dermatitis. 2007;57(1):35–9.
12. Widman TJ, Oostman H, Storrs FJ. Allergic contact dermatitis from medical adhesive bandages in patients who report having a reaction to medical bandages. Dermatitis.2008;1 9(1):32–7.
13. Marks Jr JG, Rainey MA. Cutaneous reactions to surgical preparations and dressings. Contact Dermatitis. 1984;10(1):1–5.
14. Osaki TH, Osaki MH, Belfort Jr R, Osaki T, Sant'anna AE, Haraguchi DK. Management of progressive myopathic blepharoptosis with daily application of octyl-2-cyanoacrylate liquid bandage. Ophthal Plast Reconstr Surg. 2009;25:264–6.
15. Garibaldi DC, Hindman HB, Grant MP, Iliff NT, Merbs SL. Effect of 0.5% apraclonidine on ptosis in Horner syndrome. Ophthal Plast Reconstr Surg. 2006;22(1):53–5.
16. Abdel-Latif AA, Akhtar RA, Zhou CJ. Effects of surgical sympathetic denervation on G-protein levels, alpha and beta-adrenergic receptors, cAMP production and adenylate cyclase activity in the smooth muscles of rabbit iris. Curr Eye Res. 1995;14(5):405–11.
17. Koc F, Kavuncu S, Kansu T, Acaroglu G, Firat E. The sensitivity and specificity of 0.5% apraclonidine in the diagnosis of oculosympathetic paresis. Br J Ophthalmol.2005; 89(11):1442–4.
18. Morales J, Brown SM, Abdul-Rahim AS, Crosson CE. Ocular effects of apraclonidine in Horner syndrome. Arch Ophthalmol. 2000;118(7):951–4.
19. Munden PM, Kardon RH, Denison C, Carter K. Palpebral fissure responses to topical adrenergic drugs. Am J Ophthalmol. 1991;111(6):706–10.
20. Scheinfeld N. The use of apraclonidine eyedrops to treat ptosis after the administration of botulinum toxin to the upper face. Dermatol Online J. 2005;11(1):9. http://dermatology.cdlib.org/111/pearls/iopidine/scheinfeld.html. Accessed October 15, 2009.
21. Wilkerson M, Lewis RA, Shields MB. Follicular conjunctivitis associated with apraclonidine. Am J Ophthalmol.1991; 111(1):105–6.
22. Spooner JJ. Ophthalmic disorders. In: Arcangelo VP, Peterson AM, editors. Pharmacotherapeutics for advanced practice: a practical approach. 2nd ed. Philadelphia, PA: Lippincott, Williams & Wilkins; 2006. p. 179.
23. Hennekes R. Adrenaline sensitivity of senile ptosis. Klin Monatsbl Augenheilkd. 1982;181(6):496–8.
24. Kass MA, Mandell AI, Goldberg I, Paine JM, Becker B. Dipivefrin and epinephrine treatment of elevated intraocular pressure: a comparative study. Arch Ophthalmol. 1979;97(10):1865–6. http://archopht.ama-assn.org/cgi/reprint/97/10/1865.pdf.
25. Glatt HJ, Fett DR, Putterman AM. Comparison of 2.5% and 10% phenylephrine in the elevation of upper eyelids with ptosis. Ophthalmic Surg. 1990;21(3):173–6.
26. Nunes TP, Matayoshi S. Phenylephrine 10% eye drop action in the eyelid position in healthy subjects. Arq Bras Oftalmol. 2008;71(5):639–43.
27. Mapstone R. Provocative tests in closed-angle glaucoma. Br J Ophthalmol. 1976;60(2):115–9.
28. Brans JW, Aramideh M, Schlingemann RO, Oen VM, Speelman JD, Ongerboer de Visser BW. Cornea protection in ptosis induced by botulinum injection. Ned Tijdschr Geneeskd. 1996;140(19):1031–3.
29. Fagien S. Temporary management of upper lid ptosis, lid malposition, and eyelid fissure asymmetry with botulinum toxin type A. Plast Reconstr Surg. 2004;114(7): 1892–902.

Chapter17
ExternalL evatorR esection

Morris E. Hartstein, Natan D. Kahn, and David A. Weinberg

This chapter contains a video segment which can be found at the URL:
http://www.springerimages.com

Abstract External levator resection is a ptosis procedure that can be used in both children and adults, in patients with almost any degree of levator function, and those with a negative phenylephrine test. Since a skin incision is employed, this surgical approach is easily combined with upper blepharoplasty. The surgical technique and postoperative management are described in detail.

Introduction

Ptosis repair by external levator advancement or resection is a fairly versatile procedure. Though it obviously works best in patients with good levator function (excursion of 15–20 mm), it can also be used in patients with poor levator function, e.g., congenital ptosis. This procedure has the advantage of allowing the surgeon to be able to titrate the effect on the table in patients who are awake and cooperative. In addition, it represents a "true anatomic repair" by advancing an attenuated or disinserted levator in patients with aponeurotic ptosis. The phenylephrine test (used in potential Müllerectomy patients) can be helpful in levator resection patients, as well. First, it can show the patient how the eyelid may appear postoperatively. Second, it affords the surgeon the opportunity to distinguish between ptosis (which would necessitate ptosis repair) and dermatochalasis (which would require blepharoplasty only), and, more importantly, demonstrate that to the patient to help decide which procedure to perform (either or both) Third, this test can demonstrate if there is Hering's law dependency by placing phenylephrine in one eye (the more ptotic eye) and observing the fellow eye to see if the contralateral eyelid drops. This is important in surgical planning. Finally, patients who respond well to phenylephrine generally respond well to less advancement of their levator to achieve the desired effect.

Procedure

A basic set of instruments is necessary for this procedure (Fig. 17.1). The procedure begins with marking the lid crease, optimally with a fine-tipped marking pen (Fig. 17.2). Particularly if any skin excision is planned, i.e., when concurrent blepharoplasty is performed, one should mark the patient in the upright position prior to local anesthetic injection. We prefer to use the patient's own natural crease if it is apparent and favorably positioned. If the lid crease is significantly elevated, as in many patients with involutional ptosis, or if there is no visible crease, then the incision is marked at the desired lid crease

D.A.W einberg(✉)
ConcordEye C are, Concord, NH
and
Department of Surgery (Ophthalmology),
DartmouthM edicalSc hool, Hanover, NH, USA
e-mail:da weinberg@hotmail.com

A.J. Cohen and D.A. Weinberg (eds.), *Evaluation and Management of Blepharoptosis*,
DOI 10.1007/978-0-387-92855-5_17, © Springer Science+Business Media, LLC 2011

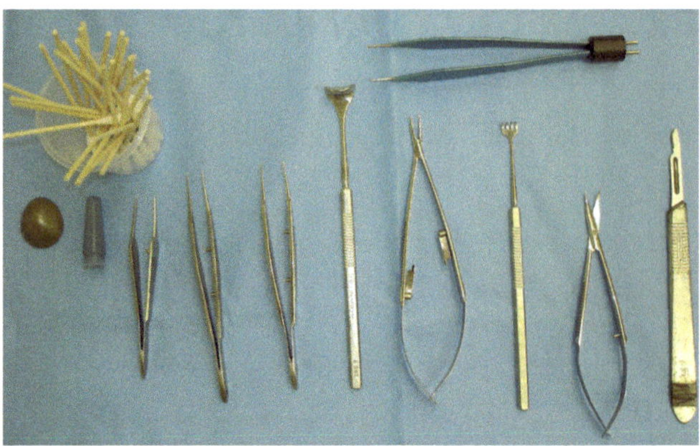

Fig. 17.1 Basicins truments et for external levator resection surgery

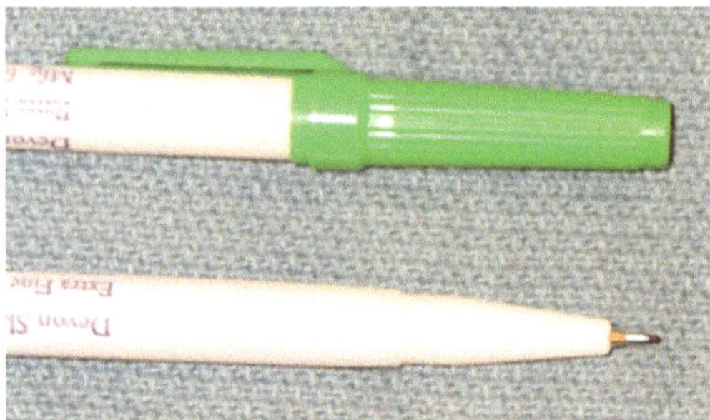

Fig. 17.2 Fine-tippedm arkingpe n

position, with the crease often being placed slightly higher in females and lower in patients of Asian heritage. Even if there is no apparent excess skin preoperatively, it is important to take into account that the ptosis repair may "produce" skin redundancy by lifting the eyelid (Fig. 17.3).

It is our preference to mark, inject, and then prep to allow time for the epinephrine to take effect. A variety of different local anesthetic solutions may be employed, e.g., 2% lidocaine with epinephrine, or a mixture of 0.5% or 0.75% bupivacaine (with or without epinephrine) mixed 50:50 with 2% lidocaine with epinephrine (1:100,000). There has been some debate as to whether or not epinephrine should be used in the local anesthetic, related to concerns over stimulation of Müller's muscle and how this may impact accuracy in eyelid positioning. However, we prefer to use epinephrine in order to facilitate hemostasis, and that seems to be the practice of most oculoplastic surgeons. The local anesthetic solution may be buffered with sodium bicarbonate.

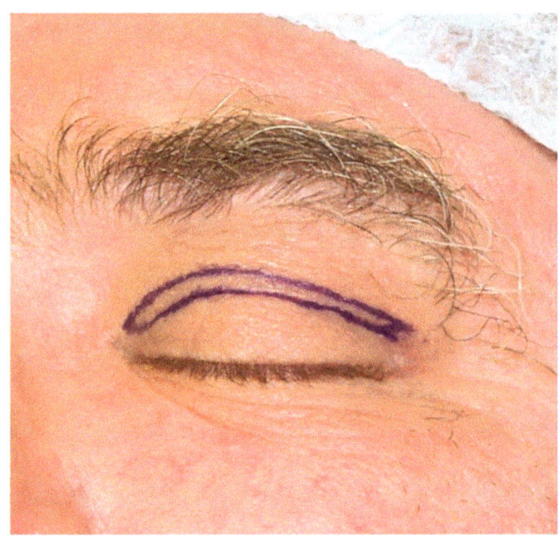

Fig. 17.3 Marking the lid crease and allowing for small amountof r edundancyc ausedbyl ide levation

Hyaluronidase should be avoided, as it may allow for inadvertent spread of the anesthetic into the levator muscle, which may weaken the muscle and impair the surgeon's ability to accurately "titrate" the ptosis repair. The local anesthetic is infiltrated just beneath the skin, with minimal volume injected (1 cc or less, unless the eyelid is very large), and intravenous sedation may reduce the pain experienced with the injection, or at least the patient's recollection of that discomfort (Fig. 17.4). Often, a small amount of local anesthetic is injected just over the central tarsus where the tarsal sutures will be passed. If IV sedation is used, it is important to make sure the effects wear off in time for the eyelid adjustment phase of surgery. While this procedure can

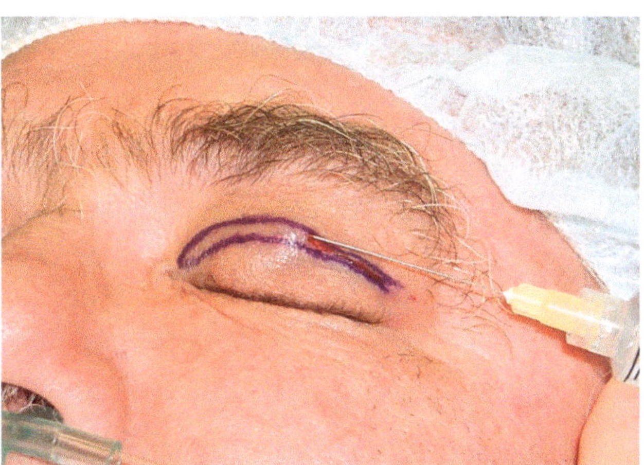

Fig. 17.4 Infiltrating local anestheticjus tbe neatht hes kin

be performed under general anesthesia, it is difficult to know how much to advance/resect the levator without patient input. If there is no choice, then a mild plication of the muscle may be safest so as not to result in an overcorrection. Thus, we strongly prefer to operate only under local or with IV sedation. The patient then undergoes a full-face prep with a head drape and split sheet to leave the entire face, or at least both eyes, exposed so that the two eyes can be compared throughout the procedure. Many patients seem to be more comfortable, and certainly less claustrophobic, with their nose and mouth left uncovered. A rigid corneal (or eye) shield, coated posteriorly with ointment, is placed, after topical anesthesia with proparacaine or tetracaine, to protect the globe while passing the tarsal sutures.

A #15c blade (smaller profile than a standard #15) is used to incise along the demarcated line(s), or one may use an alternate cutting instrument, such as Wescott scissors, Colorado needle (with cutting cautery), Ellman radiofrequency unit (Ellman International, Inc, Oceanside, NY), or CO_2 laser (Fig. 17.5). A skin or skin-muscle flap is excised (if performing a simultaneous blepharoplasty) (Figs. 17.6 and 17.7). Hemostasis is obtained with bipolar, monopolar, or thermal cautery. With an assistant retracting the superior skin edge, and the surgeon grasping the pretarsal orbicularis muscle inferiorly, dissection is carried out in a superior direction in the suborbicularis plane (Fig. 17.8). Particularly in older patients with a high crease and those with deeper superior sulci, i.e., little or no preaponeurotic fat, it is important to dissect superiorly so as not to inadvertently injure a thin levator aponeurosis when cutting the orbital septum. In addition, if one retropulses the globe, the orbital fat will prolapse forward and provide greater levator protection. The orbital septum is opened across the eyelid to expose the preaponeurotic fat, which is a useful landmark that overlies the levator aponeurosis and muscle. The adipose may be removed or contracted with cautery at this point,

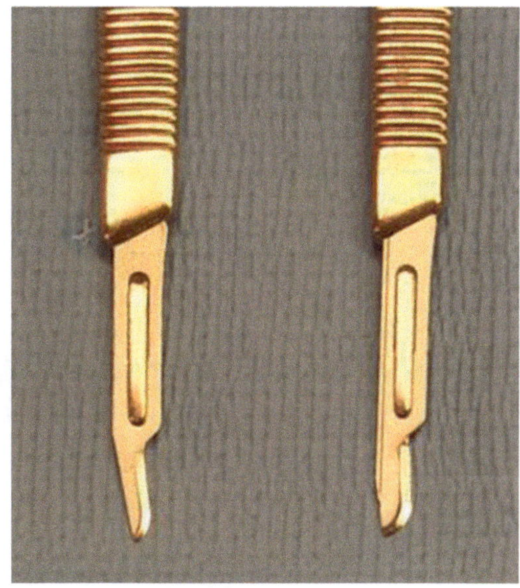

Fig. 17.5 A #15c blade is more suited to eyelid surgery thant hel arger,s tandard#15bl ade

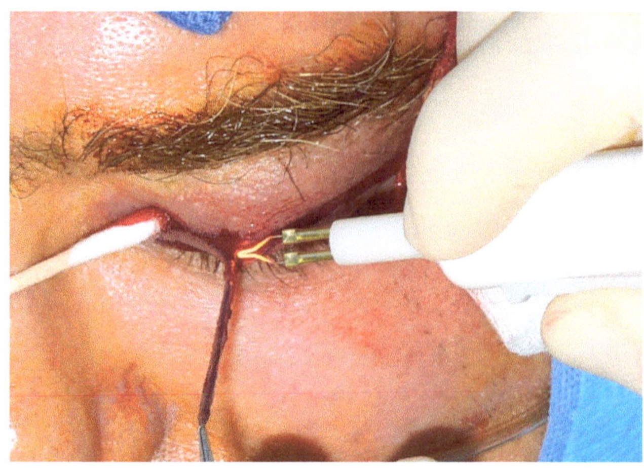

Fig. 17.6 As kin-musclefl ap is resected using a handheld cautery

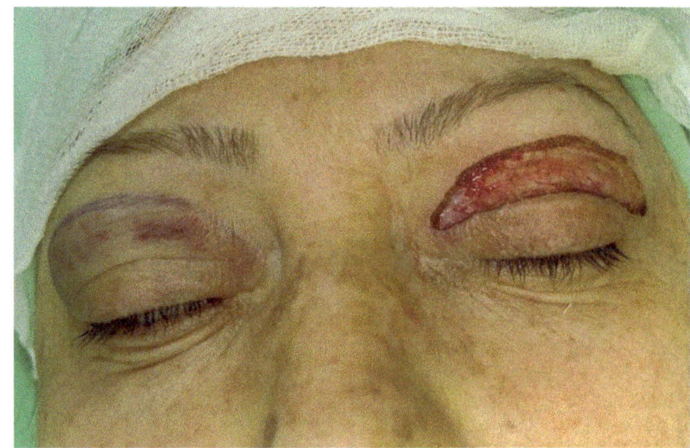

Fig. 17.7 Immediately following skin-muscle flap resection, before proceeding with dissection through deeper orbicularistis sues

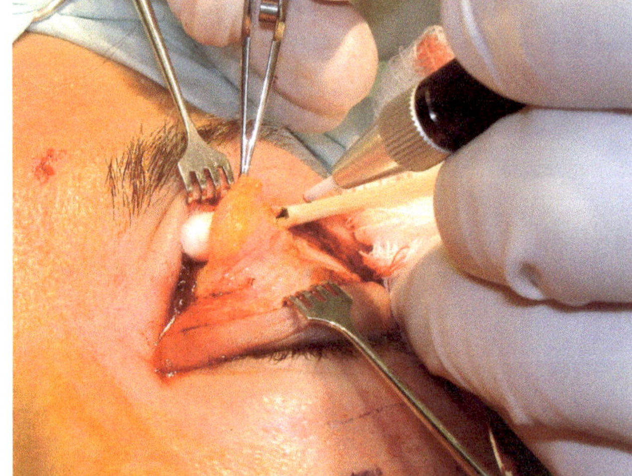

Fig. 17.8 AC O_2 laser is used to divide the orbital septum. The preaponeurotic fat – a useful landmark – sits just behind the septum, just anterior to the levator

if desired, taking care not to confuse the lacrimal gland with a lateral fat pad (lacrimal gland tends to be pinker or tanner in color and firmer in texture). In many patients with involutional ptosis there is fatty infiltration of the muscle and/or attenuation of the aponeurosis – frank disinsertion is less common. However, some studies have failed to demonstrate aponeurotic dehiscence or disinsertion in patients with involutional ptosis, raising the question as to the true etiology of this disorder.

Next, while pulling the inferior skin edge toward the patient's feet, dissection is carried in a posterior direction, down to bare tarsus over the superior half of the tarsal plate (Figs. 17.9 and 17.10). Make certain that you are working anterior to tarsus rather than superior to it as you dissect posteriorly. Some patients may have undergone a prior Hughes procedure or Fasanella-Servat procedure, and they have a vertically shortened tarsus. When dissecting posteriorly in an eyelid with vertical tarsal deficiency, there is a greater risk of injury to the globe, and in such cases usage of a rigid eye shield may be particularly helpful. It is prudent to evert the eyelid at the start of the procedure (or during the preoperative exam) to check the vertical tarsal dimension, especially if there is any uncertainty as to whether or not the patient has had prior surgeries performed. The aponeurosis is separated from the tarsal plate and from underlying Müller's muscle. As one develops the plane between levator and Müller's muscle, one must be careful to stay in that "natural" plane of diaphanous tissue, which is facilitated with traction. If the levator aponeurosis is very attenuated, it is necessary to either dissect

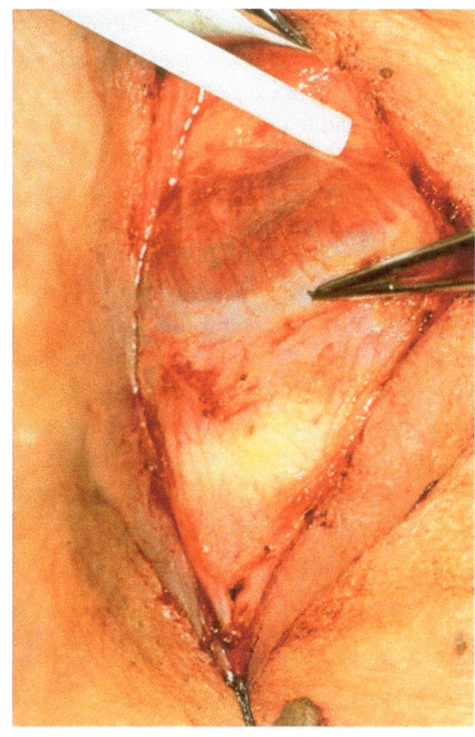

Fig. 17.10 Following dissection superiorly and inferiorly, the levator, aponeurosis, and tarsus are identified

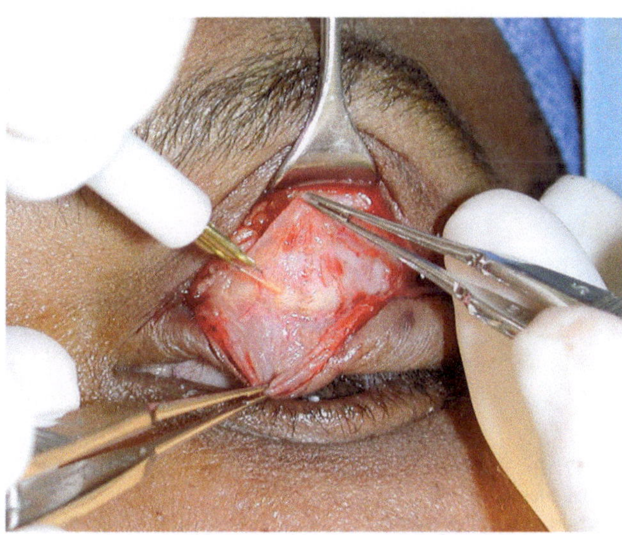

Fig.17.9 Dissectioni sc arried out down to tarsus using handheldc autery

up to the level of more healthy and robust aponeurosis or Whitnall's ligament or create a thicker, combined levator-Müller's muscle flap by instead dissecting between Müller's muscle and conjunctiva. If a suture were simply placed through a very thin area of levator aponeurosis, there would be a high likelihood of that suture cheesewiring postoperatively, resulting in an undercorrection. A narrow strip of pretarsal orbicularis muscle may be excised both for the purpose of debulking and to create a fresh edge to adhere to the tarsus, which will help form an eyelid crease with a tighter pretarsal skin platform.

There are many suture options to choose from for advancing the levator and securing it to the tarsus, including 5-0 or 6-0 absorbable polyglactin 910 or nonabsorbable polypropylene. It is important to use a spatulated needle in order to obtain a satisfactory deep lamellar suture pass through tarsus, without cutting through the tarsus anterior or posterior to that lamella. A permanent, nonbraided suture is easier to use as a "hang back" suture, if desired. A double-armed 5-0 polypropylene suture is passed partial thickness through the anterior tarsus a few millimeters below the superior tarsal border in the central/medial region of the eyelid and then both needle ends are carried through the levator aponeurosis, at least a few millimeters apart to reduce the likelihood of cheesewiring, and tied in a temporary loop knot (Figs. 17.11 and 17.12). After placing the suture in the tarsal plate, it is prudent to evert the eyelid to ensure that the suture is not full-thickness, i.e., exposed, which could cause a corneal abrasion. The suture is often passed through levator at the junction of the muscle and the aponeurosis, although one should certainly take into account the degree of ptosis and levator function when deciding where to place the suture, i.e., how much to advance the muscle. However, if there is uncertainty as to what level to pass the suture, the muscle/aponeurotic border is a good place to start (Fig. 17.13). Even in the presence of a dif-

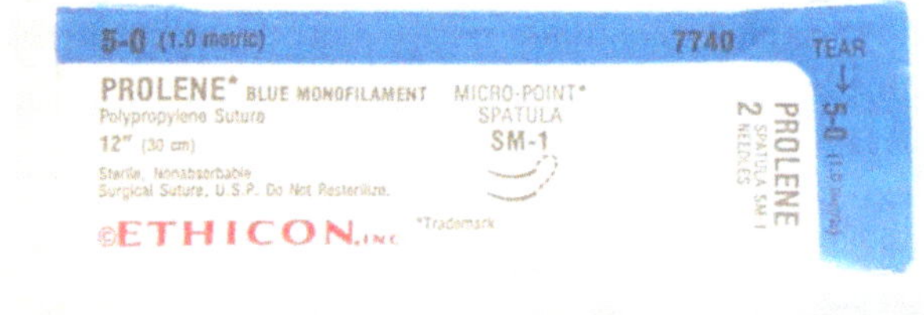

Fig. 17.11 Double-arm 5-0 prolene on spatulated needle (Ethicon, Somerville, New Jersey)

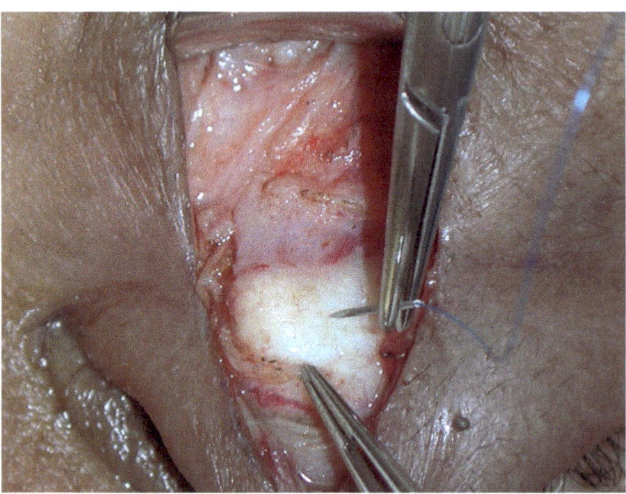

Fig.17.12 The suture is passed partial thickness through the anteriors urfaceof thet arsus

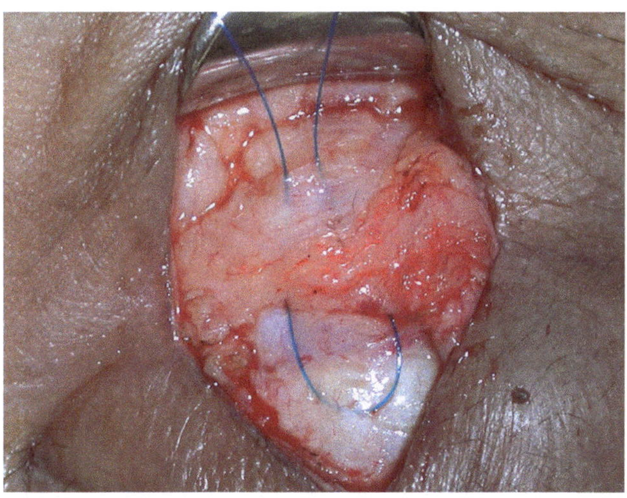

Fig.17.13 Both ends of the suture are passed through the levator with care being taken not to injure Müller's muscle, which liespos teriorly

fusely very attenuated aponeurosis, Whitnall's ligament usually provides a thickened region of the levator that should hold a suture, with less risk of cheesewiring. Care should be taken when passing this suture to avoid Müller's muscle (unless one has intentionally included Müller's in the levator flap) so as not to cause inadvertent hemorrhage, which may make it more difficult to gauge the eyelid position intraoperatively. A hematoma may also result from passing the suture through levator muscle, i.e., above Whitnall's ligament. Many surgeons avoid advancing, or resecting, levator any higher than Whitnall's ligament, with a Whitnall's suspension being the largest resection they will do. To advance levator any further will generally require cutting the medial and lateral horns of the muscle, which many colleagues prefer to avoid due to the importance of these supporting structures. If Whitnall's suspension does not raise the eyelid sufficiently, one may supplement with a superior tarsectomy. The suture can be placed though levator slightly higher than needed and then allowed to hang back if the eyelid height is overcorrected. This avoids having to remove and replace the suture higher. One suture is placed centrally at the position of the preferred high point of the eyelid margin, which is typically directly over the pupil or slightly nasal to that. An additional suture is often placed just nasal and just temporal to the central suture, as needed for contour. Even if the lid margin contour appears favorable intraoperatively with a single central suture, placement of the nasal and temporal sutures helps to stabilize the eyelid margin contour postoperatively, taking some of the tension off the central suture and reducing the chance of suture cheesewiring postoperatively. Some surgeons prefer at least three sutures to secure levator to tarsus, with the belief that this may provide the most natural eyelid contour. Nevertheless, practices vary somewhat with regard to how many sutures are placed and where they are located, and intraoperative factors will guide the surgeon.

The eye shield is removed, and the eyelid is examined with regard to its height and contour. It is commonly recommended that one place the upper eyelid slightly higher (perhaps 1–1.5 mm higher) than the desired eyelid position, as return of orbicularis muscle function and loss of epinephrine effect on Müller's muscle often lower the eyelid position postoperatively. An alert patient is critical for a reliable outcome. Therefore, it is important to reduce or discontinue IV sedation prior to evaluating eyelid position in order to have maximal patient cooperation. Bright lighting and ocular surface irritation may cause reflex blepharospasm, hence the importance of redirecting the overhead spotlights away from the patient's face and giving another drop of topical anesthetic before appraising eyelid position. It is unclear whether sitting the patient up during surgery significantly improves the accuracy of the surgical outcome. Nevertheless, many surgeons prefer to have the patient sit up intraoperatively since they believe it provides a more physiologic assessment of the eyelid position and contour, in terms of gravity and degree of patient effort.

Suture adjustments, i.e., tightening or loosening a suture, can be made in the sitting position until the desired lid height is achieved. If the suture needs to be repositioned either higher or lower in the aponeurosis, then the patient is returned to the supine position and one end of the suture is removed carefully, using the position of the remaining suture as a guide. Once the desired eyelid position and contour have been obtained, the tarsal sutures are tied down permanently and trimmed. The lid crease may be reformed, if desired, although this is often unnecessary. This may be accomplished by passing a few interrupted 6-0 absorbable sutures, in a buried interrupted fashion, through one or both edges of the wound (or just through orbicularis muscle) and the inferior edge of the levator aponeurosis (Fig. 17.14). Some surgeons will instead incorporate deep suture bites to levator during the skin closure. The skin incision may be repaired with either interrupted or running sutures, using 6-0 fast-absorbing gut or a nonabsorbable suture such as 6-0 silk, polypropylene, or braided or monofilament nylon, based upon surgeon preference. Antibiotic ointment is applied.

If eyelid laxity is contributing to poor eyelid contour or ectropion, one may need to horizontally tighten the eyelid via a lateral canthopexy suture or lateral tarsal strip procedure. Moving the tarsal sutures superiorly or inferiorly on tarsus will impact the amount of eyelid lift and the eyelid margin contour, as well as the likelihood of causing ectropion, which is greater the lower the suture is placed in tarsus. Some patients have a very thin tarsal plate, and one may need to compensate by making a longer suture pass through the thin tissue.

Cold compresses are initiated immediately after surgery and then continued at frequent intervals for the next 48 h. The patient is advised to keep his/her head elevated, such as sleeping on several pillows, in order to minimize postoperative edema. Antibiotic ointment over the wound is commonly employed, typically three times daily for up to a week, although the necessity of this practice has been questioned in the context of a sterile procedure on a healthy patient. The ointment may be used in the eye at bedtime if nocturnal lagophthalmos and exposure keratopathy are an issue. Patients should be encouraged to use artificial tears as needed, as they may suffer from increased dry eye symptoms postoperatively, which is often transient. Patients are usually seen in the office at 5–7 days postoperatively, and at

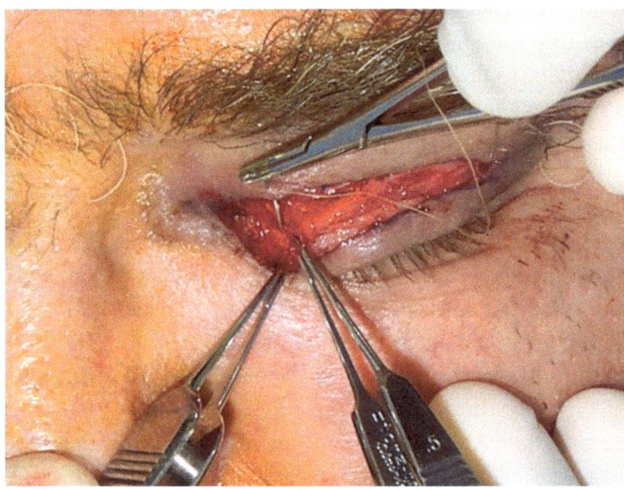

Fig. 17.14 Lidc reasei s reformed by passing a suture through skin, then levator edge, thens kin

this point, any nonabsorbable sutures may be removed. If there is an obvious under or overcorrection noted at this time, early in-office revision may be considered. For such a touch-up, the eyelid is prepped and draped in standard fashion. A small amount of local anesthetic solution is infiltrated just beneath the skin around the incision. The incision can usually be gently pulled apart without reincising. The previously placed levator advancement suture is removed and a new suture is placed to either raise or lower the lid to the desired position. Early revisions may be unwise in patients with significant postoperative edema since it may be difficult to accurately reposition the eyelid. In such cases, a short course of oral corticosteroids may improve the eyelid swelling more quickly.

In challenging cases or in reoperations, one may consider using an adjustable suture technique. The procedure is carried out as described above. After passing one polypropylene suture, a second one is passed in the same general location as the first suture, but slightly higher on the levator aponeurosis instead of tying it down, and the two suture ends are brought out through the incision and left untied. The incision is closed in standard fashion around the free suture ends, which are then steri-stripped to the forehead. When the patient is seen 5–7 days postoperatively, the option is available to cinch down the suture and tie it, thereby raising an undercorrected lid. However, if the lid height is satisfactory, the externalized suture is simply pulled out. This adjustable suture technique is only helpful when an undercorrection is present, not an overcorrection. A monofilament suture, such as polypropylene, is preferred when a suture is left exposed since there is less theoretical risk of bacterial infection than with a braided suture, which is more likely to harbor organisms.

In cases of congenital ptosis with fair to poor levator function, a maximal levator resection is usually performed. Levator muscle is often resected to the level of Whitnall's ligament and then reattached to the tarsus (Figs. 17.15 and 17.16). If levator function is poor, one should consider adding a superior tarsectomy, with care taken not to damage the peripheral vascular arcades as the lid margin is now a pedicle flap. The tarsus can be excised along the superior tarsal border or an intratarsal segment can be resected (Fig. 17.17). In congenital ptosis, the amount of levator resection and the amount of tarsus resection may be calculated by the formula: (difference in MRD1 between the two eyes) + (difference in levator function between the two eyes) + 3. For every 1 mm of levator resection not accounted for, each 1 mm of tarsal resection is equivalent to 2 mm of levator resection. In addition to tarsectomy providing extra lift, the full-thickness eyelid

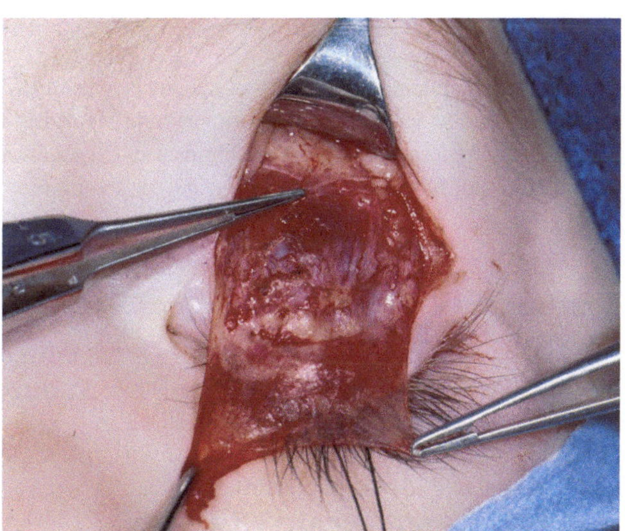

Fig. 17.15 Thinle vatori s dissected and Whitnall's ligament is identified(forceps)

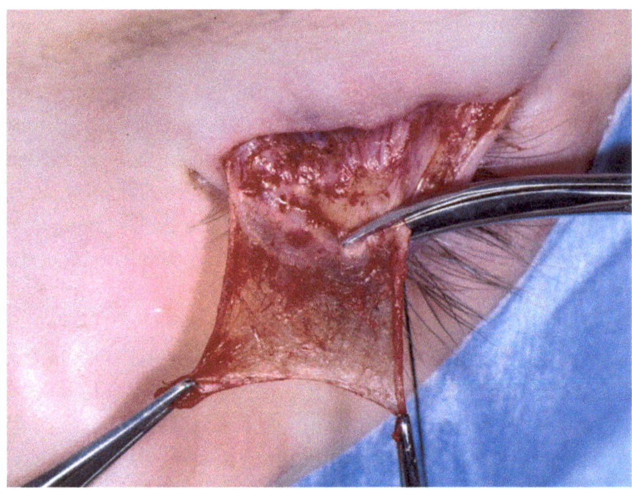

Fig.17.16 Maximal levator resectioninc ongenitalpt osis

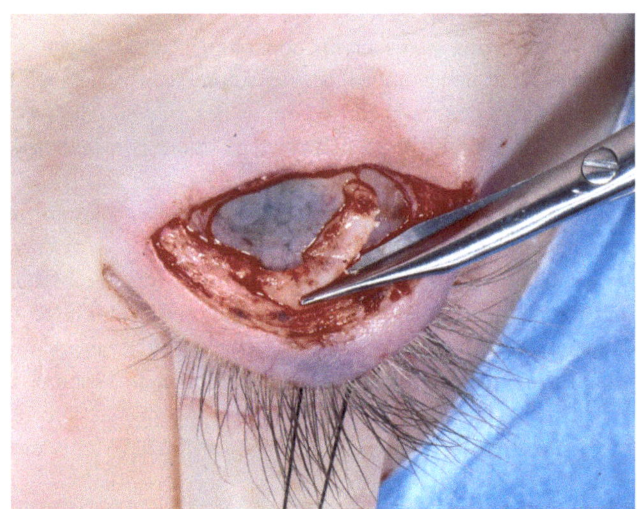

Fig.17.17 Full-thickness tarsectomy is performed. The tarsus is incised with a #15c blade (over a corneal protector) and the incision is completed withW escotts cissors

scar may help maintain the longevity of the ptosis repair. Tarsectomy can be used in primary and secondary adult ptosis surgery, especially in cases with poor levator function.

Conclusion

External levator resection is a highly versatile procedure that can be used in patients with "levator function" (eyelid excursion) ranging from excellent to poor. Lid contour abnormalities can be addressed as well. A strong knowledge of the anatomy of the upper lid as well as meticulous surgical technique is crucial. The procedure can be performed under straight local anesthetic or combined with intravenous sedation. The outline presented in this chapter should serve as a useful guide to the surgeon planning to use this approach forptos isre pair.

SuggestedR eading

Ben Simon GJ, Lee S, Schwarcz RM, McCann JD, Goldberg RA. External levator advancement vs Müller's muscle-conjunctival resection for correction of upper eyelid involutional ptosis. J Ophthalmol. 2005;140(3):426–32.

Patel SM, Linberg JV, Sivak-Callcott JA, Gunel E. Modified tarsal resection operation for congenital ptosis with fair levator function. Ophthal Plast Reconstr Surg. 2008;24(1):1–6.

Bassin RE, Putterman AM. Full-thickness eyelid resection in the treatment of secondary ptosis. Ophthal Plast Reconstr Surg. 2009;25(2):85–9.

Older JJ. Ptosis repair and blepharoplasty in the adult. Ophthalmic Surg. 1995;26(4):304–8 (review).

Erb MH, Kersten RC, Yip CC, Hudak D, Kulwin DR, McCulley TJ. Effect of unilateral blepharoptosis repair on contralateral eyelid position. Ophthal Plast Reconstr Surg. 2004;20(6):418–22.

Lucarelli MJ, Lemke BN. Small incision external levator repair: technique and early results. Am J Ophthalmol. 1999;127(6):637–44.

Demartelaere SL, Blaydon SM, Shore JW. Tarsal switch levator resection for the treatment of blepharoptosis in patients with poor eye protective mechanisms. Ophthalmology.2006; 113(12):2357–63.

McCulley TJ, Kersten RC, Kulwin DR, Feuer WJ. Outcome and influencing factors of external levator palpebrae superioris aponeurosis advancement for blepharoptosis. Ophthal Plast Reconstr Surg. 2003;19(5):388–93.

Tucker SM, Verhulst SJ. Stabilization of eyelid height after aponeurotic ptosis repair. Ophthalmology. 1999; 106(3):517–22.

Pak J, Shields M, Putterman AM. Superior tarsectomy augments super-maximum levator resection in correction of severe blepharoptosis with poor levator function. Ophthalmology.20 06;113(7):1201–8.

Baroody M, Holds JB, Sakamoto DK, Vick VL, Hartstein ME. Small incision transcutaneous levator aponeurotic repair for blepharoptosis. Ann Plast Surg. 2004;52(6):558–61.

Bartley GB, Lowry JC, Hodge DO. Results of levator-advancement blepharoptosis repair using a standard protocol: effect of epinephrine-induced eyelid position change. Trans Am Ophthalmol Soc. 1996;94:165–73; discussion 174–7.

McCord CD, Seify H, Codner MA. Transblepharoplasty ptosis repair: three-step technique. Plast Reconstr Surg.2007; 120(4):1037–44.

Espinoza GM, Holds JB. Evolution of eyelid surgery. Facial Plast Surg Clin North Am. 2005;13(4):505–10, v(review).

Holds JB, McLeish WM, Anderson RL. Whitnall's sling with superior tarsectomy for the correction of severe unilateral blepharoptosis. Arch Ophthalmol. 1993;111(9): 1285–91.

Chapter 18
Minimal Dissection, Small Incision Ptosis Correction

Bartley R. Frueh

Abstract Small-incision, minimal-dissection external levator advancement results in less disruption of the eyelid retractors. Preserving many of the levator aponeurosis attachments to the tarsus results in reduced operative time and less advancement of the levator needed to achieve satisfactory results.

Introduction

Ptosis has been corrected in many different ways, all of which have some efficacy. What makes this procedure [1] not only unique but also highly successful is the minimal dissection, which leaves many features of the eyelid lifting apparatus intact, so that extra effort is not needed to make up for the lysing of helpful attachments. The procedure is not unique for using a small incision [2, 3], and the small incision is significant, but not critical.

Principle of the Procedure

By disrupting fewer of the attachments with minimal dissection, less tucking is required to obtain the same amount of lift. The only dissection performed is in the central 10 mm of the eyelid in the following locations: 1) between the pretarsal orbicularis muscle and the underlying levator aponeurosis, and 2) between the tarsal plate and the levator aponeurosis, from the lower edge of the aponeurosis insertion on tarsus to a point superior to tarsus.

Methodology of the Procedure

Incision planning: A vertical mark is made over the center of the pupil, with the patient awake and looking in the primary position. This will be the center of the incision. The incision is marked on the lid crease, approximately 10–12 mm long, centered over the initial mark. The length of the incision is unimportant, as long as there is room to do the dissection.

Anesthesia: The patient may be sedated with a short-acting drug prior to the injection, or the injection can be made with the patient wide awake. It is important that the patient be wide awake several minutes after the injection, when the patient needs to sit up, to determine the adequacy of the elevation of the lid position accurately. The local anesthetic customarily used by the author is a 50:50 mixture of 1.0% lidocaine with epinephrine 1:100,000 and 0.75% bupivacaine. Local anesthetic is first injected under the skin of the marked incision. The needle is then placed perpendicular to the eyelid, halfway between the center of the marked incision and the lashes. It is inserted until the tarsal plate is felt with the tip of the needle, and enough anesthetic is then injected

B.R. Frueh (✉)
Department of Ophthalmology, Kellogg Eye Center, University of Michigan, Ann Arbor, MI, USA
e-mail: daweinberg@hotmail.com

A.J. Cohen and D.A. Weinberg (eds.), *Evaluation and Management of Blepharoptosis*, DOI 10.1007/978-0-387-92855-5_18, to raise a small wheal. Usually, a total of 0.6 cc of local anesthetic or less is adequate for good anesthesia.

Operative details: The skin is incised (the author prefers a sharp stitch-ribbon scissor) along the marking, staying superficial to the orbicularis, if possible, so as to minimize bleeding. Any bleeding is cauterized to make it a bloodless field. Sharp scissors are used to bluntly spread the orbicularis fibers at the incision and then aimed toward the center of the tarsal plate until the tarsal plate comes into view through the semi-transparent levator aponeurosis (Fig. 18.1). The pathway created will be about 10 mm at the skin and 8 mm at the tarsal plate (not necessary to measure – this is just an approximation to guide you). This dissection is preferably bloodless, but should there be bleeding, it is cauterized. The aponeurosis is incised with sharp scissors horizontally over the tarsal plate, just below its vertical center, under direct observation, using multiple small snips to obtain a defect that is approximately 8 mm wide (Fig. 18.2). The tarsal plate will present a clearer view than it does when viewed through the thin aponeurosis. The lower edge of the skin incision is pulled down and sharp scissors are used to bluntly dissect superiorly under the cut aponeurosis, anterior to the tarsal plate, until it is free from the underlying tarsal plate and Müller's muscle, a distance of about 12–15 mm (Fig. 18.3). An 8-mm spatula needle on a permanent single-armed 6-0 suture is then passed through this space, in line with the central vertical lid marking, as high as it will reach, and then curved forward and brought out through the upper edge of the incision, just posterior to the orbicularis oculi muscle (Fig. 18.4). The two ends of the suture are then tightly grasped and brought inferiorly, leaving a little slack in the suture. The operative lights are dimmed and the patient is requested to open his/her eyes and look up. A firm tug should be felt on the tightly held suture if the upper extent of its passage is through the aponeurosis. For the

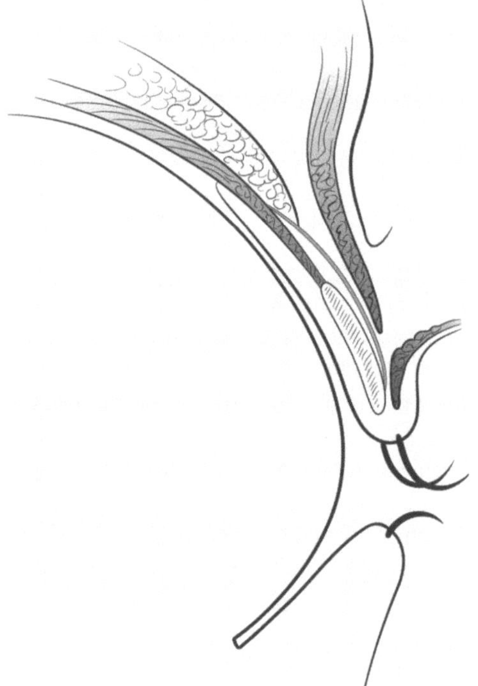

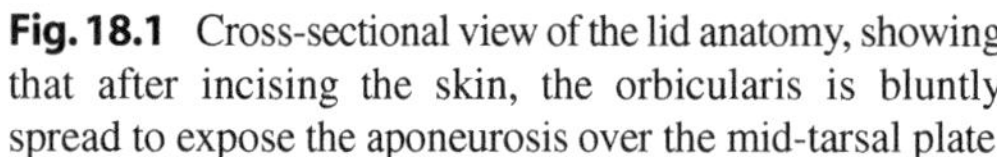

Fig. 18.1 Cross-sectional view of the lid anatomy, showing that after incising the skin, the orbicularis is bluntly spread to expose the aponeurosis over the mid-tarsal plate

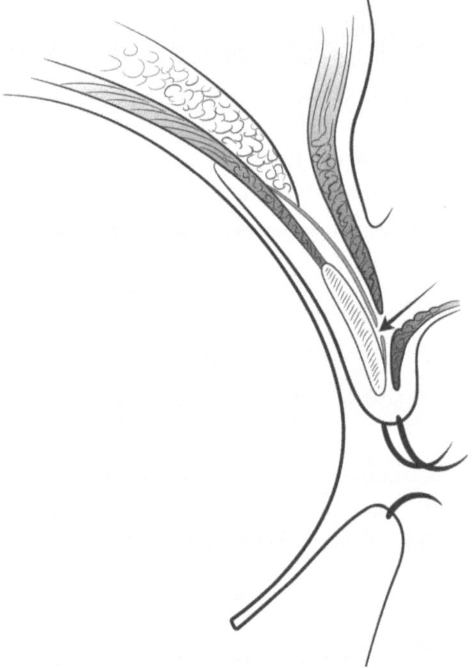

Fig. 18.2 Cross-sectional view of the eyelid with *arrow* att hea poneurosisi ncision

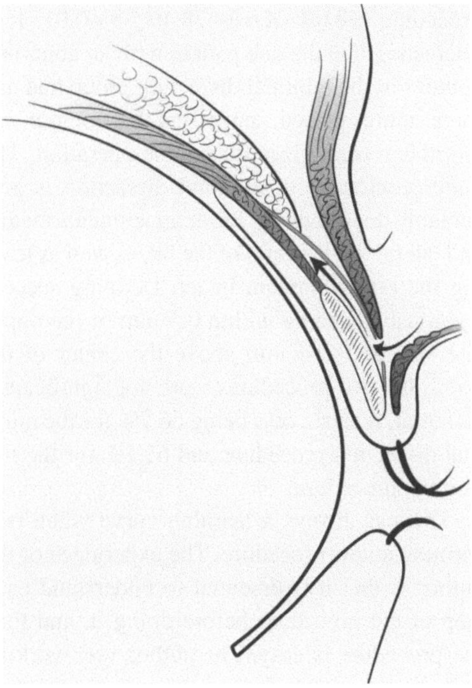

Fig. 18.3 Cross-sectional view of the eyelid with the *arrow* following the blunt dissection under the aponeurosis over the tarsal plate and the Müller's muscle

infrequent times that a firm tug is not felt (less than 5% of the time in the author's experience), the suture is re-passed and the pull on upgaze rechecked. Having demonstrated that the aponeurosis has been engaged by the suture, the tarsus is lifted from the cornea and held there, while the needle is passed horizontally through the tarsal plate in mid-tarsus, centered on the vertical central lid mark. Once the needle is placed in tarsus, the eyelid is everted to check the posterior tarsal surface, making certain that the suture is not exposed. The suture is tied with a slip knot over a surgeon's knot, leaving the suture at the correct tension that will hopefully place the eyelid at the desired position.

The patient is then asked to sit up and open his/her eyes. The eyelid height and contour are inspected. The suture tension is adjusted until the height seems optimal. If the eyelid cannot be elevated sufficiently, the suture is removed and replaced higher in the aponeurosis or lower in the tarsal plate. If the lid appears low medially or laterally, the dissection is extended in that direction by incising the skin, extending the

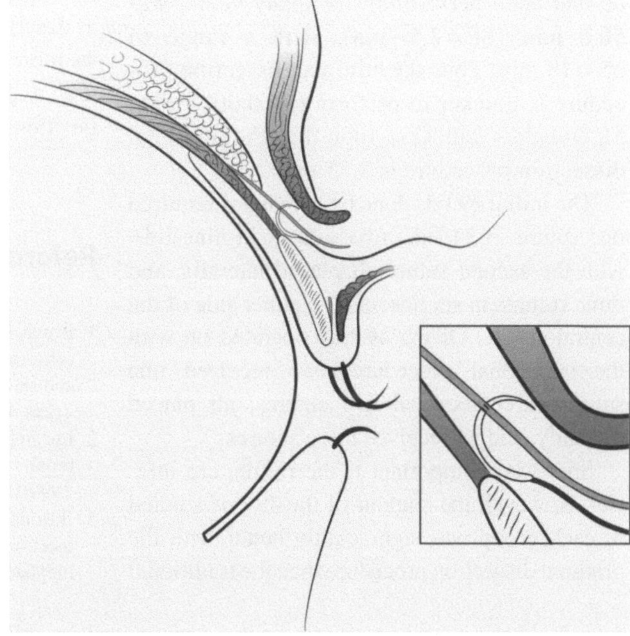

Fig. 18.4 Cross-sectional view of the eyelid showing the needle passage through the dissected space and then through the posterior surface of the aponeurosis and out of the anterior surface, posterior to the orbicularis oculi muscle

aponeurosis incision, and then spreading superiorly, as was done prior to placing the initial suture. An additional suture is similarly placed in that area and tied. When the lid position and contour seem optimal with the patient upright, the patient again assumes the supine position, and each suture is tied permanently. The skin is closed with a running suture of choice.

Why Should This Procedure Be Adopted When the One You Are Using Seems Satisfactory?

We live in an age of decreasing reimbursements and increasing examination of outcomes. If a procedure can be done more quickly and yet with greater efficacy, then it is worthy of trial.

The author's experience with this procedure, evolved by Dr. Hector McDonald of Ottowa, Canada, is that the mean time to perform it in the first 49 lids of 36 patients operated on with the minimal dissection procedure was 26.3 min (SE = 0.1 min) per eyelid, with a range of 13–68 min. The mean operating time for a random sample of 49 recent lids done on 36 patients with a traditional method, which he had been performing for many years, was 56.6 min (SE = 2.5 min), with a range of 35–119 min. Thus the minimal dissection procedure is quicker to perform ($p < 0.0001$). Dr. McDonald's quickest time for the minimal dissection procedure is 2.75 min.

The initial 49 lids done by the author required one suture in 34 lids, two sutures in nine lids, with the second suture all placed laterally, and three sutures in six lids, one on either side of the central suture. Of the 49 lids operated on with the traditional procedure, two received one suture, three received two sutures, all placed medially, and 44 received three sutures.

Speed is unimportant if the results are inferior. However, the contour of the 49 lids studied in each group was significantly better with the minimal dissection procedure than the traditional procedure, 97.6% versus 78.4%, $p < 0.01$. It is interesting that the one patient with an abnormal contour in the minimal dissection group had had three sutures placed, suggesting that contour was a problem recognized during the operation. The better contour with minimal dissection is presumably due to cutting fewer attachments medial and lateral to the center of the lid, as well as leaving the orbital septum intact. Defining success rigorously as being within 0.5 mm of the opposite side and 2–4 mm above the center of the pupil, the two procedures were not significantly different, with success being 66.7% for the minimal dissection procedure and 61.1% for the traditional procedure.

There is always a learning curve when performing a new procedure. The experience of the author is that it is essential to understand each step of the procedure before doing it, and then the procedure is easy. The author was working with two highly skilled non-eye-plastic ophthalmologists in Guatemala. These surgeons had three patients with involutional ptosis. After observing the procedure, they each operated on one eyelid of each patient. They did it perfectly and have been doing the procedure for the past 8 years successfully.

In summary, this ptosis correction procedure is simple, but the steps must be followed exactly as described. It allows the surgeon to correct ptosis more quickly, with a superior contour, with at least as good an ability to set the lid at the desired positiona sa tra ditionalproc edure.

References

1. Frueh BR, Musch DC, McDonald H. Efficacy and efficiency of a new involutional ptosis correction procedure compared to a traditional aponeurotic approach. Trans Am Ophthalmol Soc. 2004;102:199–207.
2. Lucarelli MJ, Lemke BN. Small incision external levator repair: technique and early results. Am J Ophthalmol. 1999;127(6):637–44.
3. Baroody M, Holds JB, Sakamoto DK, et al. Small incision transcutaneous levator aponeurotic repair for blepharoptosis.A nnP lastS urg.2004; 52(6):558–61.

Chapter19
Müller's Muscle-Conjunctival Resection (PosteriorA pproach)

Adam J. Cohen and David A. Weinberg

Abstract Müller's muscle-conjunctival resection is a reliable, time-proven, and relatively easy technique for correction of mild-to-moderate blepharoptosis with good levator function.

Putterman and Urist first described Müller's muscle-conjunctival resection (MMCR) in 1975 [1]. MMCR is traditionally used in selected cases of blepharoptosis with good levator function responding positively to pharmacologic sympathetic stimulation with phenylephrine [1]. Favorable response to MMCR has rarely been found in patients with poor to fair levator function [2, 3].

Müller's muscle is a sympathetically innervated eyelid elevator. Originating from the undersurface of the levator palpebralis superioris, it is approximately 12 mm in length and inserts on the superior tarsal border. When approached from the posterior surface of the eyelid, Müller's muscle lies directly beneath the conjunctiva just cephalad to the superior tarsal border. Stimulation of Müller's muscle results in upper eyelid elevation of approximately 2–3 mm [4]; hence, oculosymphathetic paresis (Horner's syndrome) seldom produces ptosis of more than 2–3 mm.

The decision to perform MMCR usually rests on elevation of the eyelid in response to sympathetic agents. The marginal reflex distance (MRD_1) should be measured prior to and 5 min following instillation of phenylephrine eye drops [5] or 0.5% apraclonindine solution [6]. Glatt et al. reported a statistically significant but clinical insignificant difference in eyelid position when comparing 2.5 and 10% phenylephrine [7]. Several colleagues have described cardiovascular side effects with the use of 10% phenylephrine [8, 10]. These reports have prompted the use of 2.5% phenylephrine by the authors and many colleagues.

There have been studies of successful outcomes with MMCR in patients with poor responsetophe nylephrinec hallenge [9].

The patient is instructed to look down, and one drop of the medicine is placed in the superior fornix. An additional drop is placed 1 min later, and the upper eyelid position is assessed 5 min after that. A positive response is somewhat subjective and is defined as satisfactory eyelid elevation to correct the blepharoptosis from an esthetic and functional standpoint.

One simple approach to quantifying the necessary amount of tissue resection to achieve the desired lid position is as follows. If the ptosis is unilateral, then the affected eyelid is compared to the opposite, "normal" eyelid after instillation of the phenylephrine. The same is true for bilateral asymmetric ptosis when the goal is to bring the height of the more ptotic lid up to the level of the higher lid. An 8-mm resection is performed when the ptotic lid raises to the height of the opposite lid, while the amount of resection is increased (often to 9–10 mm) if the lid is a bit

A.J.C ohen(✉)
TheA rtof Eye s, Skokie, IL, USA
e-mail:a cohen@theartofeyes.com

A.J. Cohen and D.A. Weinberg (eds.), *Evaluation and Management of Blepharoptosis*,
DOI 10.1007/978-0-387-92855-5_19, © Springer Science+Business Media, LLC 2011

low or decreased (often to 6–7 mm) if the lid is a bit too high after phenylephrine eyedrops. For bilateral ptosis, there is usually a symmetric response to the phenylephrine drops bilaterally. The amount of resection may be adjusted to address any preoperative asymmetry between the upper lids and to adjust for the degree of response to the phenylephrine.

Several authors have described various algorithms to predict the amount of tissue resection needed to correct various degrees of ptosis. Putterman described an 8.25-mm MMCR when normal eyelid height was achieved in response to 10% phenylephrine [11]. Weinstein [12] described a 4:1 ratio of tissue resection to the amount of eyelid elevation. This linear relationship began with 8 mm of resection to achieve 2 mm of eyelid elevation. Adding or subtracting 1 mm of tissue resection will result in a 0.25-mm difference in eyelid height, according to that formula.

Dresner [13], using a modified technique, also studied the relationship between the amount of resection and postoperative eyelid height. He did *not* find a linear relationship between the preoperative response to phenylephrine and postsurgical eyelid height. His algorithm supported 4 mm of resection for 1.0 mm of eyelid elevation, 6 mm of resection for 1.5 mm of elevation, 10 mm of resection for 2 mm of elevation, and 11–12 mm of resection to achieve 3 mm or greater of ptosis correction. His algorithm was dependent on a preoperative response to phenylephrine of 2 mm or greater of eyelid elevation.

Mercandetti et al. [14] constructed a linear regression algorithm that found an approximate 3:1 ratio of resection to eyelid elevation. They also suggested tailoring the resection based upon clinical outcomes with the MMCR.

Perry et al. [15] supported a 9-mm MMCR to achieve the same amount of eyelid elevation after maximal stimulation with 10% phenylephrine. His algorithm advised 9 mm of MMCR + 1 mm of tarsal resection for each millimeter of undercorrection with phenylephrine. One should find a 1:1 ratio between the amount of tarsal resection and the amount of eyelid elevation. It has been recommended that no more than 2.5 mm of tarsus be resected to prevent eyelid instability.

Ben Simon et al. [16] found a 40% underestimation of postoperative eyelid elevation with 10% phenylephrine stimulation. They concluded that a simple linear relationship did not exist based on the analysis of their data.

Ayala et al. [17] described an approximate 5:1 ratio of resection to amount of lift in patients with moderate ptosis, good levator function, and positive response to phenylephrine. Thus, the quantitative relationship between Müller muscle resection and degree of ptosis correction remains somewhat unclear and is probably quite technique-dependent, although there could be patient-related variables at work. Therefore, surgeons should develop their own regression formula to establish the amount of tissue resection needed to achieve a given amount of ptosis correction in their hands.

Technique [5]

Prior to surgery, the surgeon should review the preoperative plan, and it is recommended to have the planned amount of MMCR resection written down in a visible location and the patient's preoperative photograph for reference during surgery.

MMCR can be performed with local anesthetic alone or with monitored anesthesia care (MAC). In fact, this procedure may be done under general anesthesia, if so desired, since patient cooperation is unnecessary. A frontal or supraorbital nerve block provides excellent anesthesia without eyelid distortion. The frontal nerve block involves an intraorbital injection, which does carry some risk, although complications are rare when carefully performed. MAC reduces the chance of sudden patient movement during injection that can place the globe and surrounding structures at risk for injury, as well as providing greater patient comfort during the injection.

Frontal nerve block (technique utilized by one of the authors, AJC) – Once the patient has been adequately sedated, a 25-gauge, 1½ in. sharp needle is passed below the midsuperior orbital rim with the needle lumen facing the orbital roof (bevel up), with the needle orientation parallel to the orbital roof. One should carefully slide along the orbital roof to a depth of 1½ in. One and one half to 2 ml of anesthetic solution is infiltrated followed by gentle digital pressure [17]. Two percent lidocaine with epinephrine and/or 0.5–0.75% bupivicaine is often used, and this varies based upon surgeon preference. If the patient is adequately blocked, complete ptosis will result [18].

Supraorbital Nerve Block- A short 27- or 30-gauge needle is used to inject approximately 1 cc of a local anesthetic solution just inside the superior orbital rim adjacent to the supraorbital notch.

To enhance intraoperative comfort, local anesthetic may also be infiltrated just inside the superolateral orbital rim to anesthetize the lacrimal nerve. If additional local anesthesia is needed, subconjunctival infiltration above the superior tarsal border can be given. Subconjunctival infiltration is best performed following the placement of the Putterman clamp to avoid tissue distortion and altering the quantitative predictability of the procedure.

The eyelid is everted over a Desmarres lid retractor (Fig. 19.1), and this may be facilitated by an optional 4-0 silk suture passed through the eyelid margin. A caliper is used to demarcate a point cephalad to the superior tarsal border where traction sutures will be placed (Fig. 19.2). This distance should equal the preoperative-determined amount of resection divided by two. Traction sutures (the authors often employ 4-0, 5-0, or 6-0 silk) are then passed through conjunctiva and Müller's muscle at the desired height above tarsus using two contiguous sutures medially and laterally, or sometimes three sutures medially, centrally, and laterally (Fig. 19.3). The sutures should be placed with a long and relatively shallow needle pass, deep enough to engage Müller's muscle but not levator. If one prefers to use a single suture, a double-armed silk suture may be used. After a central bite of tissue is secured, one arm of the suture is passed from central to medial, while the other end is passed from central to lateral. These lateral and medial passes are placed equidistant and parallel to the central pass.

As an alternative to silk traction sutures, the conjunctiva can be marked at the desired height with gentle handheld cautery or methylene blue. If using cautery, the surgeon should be cognizant that the heat can produce a welding effect, potentially joining Müller's muscle to the underlying levator aponeurosis, which could result in

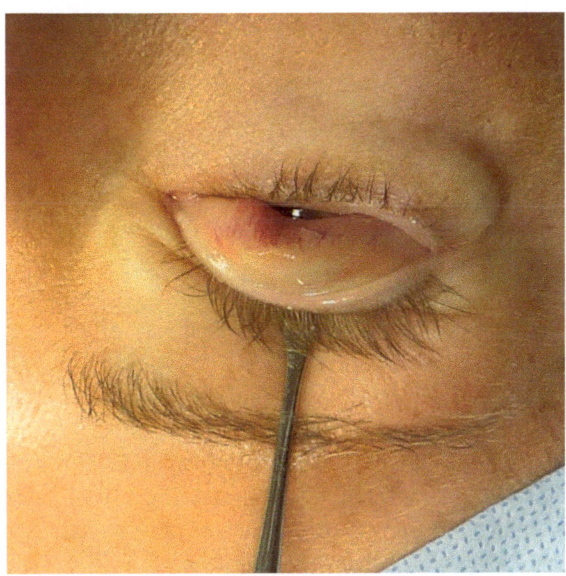

Fig.19.1 Theuppe re yelid is everted over a Desmarres retractor, exposing the superiort arsalbor der

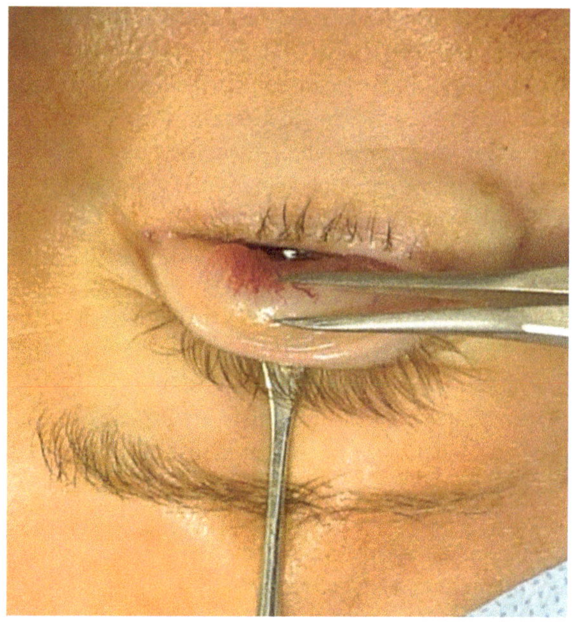

Fig. 19.2 Calipersa reus ed to measure the desired distance above tarsus that the traction sutures will be place. This distance is half the amount of intended tissue resection, e.g. 4 mm for a planned8m mr esection

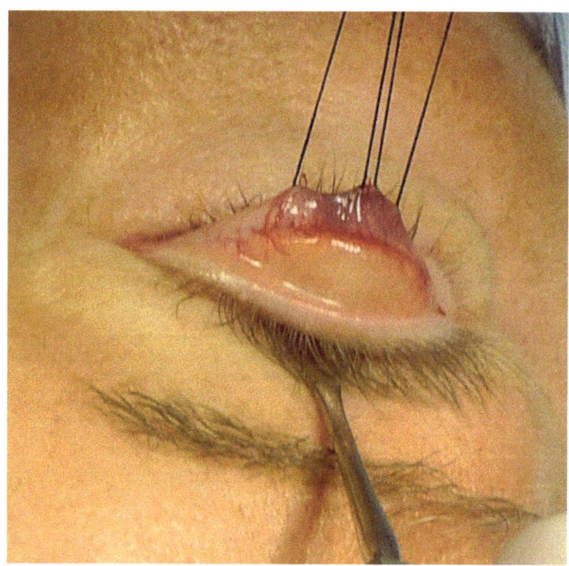

Fig. 19.3 Two4-0s ilk traction sutures have been placed through conjunctiva and Müller's muscle medially andl aterally

unintentional levator resection that may affect the final eyelid position.

A Putterman Müller's muscle–conjunctiva resection clamp (Ambler Surgical Corp, Exton, PA, USA) is used to secure the proper amount of conjunctiva and Müller's muscle (Fig. 19.4). Conjunctiva and Müller's muscle are pulled anteriorly with either the traction suture or forceps while applying the clamp. Anterior traction on these tissues facilitates clamp placement and aids in separating Müller's muscle from the levator aponeurosis. There has been some debate over whether the clamp should be centered over the pupil or tarsal plate since lateral shifting of the tarsus may occur with eyelid laxity – the authors usually center the clamp over the tarsal plate to achieve the optimal eyelid margin contour. The clamp is advanced to the superior edge of tarsus and then locked. The clamp is held while forceps are used to gently tug on the preseptal eyelid skin to be assured that skin and levator aponeurosis are not caught within the clamp. The skin should easily tent upwards, signifying that the proper structures (conjunctiva and Müller's muscle) are engaged in the clamp.

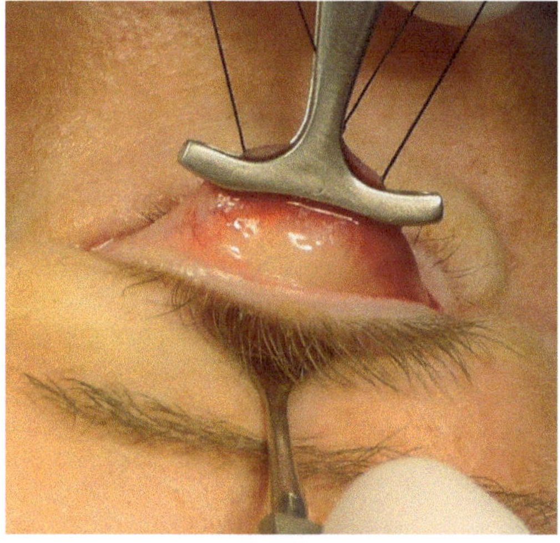

Fig. 19.4 The traction sutures are placed on upward stretch, and a Putterman clamp is applied and advanced to the superior tarsal border. Care is taken to be certain that levator aponeurosis and skin are not secured within thec lamp

There are a variety different ways that have been described to place a suture. One way is to use a 5-0 or 6-0 double-armed, plain gut suture on a G-3 needle (Ethicon, Inc. Skillman, NJ, USA), which is passed approximately 0.5–1 mm below the clamp to avoid cutting the suture when excising tissue within the clamp. The suture is placed lateral to medial in a horizontal mattress, running fashion, resulting in plication of the conjunctiva and Müller's muscle directly beneath the clamp (Fig. 19.5a, b). Once the medial most aspect of the clamped tissue is reached, the suture may be run in a lateral fashion prior to using a 15 blade to excise the tissue and suture trapped within the clamp (Fig. 19.6). To minimize the risk of cutting the previously placed plain gut suture, the blade is angled with the sharp surface directly abutting the clamp at a 45° angle (Fig. 19.7). If the suture has not been passed laterally prior to tissue excision (Fig. 19.8), the wound is then closed beginning medially by approximating the edges of conjunctiva and Müller's muscle. Although bleeding can occur, it tends to be self-limited once the conjunctiva is closed. At the lateral most aspect, the suture is cinched, and one of the needles is passed through the conjunctiva in the cephalad portion of the upper eyelid and trimmed at the surface. This completely buries the knot and the end of the suture, avoiding

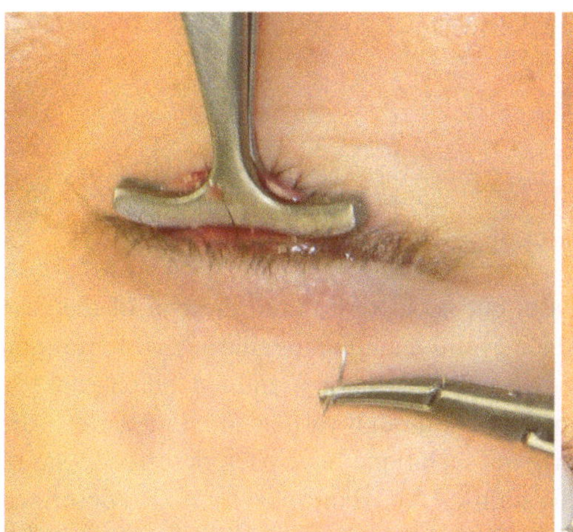

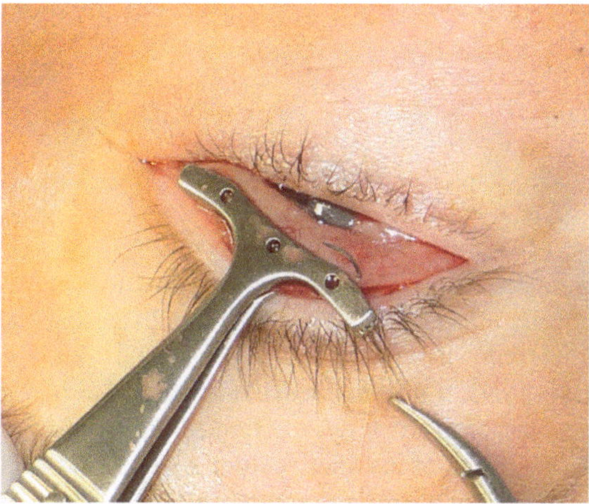

Fig. 19.5 (**a**) A 6-0 plain gut suture is introduced through skin laterally and placed through full-thickness eyelid, exiting conjunctiva at the lateral end of the clamp (**b**)

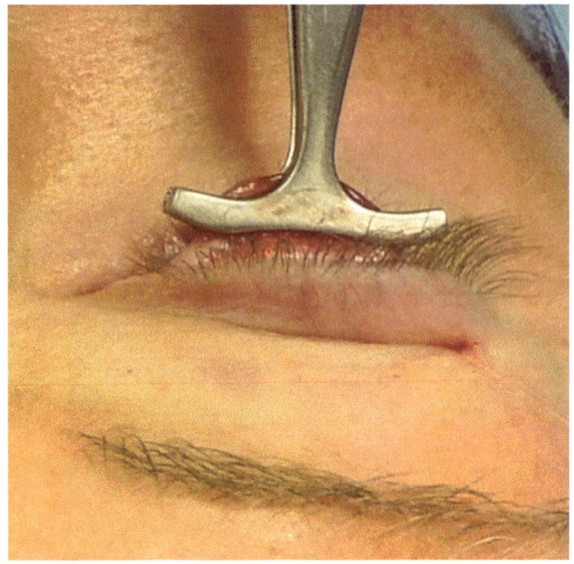

Fig. 19.6 The 6-0 plain gut suture has already been placed as a running suture, woven through the tissue just below the clamp, going from lateral to medial and then back from medial to lateral, exiting skin adjacent to the entrypoi nt

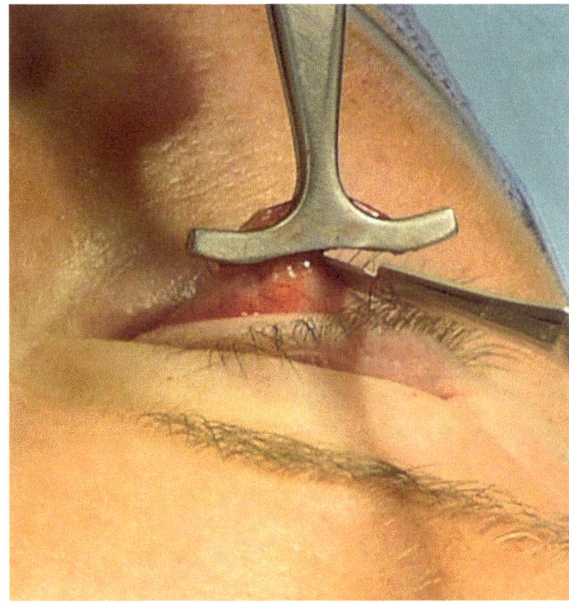

Fig. 19.7 A #15 blade is used to divide the tissue between the clamp and the running suture, with the blade angled 45° toward the clamp, in order to avoid cutting the suture. One should try to place the suture 0.5–1 mm away from the clamp to allow roomf ort hisi ncision

irritation to the globe. Other surgeons use an equally effective technique – externalizing the knot onto the lateral preseptal eyelid skin (Fig. 19.9). If the knot is externalized and concomitant blepharoplasty is performed, one should be cognizant of the knot position to avoid cutting the suture during skin removal. In cases of combined upper blepharoplasty and MMCR, often the skin is resected at the beginning of the case, but not sutured until the end of the case since eyelid manipulation during MMCR might cause dehiscence of a sutured blepharoplasty incision. Although various modifications of the original technique have been described, one of the authors (AJC) has found the earlier described technique with a slight modification of burying the suture beneath the conjunctiva to provide reliable results.

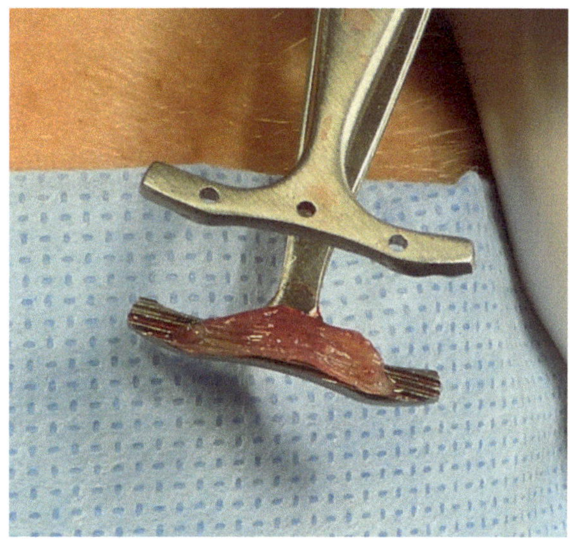

Fig. 19.8 Notethe e xcised tissue within the Putterman clamp

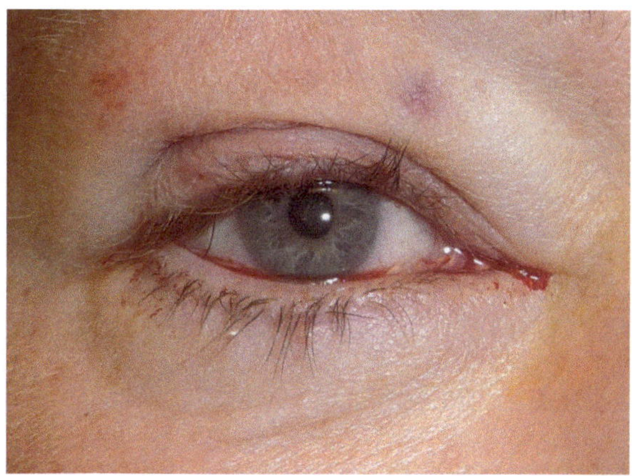

Fig. 19.9 Immediately following surgery. Note the dimple along the lateral eyelid crease, where the suturew astie de xternally

Typically, an equal amount of tissue is excised medially and laterally. However, one may address an eyelid contour deformity, e.g., ptosis that is greater temporally, by an asymmetric resection, i.e., placing the traction sutures higher and resecting more tissue in the more ptotic region of the eyelid.

Some surgeons prefer placement of a bandage contact lens at the end of the procedure to prevent ocular surface irritation if the suture becomes exposed. In our experience, suture exposure with resultant eye irritation is less of an issue when exteriorizing the suture knot on the skin. A combination antibiotic–steroid drop or ointment may be instilled at the end of the case, and the patient is asked to use this eye medication four times daily for 1 week, along with artificial tears as needed.

Complications are uncommon and include over- or undercorrection of the ptotic eyelid, eyelid asymmetry, corneal epitheliopathy or ulceration, hemorrhage, and rarely intraoperative injury to the globe. Eyelid margin contour deformity is less common with MMCR than with levator resection, and symblepharon formation is rare.

MMCR may be safely performed in patients with glaucoma filtering blebs [19, 20], although one certainly needs to be careful in a patient with an elevated, thin-walled, cystic bleb. Dry eye has been suggested to be a risk due to resection of accessory lacrimal glands of Wolfring. However, Dailey et al. found no significant effect on tear productionre sultingfromM MCR [21].

Advantages of MMCR include: (1) very quick procedure, (2) very predictable (although it has been suggested that it may be less reliable in congenital ptosis), (3) does not require any intraoperative patient cooperation, (4) the eyelid can be completely anesthetized since it is a prequantified procedure that is not titrated intraoperatively, (5) postoperative eyelid contour problems are rare, and (6) no visible skin incision or resultant scar, unless concurrent upper blepharoplasty is performed. Contraindications to MMCR include: (1) a shallow superior fornix, (2) poor or fair levator function, except in the rare patient with a positive phenylephrine test. MMCR also may not be the procedure of choice in patients with greater than 3-mm ptosis.

MMCR continues to be a useful technique since its original description and should be included in one's surgical repertoire for blepharoptosis repair, particularly in patients with mild-to-moderate ptosis and good-to-excellent levator function, whether or not they respond to phenylephrine preoperatively. Despite criticism that MMCR does not directly address the presumed site of pathology in involutional ptosis, i.e., the levator muscle and aponeurosis, MMCR remains a quick, easy and highly effective procedure in appropriate patients with ptosis (Figs. 19.10a nd 19.11).

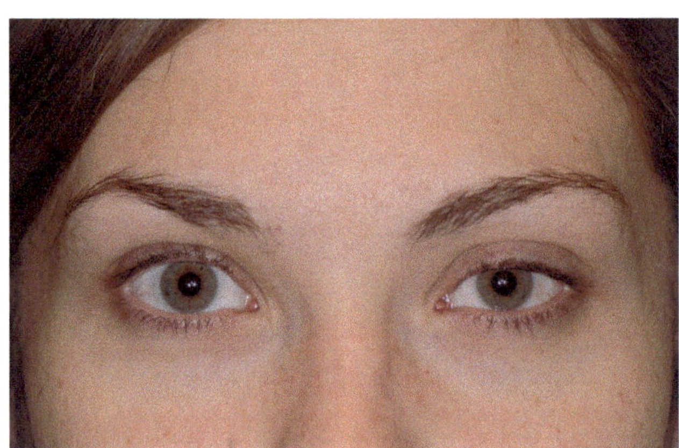

Fig.19.1 0 Preoperative image of left upper eyelid ptosis

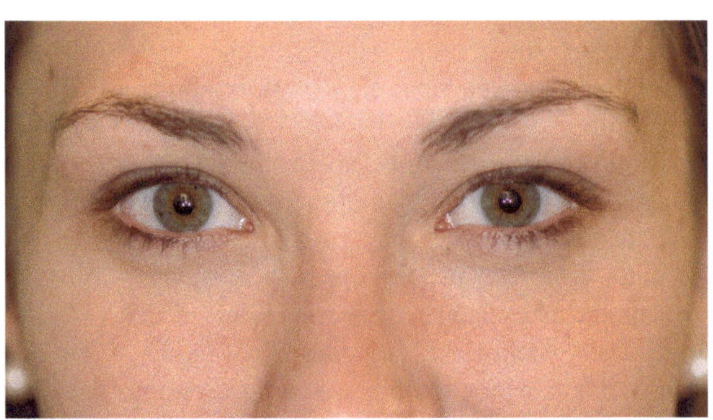

Fig.19.11 Postoperative image of left upper eyelid followingM MCR

References

1. Putterman AM, Urist M. Müller's muscle-conjunctival resection: technique for treatment of blepharoptosis. Arch Ophthalmol. 1975;93:619–23.
2. Cohen AJ, Weinberg DA. Müller's muscle-conjunctival resection for blepharoptosis with poor levator function. Ophthalmic Surg Lasers. 2002;33:491–2.
3. Georgescu D, Epstein G, Fountain T, Migliori M, Mannor G, Weinberg D. Müller's muscle conjunctival resection for blepharoptosis in patients with poor to fair levator function. Ophthalmic Surg Lasers Imaging.2009;40(6):597–9.
4. Cohen AJ, Mercandetti M. Ptosis, adult.eMedicine from WebMD. http://emedicine.medscape.com/article/1212082-overview.A ccessed18N ov2009.
5. Cohen AJ, Bernstein JA. Müller's muscle-conjunctival resection for blepharoptosis repair. Techniques in ophthalmology. 2002;33(6):`491–2.
6. Yazici B. Use of 0.5% aproclonindine solution in evaluation of blepharoptosis. Ophthal Plast Reconstr Surg.2008;24(2):2 99–301.
7. Glatt HJ, Fett DR, Putermann AM. Comparison of 2.5% and 10% phenylephrine in the elevation of upper eyelids with ptosis. Ophthalmic Surg. 1990; 21(3):173–6.
8. Miller SA, Mieler WF. Systemic reactions to subconjunctival phenylephrine. Can J Ophthalmol. 1978; 13(4):290–3.
9. Baldwin HC, Bhagey J, Khooshabeh R. Open sky Müller muscle-conjunctival resection in phenylephrine test-negative blepharoptosis patients. Ophthal Plast Reconstr Surg. 2005;21(4):276–80.
10. Fraunfelder FW, Fraunfelder FT, Jensvold B. Adverse systemic effects from pledgets of ocular topical phenylephrine 10%. Am J Ophthalmol. 2002;134(4): 624–5.
11. Putterman AM, Fett DR. Müller's muscle in the treatment of upper eyelid ptosis; a ten year study. Ophthalmic Surg. 1986;17:354–60.
12. Weinstein GS, Buerger GF. Modification of the Müller's muscle-conjunctival resection operation for blepharoptosis. Am J Ophthalmol. 1982;93(5):647–51.
13. Dresner SC. Further modifications of the Müller's muscle-conjunctival resection procedure for blepharoptosis. Ophthal Plast Reconstr Surg. 1991;7:114–22.
14. Mercandetti M, Putterman AM, Cohen ME, Mirante JP, Cohen AJ. Internal levator advancement by Müller's muscle-conjunctival resection: technique and review. Arch Facial Plast Surg. 2001;3(2):104–10.
15. Perry JD, Kadakia A, Foster JA. A new algorithm using conjunctival Müller's muscle resection with or without tarsectomy. Ophthal Plast Reconstr Surg. 2002;18(6):426–29.
16. Ben Simon GJ, Lee S, Schwarcz RM, McCann JD, Goldberg RA. Müller's muscle-conjunctival resection for correction of upper eyelid ptosis. Arch Facial Plast Surg. 2007;9(6):413–17.
17. Ayala E, Galvez C, Gonzalez-Candial M, Medel R. Predictability of conjunctival-müllerectomy for blepharoptosis repair. Orbit. 2007;26:217–22.
18. Cohen AJ. Oculoplastic and orbital surgery. Ophthalmol Clin North Am. 2006;19(2):257–67.
19. Georgescu D, Cole E, Epstein G, Fountain T, Migliori M, Nguyen Q, et al. Müller muscle-conjunctiva resection for blepharoptosis in patients with glaucoma filtering blebs. Ophthal Plast Reconstr Surg. 2007;23: 285–7.
20. Michels KS, Vagefi MR, Steele E, Zwick OM, Torres JJ, Seiff SR, et al. Müller muscle-conjunctiva resection to correct ptosis in high-risk patients. Ophthal Plast Reconstr Surg. 2007;23:363–6.
21. Dailey RA, Saulny SM, Sullivan SA. Müller's muscle-conjunctival resection-effect on tear production. OphthalP lastR econstrS urg.2002; 18(6):421–25.

Chapter20
Open-Sky (Anterior Approach) Müller's Muscle Resectionf ort heC orrectiono fB lepharoptosis

Heather Baldwin

Abstract Aponeurotic blepharoptosis may be safely and effectively corrected by resection of Müller's muscle. This surgery is thought to raise the upper lid by advancement of the levator muscle and aponeurosis. A particular feature of the technique is a consistently good postoperative eyelid contour, achieved through high placement of sutures on the tarsal plate. The open-sky technique offers advantages over other ptosis surgeries, including direct visualization of Müller's muscle, opportunity for adjustment of lid height, the potential for preservation of conjunctival tissue, and efficacy in patients who do not demonstrate a positive phenylephrine test.

Introduction

Müller's muscle is a small smooth muscle arising from the striated levator muscle along with the aponeurosis at or slightly above the level of the superior fornix. The body of Müller's muscle extends forward and downward for about 10 mm, enclosed in a rich vascular sheath. It is firmly attached to the conjunctiva, but easily separated from the aponeurosis. Its nerve supply is from the cervical sympathetic chain. The muscle helps to maintain the tone of the raised eyelids, contributing to the final 2 mm of lid elevation. This is based on clinical observation of patients with Horner's syndrome who are often found to have a mild ptosis of around 2 mm.

Müller's muscle inserts onto the upper border of the tarsal plate through a 0.5–1.5 mm tendon. The attachment of the levator aponeurosis to the tarsal plate is less well defined. It has been proposed that aponeurosis fibers insert into the anterior surface of the tarsal plate, as well as into orbicularis fibers forming the skin crease. Proponents of this theory support the aponeurosis as the main transmitter of levator contraction and, therefore, principally responsible for eyelid height [1, 2]. Based on this theory, traditional techniques for the correction of ptosis use aponeurosis advancement or resection to elevate the lid. By contrast, others propose that the levator aponeurosis ends blindly in a transverse ridge 2–3 mm above the tarsal plate [3–5], and that the aponeurosis supports the skin, the orbicularis, and the lashes, whereas the main upward pull of the tarsal plate is relayed by Müller's muscle. An extrapolation of this proposal is that Müller's muscle may be acting as a spindle in a stretch reflex [6].

These theories place emphasis on the role of Müller's muscle in determining eyelid height, and support the option of Müller's muscle resection for the correction of ptosis. Since a strip of muscle remains in place, there is preservation and even augmentation of changes in eyelid height associated with emotion and other autonomically mediated facial expressions.

Correction of blepharoptosis using Müller's muscle-conjunctival resection was originally described by Putterman, who used a modified clamp designed for the Fasanella–Servat procedure.

H.B aldwin (✉)
PrincessM argaretH ospital Windsor, UK
e-mail:he athercbaldwin@hotmail.com

A.J. Cohen and D.A. Weinberg (eds.), *Evaluation and Management of Blepharoptosis*,
DOI 10.1007/978-0-387-92855-5_20, © Springer Science+Business Media LLC, 2011

He bluntly separated the conjunctiva and Müller's muscle from the underlying levator aponeurosis by a posterior approach [7]. Müller's muscle-conjunctival resection has been reported to give excellent results in terms of adequate and predictable lid elevation and contour [7–15]. This chapter describes a modification of this technique, in which direct visualization of Müller's muscle is obtained before its dissection and resection, and sutures are passed through the skin crease [16–18].

SurgicalT echnique

As with all the surgeries to correct blepharoptosis, this procedure may be carried out under local anaesthesia or general anaesthesia, and the considerations taken into account are the same. When local anesthesia is employed, adrenaline may be omitted to avoid stimulation of Müller's muscle, thereby influencing the height of the eyelid. Minimal amounts are injected to avoid tissue distortion. The skin crease is marked, and any excess skin is removed if a simultaneous blepharoplasty is being performed. Next the lid is everted over a Desmarres retractor. This may be held in place by traction using a lid margin suture. On the posterior lid surface, an incision is made along the upper border of the tarsal plate and then Müller's muscle and conjunctiva are lifted together from the levator aponeurosis. A subtotal resection of the conjunctiva and Müller's muscle is performed, preserving a 1–2 mm stump of Müller's muscle. Three double-ended 5/0 silk sutures are passed through the cut edge of forniceal conjunctiva, Müller's muscle, and the upper border of the tarsal plate, and finally through the skin crease marked at the beginning of the operation. The first suture is placed at the midpoint of the lid over the pupil, slightly medially in adults, and the other two sutures are placed at approximately equal distances on each side, 3–5 mm from the middle suture, but adjusted according to the age of the patient and the lid contour on the table. The central suture is tied in a loop so that the lid height may be assessed and adjusted as needed. The other two sutures are tied after assessment of the lid contour.

The wound is dressed according to the surgeon's preference, and if silk sutures are used, they may be removed between 5 and 21 days postoperatively. If the lid margin is on or above the upper limbus, the sutures may be removed in the earlier stages and a regime of lash traction three times daily is applied; if below the limbus, the sutures may be removed later.

Preservation of the Conjunctiva

A modification of the open-sky technique involves resection of Müller's muscle alone (Fig. 20.1), thereby preserving healthy conjunctival tissue in its anatomical position [18]. It may be desirable to preserve healthy conjunctival tissue for two principal reasons. First, concern has previously been raised that excision of part of the tarsal conjunctiva, and therefore a proportion of goblet cells, might lead to dry eyes following this procedure. In fact, it appears that none of the elements necessary for a healthy tear film, including mucin secretors (goblet cells), lacrimal secretors (accessory lacrimal glands), and lipid secretors (meibomian glands), are significantly affected [19]. However, there are no long-term follow-up data available, and it may be that their tear film could be compromised in later years. Patients with a history of dry eye are traditionally thought to be unsuitable for Müller's muscle–conjunctival resection, but may be able to benefit from the same procedure with preservation of the conjunctiva. The preservation of the conjunctiva also has anatomical advantages. Although Putterman has reported safe use of his technique in 35 anophthalmic patients [11], preservation of conjunctiva would decrease the risk of fornix shallowing in these patients.

In order to use this modification, the conjunctiva and Müller's muscle are incised just above the upper border of the tarsal plate. The plane between Müller's muscle and the levator aponeurosis is identified, and blunt dissection on this plane is extended upward until a rolled white band is seen (folded aponeurosis). Müller's muscle is then lifted off the conjunctiva up to the level of the fornix. At this stage, a subtotal Müller's muscle resection is performed, leaving a 2–3 mm stump,

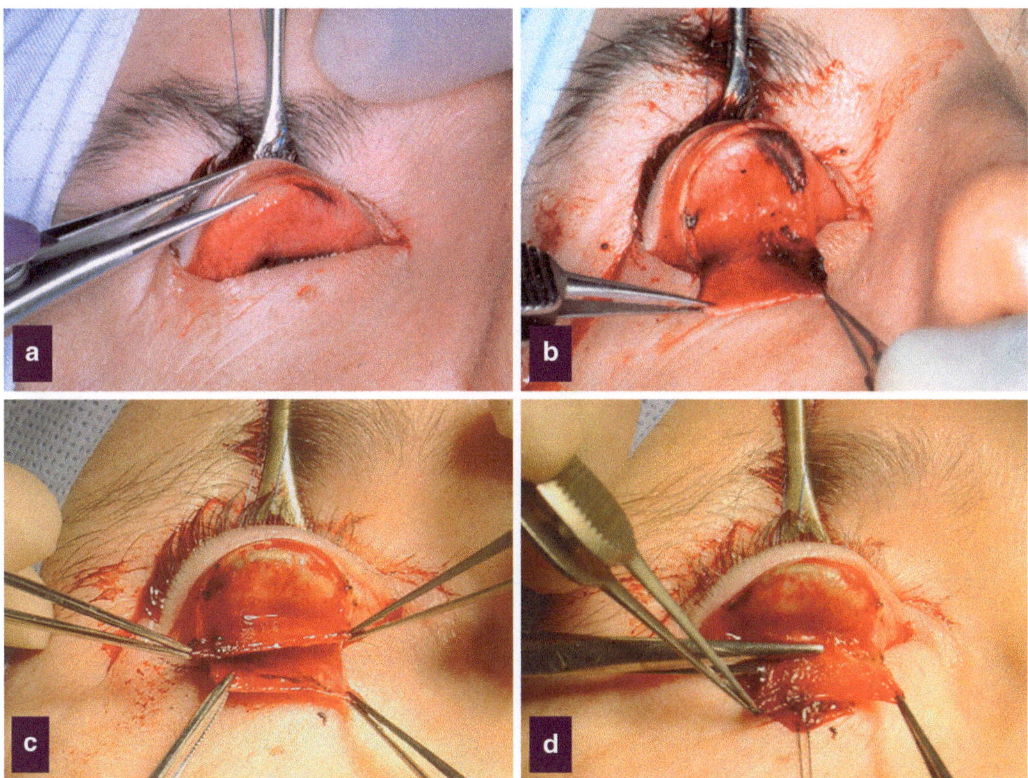

Fig. 20.1 Surgical technique for isolated (conjunctiva-sparing) Müller muscle resection. (**a**) The lid is everted, and conjunctiva and Müller's muscle incised just above the upper border of the tarsal plate. (**b**) Blunt dissection is performed in the plane between Müller's muscle and the levator aponeurosis. (**c**) Müller's muscle is lifted off the conjunctiva up to the level of the fornix. (**d**) A subtotal Müller's muscle resection is performed, leaving a 2–3 mm stump

as in the technique described above. A double-ended 5/0 silk suture is placed through the conjunctiva at the level of the initial incision, through the stump of Müller's muscle, through the upper border of the tarsal plate, and finally out through the marked skin crease. This suture is tied on a loop, and eyelid height and contour checked. Two further sutures are placed through the same structures medially and laterally, and also tied on loops. Height and contour are then checked before tying the sutures on the skin crease.

Open-Sky Müller's Muscle Resection and the Phenylephrine Test

Müller's muscle is an unusual smooth muscle due to its innervation by the sympathetic rather than the parasympathetic nervous system. It is therefore susceptible to stimulation by phenylephrine, a direct-acting alpha-1 adrenergic agonist. Interestingly, however, alpha-2 receptors have been found to be the predominant adrenergic receptors in Müller's muscle, and beta-1 receptor subtypes predominant in the levator muscle [20]. This raises the question of whether the phenylephrine test allows a complete representation of Müller muscle action; it is probably accurate for alpha-1 receptors, but it does not include assessment of alpha-2 receptors.

A positive phenylephrine test has traditionally been used as an indication that resection of Müller's muscle will raise the lid margin. Topical applications of phenylephrine have been used in either the 2.5% or 10% preparations [7, 8, 10–12, 21]. Phenylephrine is a direct acting sympathomimetic drug that stimulates the sympathetic innervation of Müller's muscle, causing it to contract and shorten, thereby elevating the eyelid. The degree of elevation produced by the topical

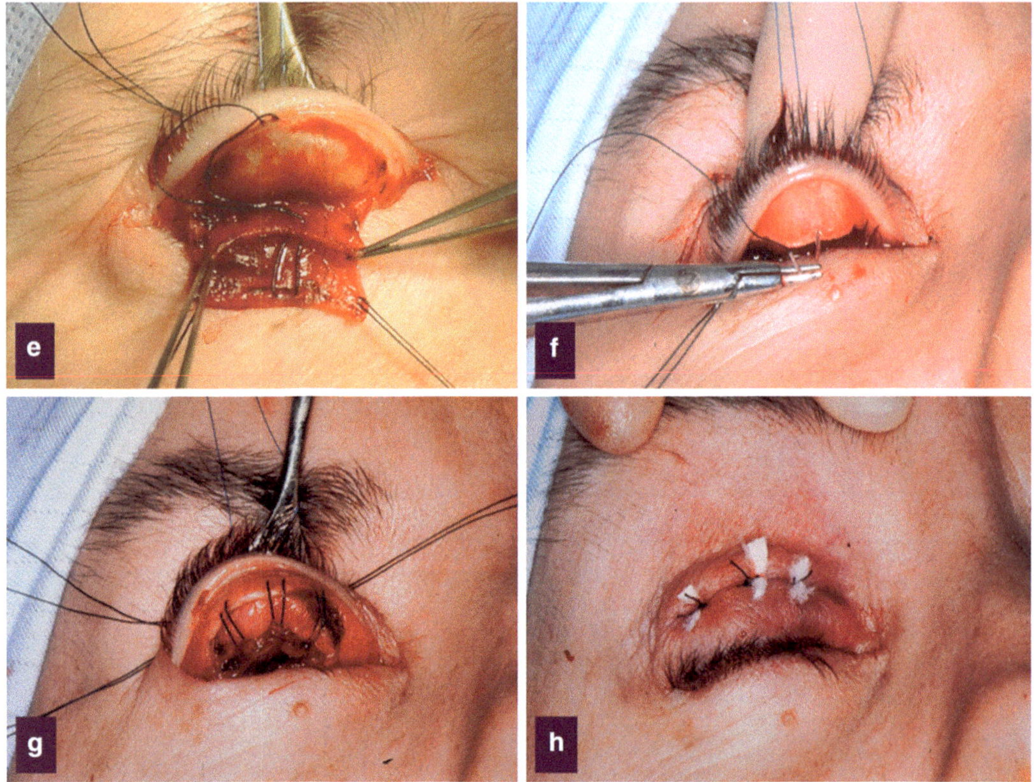

Fig. 20.1 (continued) (**e**) Adouble-ended 5/0 silk suture is placed through the conjunctiva at the level of the initial incision, through the stump of Müller's muscle, (**f**) through the upper border of the tarsal plate and finally out through the marked skin crease. (**g**) This suture is tied on a loop, and eyelid height and contour are checked before placing the other two sutures. (**h**) The eyelid at the end of theope ration

phenylephrine has also been used to calculate the amount of tissue to be resected [7, 8, 10]. If the lid has no response or an extremely poor response to the instillation of phenylephrine, an alternative technique, such as a direct levator tuck, resection, or advancement, is traditionally performed.

However, the most likely explanation for the efficacy of the open-sky Müller's muscle– conjunctival resection technique is that the surgery results in advancement of the levator muscle. This explains how the technique, therefore, works in patients *without* a positive response to topical phenylephrine.

Discussion

There are two possible explanations for the success of Müller's muscle–conjunctival resection in raising the lid margin. First, resection of Müller's muscle might enhance the stretch reflex transmitted to the levator muscle, and thereby increase the tone in that muscle. However, the clinical results suggest that it is more likely that this technique works by simple advancement of the levator muscle itself, along with the aponeurosis. Suturing muscular and vascular tissue such as Müller's muscle to the tarsal plate may provide a more stable and durable adhesion than suturing the levator aponeurosis when it has been affected by fibro-fatty degeneration. The mechanism by which Müller's muscle resection alleviates ptosis would, therefore, be by transmitting the contraction force of levator muscle directly to the tarsal plate instead of transmitting through its aponeurotic attachment. This would occur irrespective of the level of the aponeurotic defect.

The technique presented here is significantly different from other techniques that aim to correct ptosis by excising conjunctiva, tarsal plate, and/or Müller's muscle. The Fasanella–Servat procedure probably does not depend on a Müllerectomy, but is effective due to posterior lamellar shortening, or advancement of the levator aponeurosis complex on the tarsus. It has been shown that the technique was effective in a series of ptosis patients despite histological evidence that absent or minimal smooth muscle resection was performed [22]. The traditional Müller's muscle–conjunctival resection also relies on a closed-clamp technique, in which the actual amount of smooth muscle resected is not visibly measurable, and may be effective by the same mechanisms as the Fasanella–Servat procedure [23]. The open-sky technique may provide specific advantage for ptosis repair in phenylephrine test-negative patients, as the technique allows for maximal resection of Müller's muscle under direct visualization to provide for more powerful levator advancement [17].

The open-sky technique for Müller's muscle–conjunctival resection without the use of the clamp has several advantages over the closed technique originally described by Putterman. First, the technique is performed under direct visualization of the relevant eyelid structures. Second, there is opportunity for intraoperative adjustment by placement of sutures higher up in the residual stump of Müller's muscle or by resection of a strip of tarsal plate, if necessary. In the event of adequate height still not being achieved, the procedure may easily be converted to a posterior approach levator resection as described by Collin [2]. The timing of removal of "pull-out" silk sutures, also described by Collin in the same paper, allows some postoperative manipulation of lid height. Third, attachment of Müller's muscle directly to the skin augments the skin crease, which is not the case in other types of posterior approach ptosis surgery. Fourth, the technique is easily modified to allow preservation of the conjunctiva [18]. Finally, the technique has been shown to be effective in phenylephrine test-negative as well as phenylephrine test-positive patients [17], making it a safe and effective method for correction of ptosis in many patients with mild to moderate ptosis (Figs. 20.2–20.4).

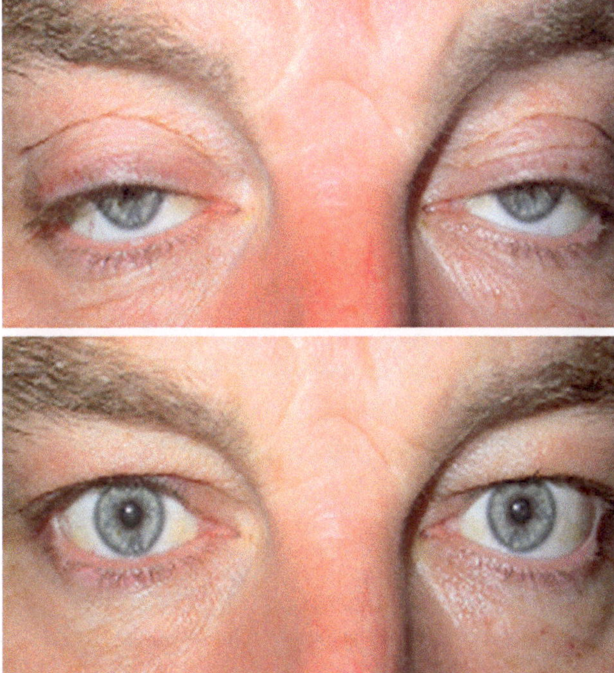

Fig.20.2 Bilateralpt osis corrected with isolated Müller's muscler esection

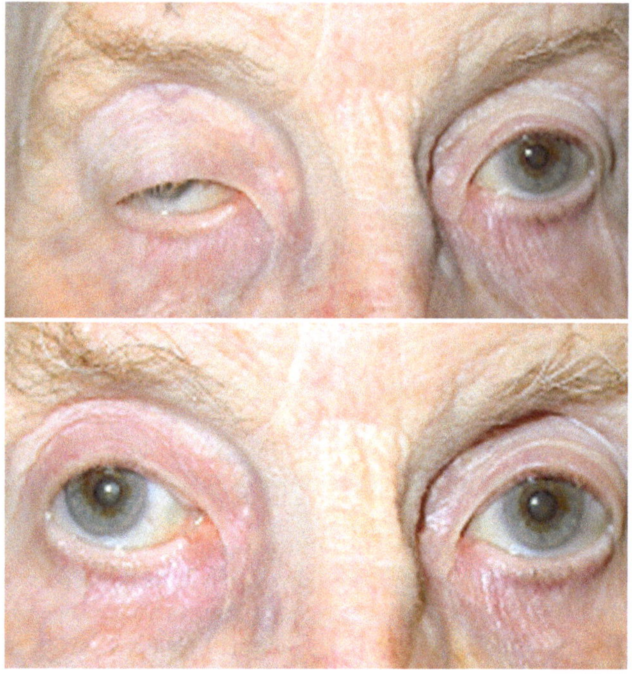

Fig.20.3 Unilateralpt osis corrected with isolated Müller's muscler esection

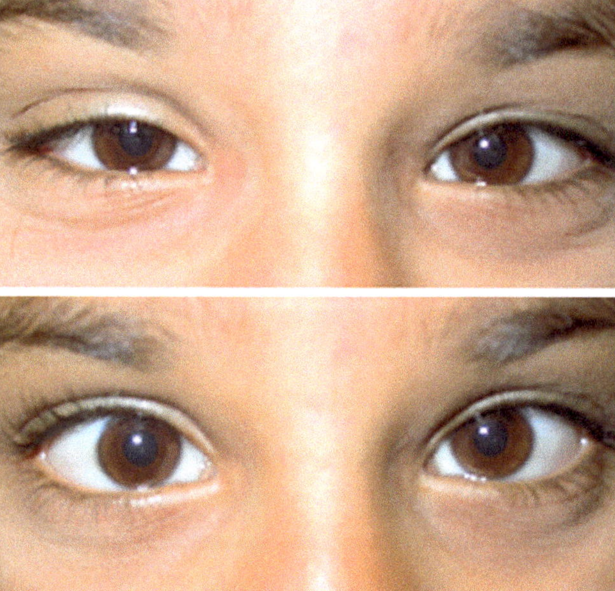

Fig.20.4 Congenitalpt osis (right eye) corrected with isolated Müller's muscle resection

References

1. Beard C. Müller's superior tarsal muscle; anatomy, physiology, and clinical significance. Ann Plast Surg. 1985;14:324–33.
2. Collin JRO. Ptosis repair of aponeurotic defects by the posterior approach. Br J Ophthalmol. 1979;63(8): 586–90.
3. Berke RN, Wadsworth JAC. Histology of levator muscle in congenital and acquired ptosis. Arch Ophthalmol.1955; 53:413.

4. WerbA .Ptos is.A ustJ O phthalmol.1976; 4:40.
5. Bang YH, Park SH, Kim JH, et al. The role of Müller's muscle reconsidered. Plast Reconstr Surg. 1998; 101(5):1200–4.
6. Kiyoshi M. Stretching of the Müller muscle results in involuntary contraction of the levator muscle. Ophthal Plast Reconstr Surg. 2002;18(1):5–10.
7. Putterman AM, Urist MJ. Müller muscle-conjunctiva resection for treatment of blepharoptosis. Arch Ophthalmol.1975 ;93:619–23.
8. Putterman AM, Urist MJ. Müller muscle-conjunctiva resection ptosis procedure. Ophthalmic Surg. 1978;9: 27–32.
9. Weinstein GS, Buerger Jr GF. Modifications of the Müller's muscle-conjunctiva resection operation for blepharoptosis. Am J Ophtahlmol. 1982;93:647–51.
10. Putterman AM, Fett DR. Müller's muscle in the treatment of upper eyelid ptosis – a ten year study. Ophthalmic Surg. 1986;17:354–60.
11. Karesh JW, Putterman AM, Fett DR. Conjunctiva-Müller's muscle excision to correct anophthalmic ptosis. Ophthalmology. 1986;93(8):1068–71.
12. Guyuron B, Davies B. Experience with the modified Putterman procedure. Plast Reconstr Surg. 1988;82: 775–80.
13. Glatt HJ, Putterman AM, Fett DR. Müller's muscle-conjunctival resection procedure in the treatment of ptosis in Horner's syndrome. Ophthalmic Surg. 1990;21:93–6.
14. Dresner SC. Further modifications of the Müller's muscle-conjunctival resection procedure for blepharoptosis. Ophthal Plast Reconstr Surg. 1991;7:114–22.
15. Press UP, Schayan-Araghi K, et al. Die Müller-Muskel-Resection: Indication, Technik und Ergebnisse. Ophthalmologe. 1994;91:533–5.
16. Lake S, Mohammad-Ali FH, Khooshabeh R. Open sky Müller's muscle-conjunctiva resection for ptosis surgery. Eye. 2003;17(9):1008–12.
17. Baldwin HC, Bhagey J, Khooshabeh R. Open sky Müller's muscle-conjunctival resection in phenylephrine test negative blepharoptosis patients. Ophthal Plast Reconstr Surg. 2005;21(4):276–80.
18. Khooshabeh R, Baldwin H. Isolated Müller's muscle resection for the correction of blepharoptosis. Eye (Lond).2008; 22(2):267–72.
19. ShieldsM ,P uttermanA .M üllerm uscle-conjunctival resection: effect on tear production (Comment). Ophthal Plast Reconstr Surg. 2003;19:254–5.
20. Esmaeli-Gustein B, Hewlett BR, Pashby RC, et al. Distribution of adrenergic receptors subtypes in the retractor muscles of the upper eyelid. Ophthal Plast Recontr Surg. 1999;15:92–9.
21. Glatt HJ, Fett DR, Putterman AM. Comparison of 2.5% and 10% phenylephrine in the evaluation of upper eyelids with ptosis. Ophthalmic Surg. 1990;21: 173–6.
22. Buckman G, Jacobiec FA, Hyde K, et al. Success of the Fasanella-Servat operation independent of Müller's smooth muscle excision. Ophthalmology. 1989;96:413–8.
23. Mercadetti M, Putterman AM, Cohen ME, et al. Internal levator advancement by Müller's muscle-conjunctival resection: technique and review. Arch FacialP lastS urg.2001; 3(2):104–10.

Chapter21
TheFas anella–ServatPr oceduref orPt osis

Kim Jebodhsingh, James Oestreicher, and John T. Harvey

Abstract The Fasanella–Servat procedure is useful in correcting ptosis of the upper eyelid. It does so by removing conjunctiva, Müller's muscle, and tarsus using a posterior eyelid approach. A graded algorithm provides a high success rate in patients who have ptosis with good levator muscle function. The surgery is quick and atraumatic and can be used in frail and elderly patients. The surgery can be used to correct upper eyelid contour abnormalities.

History

Dr. Fasanella and Dr. Servat met in 1959 when the young Peruvian, Dr. Servat, went to New Haven, Connecticut, for his ophthalmology residency at Yale University under the mentoring of Dr. Rocko M. Fasanella, the Chief of the Eye Service. It was here, on a busy surgical day in 1960, where they operated on a child with ptosis who had Cooley anemia requiring multiple transfusions. Speed was essential, and on that day, the Fasanella–Servat procedure was created [1]. In 1961, Fasanella and Servat [2] described their procedure for correcting small amounts of ptosis in patients with normal levator function. The procedure, as they described it, involved everting the upper eyelid and infiltration of local anesthetic into the subconjunctival space above the tarsal plate, placing two curved hemostats no more than 3 mm from the upper border of the tarsus, then placing 5-0 chromic sutures in a horizontal mattress fashion above the two curved hemostats. The tissue in the hemostats was excised, and two Frost sutures were placed to prevent corneal abrasion. The procedure was described as the removal of tarsus, conjunctiva, Müller's muscle, and levator palpebrae superioris.

Mechanismo fA ction

Over the years, there have been a number of suggestions as to the mechanism by which this procedure works. Fasanella and Servat proposed that it was the shortening of the levator, Müller's muscle, tarsus, and conjunctiva that caused the eyelid elevation [2]. However, Beard proposed that it was the shortening of the tarsus [3], and he showed in pathologic studies that excised tissues consisted of only conjunctiva, Müller's muscle, and tarsus and without levator muscle present [3]. Beard correctly noted that retraction of the aponeurosis prevented its inclusion in hemostats, and this was later confirmed by Putterman. Putterman concluded that resection and advancement of Müller's muscle was the basis for success in the Fasanella–Servat procedure [4]. He found that when an external levator resection was performed with a Putterman clamp in place, the levator aponeurosis was easily accessible and not found to be trapped by the clamp [5]. Furthermore, Putterman pointed out that there is

J.T.H arvey(✉)
Department of Ophthalmology, McMaster University
MedicalC entre, Hamilton, ON, Canada
e-mail:jtha rvey@mcmaster.ca

A.J. Cohen and D.A. Weinberg (eds.), *Evaluation and Management of Blepharoptosis*,
DOI 10.1007/978-0-387-92855-5_21, © Springer Science+Business Media, LLC 2011

no eyelid elevation in tarsoconjunctival grafts taken from the upper eyelid. In 1989, Buckman et al. [6] performed a histopathology study that showed that 87.5% of specimens displayed minimal or no smooth muscle, and they concluded that Müller's muscle resection had little, if any, effect. However, it was further stated that no correlation was found between the amount of tarsus excised and the degree of eyelid elevation achieved. The mechanism of action of the Fasanella–Servat procedure has remained inconclusive.

Indications

The Fasanella–Servat procedure is suited for no more than 3 mm of ptosis with levator function greater than 10 mm [2, 4, 7]. Ideally, it is used for 1.5–2 mm of ptosis with levator function of 13–15 mm. The procedure has been used for congenital, neurogenic, myogenic, traumatic, bilateral ptosis as well as correction of eyelid contour abnormality from previous surgery or trauma. It is contraindicated in patients with significant posterior lamellar scarring or shortened tarsus (congenital, surgical, or traumatic). It is generally recommended that this procedure should not be repeated if unsuccessful on the first attempt as this could cause shortening of the tarsus and eyelid instability. To our knowledge, there have not been any studies that look specifically at complications after a Fasanella–Servat procedure in patients with corneal disease or following corneal surgery. However, it has been shown that in high-risk patients with glaucoma filtering blebs, Müller muscle–conjunctiva resection can provide an effective and safe means for ptosis repair [8].

It has been suggested that the absence of eyelid elevation following instillation of phenylephrine indicates poor response of Müller's muscle to adrenergic stimulation, indicating that a tarsoconjunctiva-Müllerectomy (Fasanella procedure) or an anterior approach (levator advancement surgery) may prove more beneficial than a pure conjunctivo-Müllerectomy [5]. However, in 2007, Skibell et al. showed that the Fasanella–Servat and Putterman procedures have equal outcomes,inde pendentofa drenergicre ceptors [9].

Procedure

There have been multiple variations of the original procedure described by Dr. Fasanella and Dr. Servat. Beard modified the technique in 1969 using a running suture of catgut and externalizing the knot in the temporal crease [3]. In 1972, Putterman developed a clamp to supplant the use of curved hemostats for the Fasanella–Servat procedure [5]. The clamp was placed over the superior 3 mm of tarsus and Müller's muscle, and a double-armed 6-0 plain gut suture is placed in a running fashion above the clamp. This clamp is best known today for its use in the Müller's muscle conjunctival resection procedure. In 1973, Crawford used a Demarres retractor to evert the eyelid [10]. Bodian [11] used a 5-0 running nylon suture that he exteriorized with bolsters to the eyelid. In an effort to end the cut-and-sew technique, Fox [12] excised all eyelid tissue above the hemostats and placed a running 5-0 plain gut suture across the inner eyelid. Lauring, [13] in 1977, described a sutureless method, in which two curved hemostats were placed on the everted eyelid for 1 min. Iris scissors were used to cut down the broad groove left by the clamps after the hemostats were then removed. There have also been others that have described a sutureless technique [14]. In 1983, Betharia et al. [15] used sutures instead of curved hemostats to isolate the eyelid tissue to be excised.

Since its inception in 1961, the Fasanella–Servat procedure has become more refined. Beard and Putterman were responsible for two major advances in technique. Beard advocated a simplified suturing approach, and the Putterman clamp increased efficiency.

Description of the Procedure

The patient is positioned in the usual fashion, topical anesthesia is placed into the conjunctival sac, and the upper eyelid is infiltrated with local anesthetic in the usual way.

The patient is instructed to "look down." This aids in everting the eyelid over the Desmarres

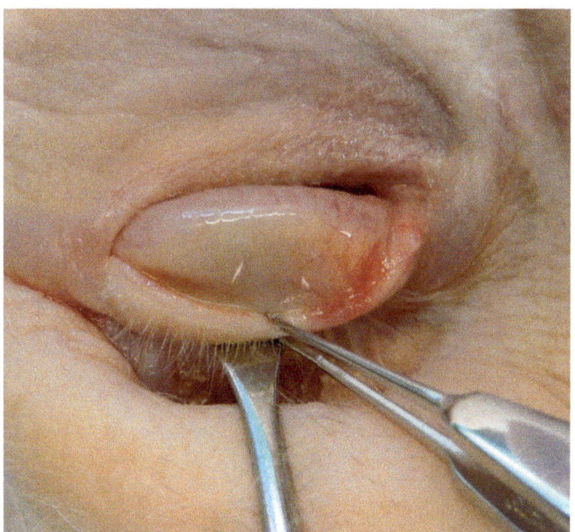

Fig. 21.1 The upper eyelid is everted over a Desmarres retractor

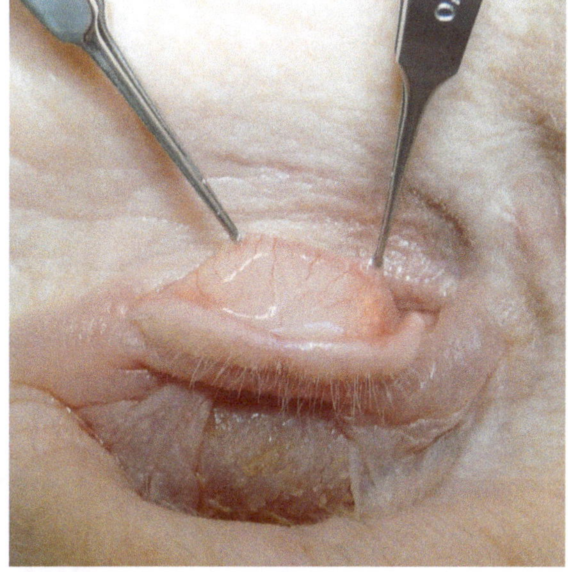

Fig. 21.2 Theta rsusi s grasped at the "corners." The "corner" is the arbitrary location at the junction of the "horizontal" superior tarsal border and the "vertical" medial(orl ateral)bor der

retractor (Fig. 21.1). With toothed forceps the tarsus is grasped at the medial and lateral "corners" (Fig. 21.2). The "corners" are an arbitrary location where the horizontal and vertical portions of the tarsus meet. (If one thinks of the tarsus as a rectangle, then the superior border is the horizontal edge and the medial and lateral borders of the tarsus are the vertical edges. Where these meet is the "corner.") Grasping too narrow a portion of tarsus will give a peaked eyelid contour. The Putterman clamp is applied (Fig. 21.3). The placement of the clamp determines the amount of eyelid elevation that will occur. Small (1 mm), medium (2 mm), and large resections (3 mm) correspond to one clamp width, two clamp widths, or three clamp widths of resection, respectively. The original description of the procedure called for two curved hemostats, and this can be used instead of the Putterman clamp (Fig. 21.4). A double-armed absorbable suture is placed full thickness "back and forth" superior to the clamp (Figs. 21.5 and 21.6).

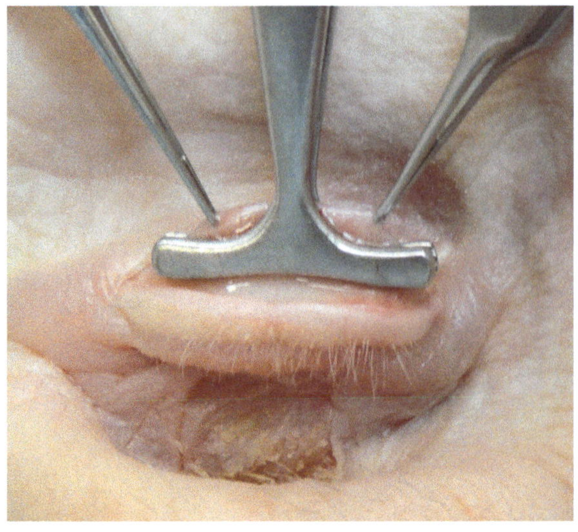

Fig. 21.3 ThePutte rman clamp is placed. The amount of tarsus included in the clamp will determine the amountof l ide levation

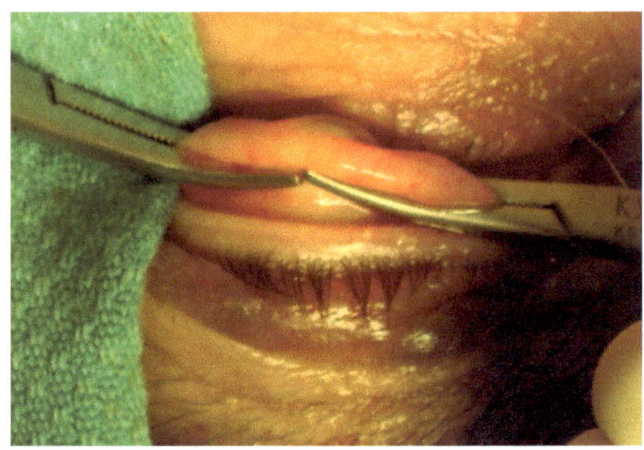

Fig. 21.4 Asa na lternative, *curved* hemostats can be used to clamp the tarsus. This is how the surgery was originally described by Fasanellaa ndSe rvat

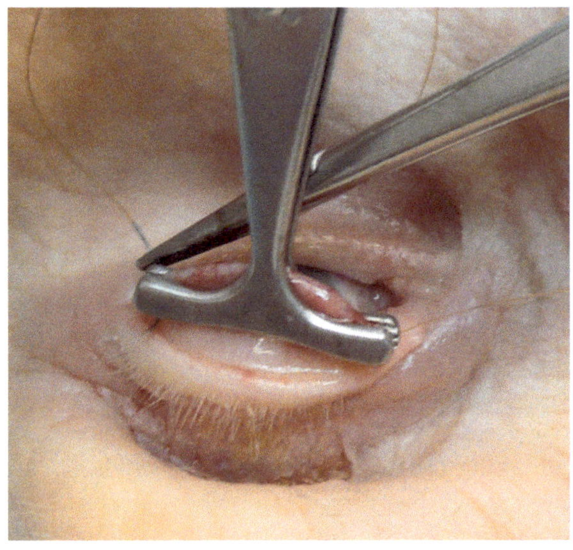

Fig. 21.5 A5-0c hromic suture is passed “back and forth”s uperiort ot hec lamp

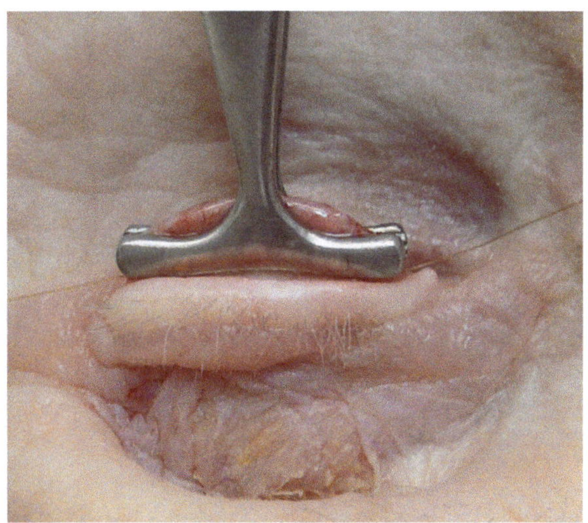

Fig. 21.6 Thes utureha s beenpl aced

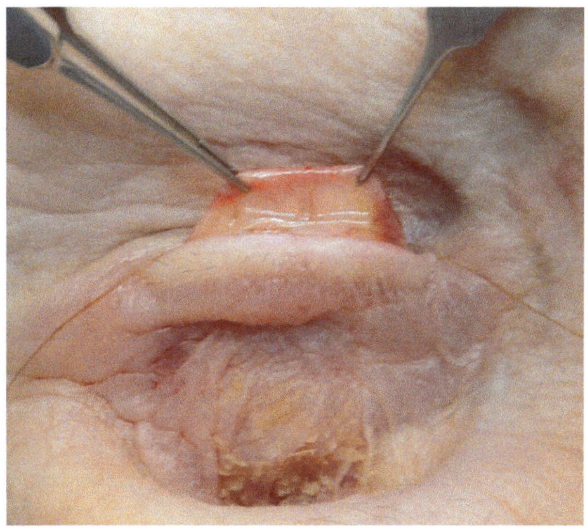

Fig. 21.7 ThePutte rman clampi sr emoved

The clamp is removed, and the "corners" are once again grasped (Fig. 21.7). The tarsus with attached conjunctiva is resected (Figs. 21.8 and 21.9). The suture is tested to ensure that it has not been accidentally cut (Fig. 21.10). The lateral arm of the suture is passed from the conjunctival side through to the skin side of the eyelid where it is tied (Figs. 21.11 and 21.12). The medial end is handled likewise (Fig. 21.13). Thee yeis dre ssedinthe us ualf ashion.

Complications

Complications of the Fasanella–Servat procedure include under or overcorrection, contour abnormalities, contralateral ptosis secondary to Hering's law (which is a "risk" with any type of unilateral ptosis procedure), duplicate eyelid creases, suture allergies, corneal abrasions, dry eye syndrome, hematomas, wound dehiscence, pyogenicgra nulomas,a ndble eding [7, 16].

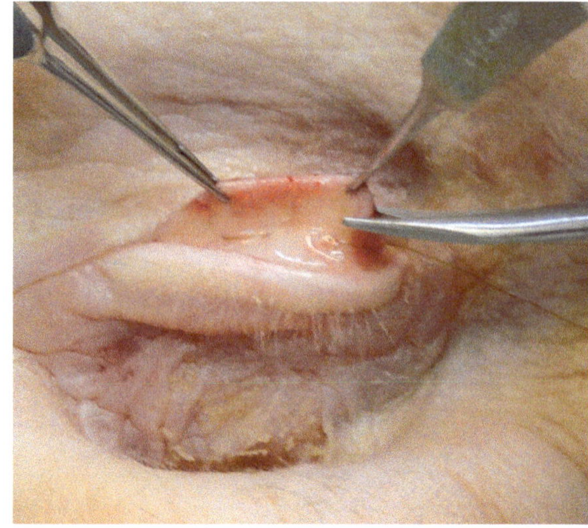

Fig. 21.8 The tarsus and reflected conjunctiva/Müller's muscle are removed

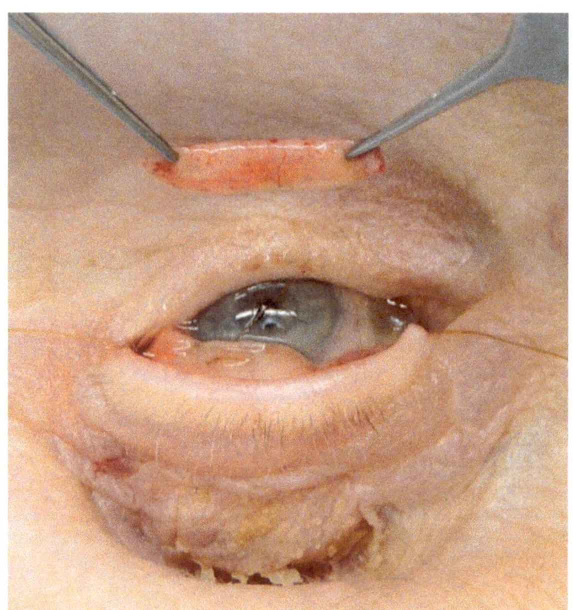

Fig. 21.9 Here is shown the removed fragment of tarsus with reflected conjunctiva. Bleeding is minimal from the cut edge due to the hemostatic effect of the clamp

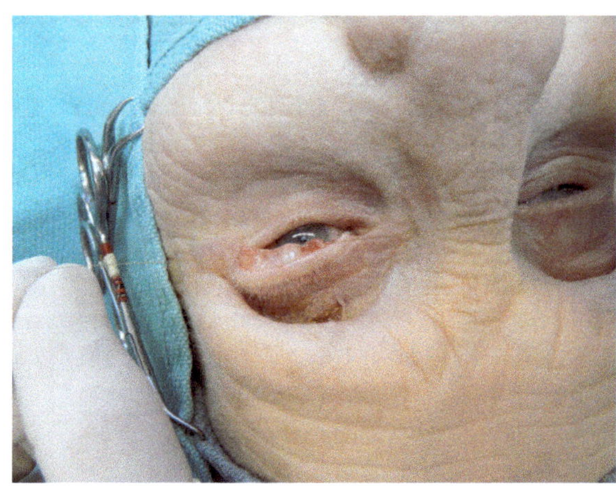

Fig. 21.10 The suture is pulled taut to ensure that it has not been inadvertently cut

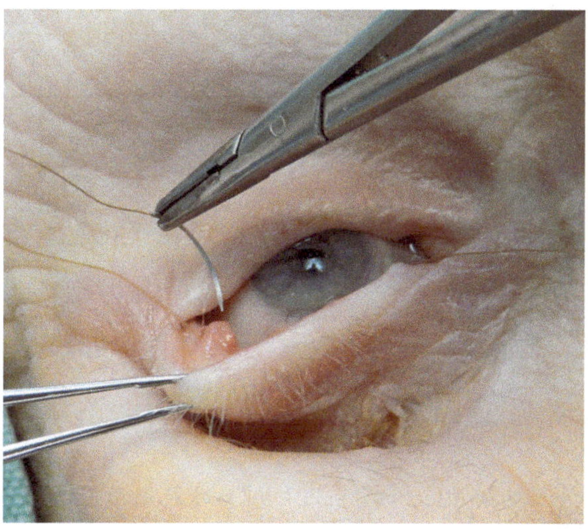

Fig. 21.11 Thedoubl e-armed ends of the suture are passed from the ends of the conjunctival wounds out to thes kins urfaceof thel id

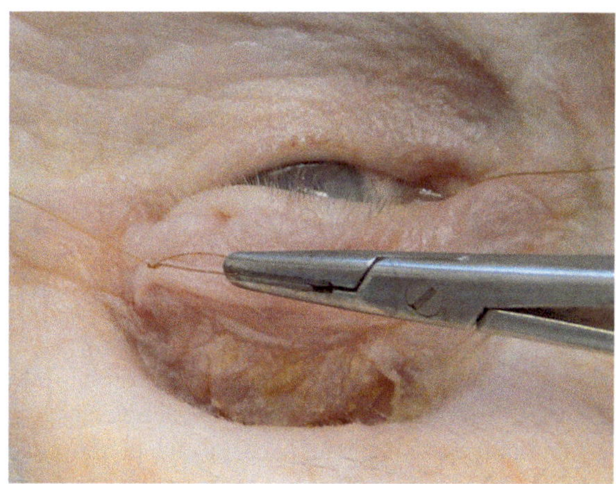

Fig. 21.12 Thes uturei s passed through skin and knottede xternally

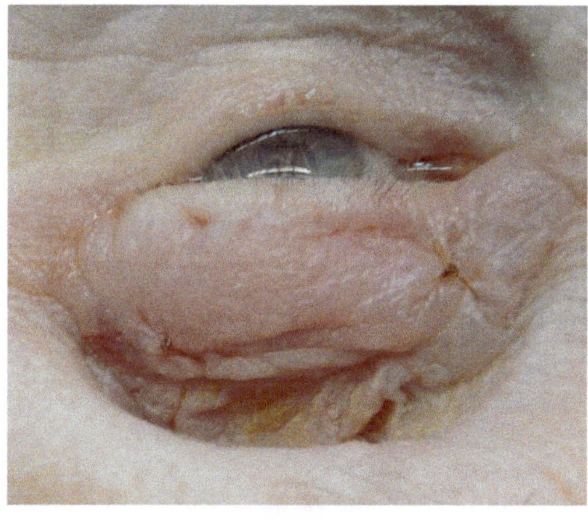

Fig. 21.13 Both the medial and lateral ends of the suture havebe enknot tedont hes kins urface

Undercorrection can be avoided by selecting patients with minimal ptosis and sufficient levator function. Eyelid peaking can be prevented by careful placement of the hemostat or the Putterman clamp and precise suture placement. The insertion of a bandage contact lens can help avoid postoperative keratopathy. There is the potential for postoperative dermatochalasis and double eyelid crease [17]. To prevent bleeding and hematoma formation, it may be necessary to preoperatively stop anticoagulants.

There are a few recommendations for postoperative adjustments for contour and height abnormalities. Beard [18] described using local anesthesia and without suture removal, "stretching" the eyelid. For overcorrection, eyelid massage

Table21.1 Summarizedr esults–P ange ta l. [7]

Typeofptos is	*n*	Success rate (%)	Preoperativept osis (mean, in mm)	Amounte xcised (mean, in mm)	Levatorf unction (mean, in mm)
Involutional	57	87.7	1.96	1.89	13.3
Postintraoculars urgery	53	92.4	2.33	2.10	12.5
Horner'ss yndrome	8	100	1.93	2.12	13.6
Congenital	17	76.4	1.56	1.91	10.5
Followingpre vious surgery or contour abnormality	11	100	1.58	Variable	13.3
Myogenic/other	7	85.2	1.20	1.36	10.7
Total(ora verage)	153	89.5	1.76	1.88[a]	12.3

[a]Excludes cases of eyelid contour correction

can also be effective [19, 20]. In 2009, Rosenburg et al. [21] described an office procedure without anesthetic that causes minimal discomfort to the patient. Six days postoperatively (when much of the edema has resolved but tissues have not yet densely fibrosed), gentle downward tugging is performed in the desired area of adjustment from the lashes or eyelid margin.

Discussion

This procedure has the advantage of high reliability with appropriate preoperative criteria and is minimally invasive. The success rate of the Fasanella–Servat procedure has been reported to range from 28 [22] to 95% [14] for most types of ptosis.

In 2007, Pang et al. [7] found a success rate of 89.5% of cases (137/153). The authors retrospectively reviewed 169 charts of two surgeons (JTH and JHO) from 1988 to 1996. Among subgroups, success was highest at 100% in Horner's syndrome (8/8) and postlevator surgery (11/11) and lowest in congenital ptosis at 76.4% (13/18). Seventy-five percent of failures were undercorrections. These results are summarized in Table 21.1.

The procedure is generally quick so that it can be done in frail patients relatively safely with local anesthetic in a treatment room. It is less likely to cause overcorrection or contour abnormalities than levator advancement surgery. The operation is very useful for small degrees of ptosis, and the likelihood of overcorrection is low. In cases where there is scarring in the eyelid skin crease from trauma or previous surgery, it can bypass the scar by working posteriorly.

Like any operation, proper patient selection is the key, and in the average oculoplastic practice, up to 75% of ptosis repairs can be done using this method. It can be combined with blepharoplasty, but this creates two wounds unnecessarily. So, we prefer levator advancement in the setting of blepharoplasty surgery.

Contour abnormalities can be addressed by skewing the clamp to one side. In other words, if the medial portion of the eyelid is low, but the lateral side has good height, then the clamp can be placed on the medial ½ of the eyelid to elevate only one side of the eyelid. This is especially valuable in a reoperation situation.

In summary, this operation is one of the great creations of oculoplastic surgery. Many people have used their ingenuity to enhance and perfect thiste chnique.

References

1. Fasanella RM, Shields MB. Obituaries – Javier Servat, MD. Arch Ophthalmol. 2002;120:104.
2. Fasanella RM, Servat J. Levator resection for minimal ptosis: another simplified operation. Arch Ophthalmol.1961; 65:493–6.
3. Beard C. Ptosis. 3rd ed. St. Louis: The C.V. Mosby Company; 1981. p. 232–66.

4. Putterman AM, Urist MJ. Müller's muscle-conjunctival resection ptosis procedure. Ophthalmic Surg. 1978;9(3):27–32.
5. Putterman AM. A clamp for strengthening Müller's muscle in the treatment of ptosis. Modification, theory, and clamp for the Fasanella-Servat ptosis operation. Arch Ophthalmol. 1972;87(6):665–7.
6. Buckman G, Jakobiec FA, Hyde K, et al. Success of the Fasanella-Servat operation independent of Müller's smooth muscle excision. Ophthalmology. 1989;96:413–8.
7. Pang NK, Newsom RW, Oestreicher JH, Chung HT, Harvey JT. Fasanella-Servat procedure: indications, efficacy, and complications. Can J Ophthalmol. 2008;43(1):84–8.
8. Georgescu D, Cole E, Epstein G, Fountain T, Migliori M, Nguyen Q, et al. Müller muscle-conjunctiva resection for blepharoptosis in patients with glaucoma filtering blebs. Ophthal Plast Reconstr Surg. 2007;23(4):285.
9. Skibell BC, Harvey JH, Oestreicher JH, Howarth D, Gibbs A, Wegrynowski T, et al. Adrenergic receptors in the ptotic human eyelid: correlation with phenylephrine testing and surgical success in ptosis repair. Ophthal Plast Reconstr Surg. 2007;23(5):367–71.
10. Crawford JS. Repair of blepharoptosis with a modification of the Fasanella-Servat operation. Can J Ophthalmol.1973; 8(1):19–23.
11. Bodian M. A revised Fasanella-Servat ptosis operation. Ann Ophthalmol. 1975;7(4):603–5.
12. Fox SA. A modified Fasanella-Servat procedure for ptosis. Arch Ophthalmol. 1975;93(8):639–40.
13. Lauring L. Blepharoptosis correction with the sutureless Fasanella-Servat operation. Arch Ophthalmol. 1977;95:671–4.
14. Gupta VP, Aggarwal R, Mathur SP. Blepharoptosis repair by modified sutureless Fasanella-Servat Operation (F.S.O.) – a large series of 50 cases. Indian J Ophthalmol. 1992;40:86–9.
15. Betharia SM. Transconjunctival levator resection: a modified simple technique. Ann Ophthalmol. 1988;20(6):234–8.
16. Carroll RP. Preventable problems following the Fasanella-Servat procedure. Ophthalmic Surg. 1980;11:44–51.
17. PersonalC ommunication,D r.J .O estreicher.
18. Beard C. Blepharoptosis repair by modified Fasanella-Servat operation. Am J Ophthalmol. 1970;69(5):850–7.
19. Dortzbach RK, Kronish JW. Early revision in the office for adults after unsatisfactory blepharoptosis correction. Am J Ophthalmol. 1993;115:68–75.
20. Jordan DR, Anderson RL. A simple procedure for adjusting eyelid position after aponeurotic ptosis surgery. Arch Ophthalmol. 1987;105:1288–91.
21. Rosenberg C, Lelli Jr GJ, Lisman RD. Early postoperative adjustment of the Fasanella-Servat procedure: review of 102 consecutive cases. Ophthal Plast Reconstr Surg. 2009;25(1):19–22.
22. Sampath R, Saunders DC, Leatherbarrow B. The Fasanella-Servat procedure: a retrospective study. Eye.1995; 9(Pt1) :124–5.

Chapter22
Full-Thickness Eyelid Resection forB lepharoptosisC orrection

Shu-Hong Chang and Norm Shorr

Abstract Full-thickness eyelid resection offers predictable correction of blepharoptosis in scarred, multioperated eyelids. Two surgical techniques, the lamellar and en bloc techniques, are described in detail. Both techniques rely on removal of tarsus, and/or scar tissue replacing tarsus, in a millimeter-for-millimeter fashion to achieve the desired amount of correction. Results are highly predictable because the scarred, multioperated eyelid loses distensibility and fluidity between tissue planes such that the amount of tissue resection corresponds exactly to the amount of eyelid elevation. Ways to address asymmetric tarsal platform show and contour deformitya rea lsopre sented.

The concept of full-thickness eyelid resection was first introduced by Hervouet and Tessier in 1956 [1], then popularized in the 1970s [2]. In 1975, McCord described an external approach tarsoaponeurectomy for initial blepharoptosis surgery in which pretarsal orbicularis muscle is excised and a formula is then used to determine the extent of removal of underlying levator muscle aponeurosis, tarsus, Müller's muscle, and conjunctiva [3]. Mustarde developed the split-level full-thickness eyelid resection, in which the anterior skin–orbicularis resection is performed at a level superior to the tarsoconjunctival resection, with the goal of tissue preservation by tucking the levator aponeurosis-Müller's muscle complex [4]. While Mustarde reported satisfactory results on patients with mild-to-moderate blepharoptosis, Karesh expanded this technique for use on patients with severe blepharoptosisw ithpoorle vatorfunc tion [5].

We define full-thickness eyelid resection for blepharoptosis correction as the external approach removal of all or some tissue layers from both the anterior and posterior eyelid lamellae but always with tarsus (and/or scar tissue replacing tarsus) resection in a millimeter-for-millimeter ratio to achieve the desired amount of correction. This approach is recommended for secondary correction of residual blepharoptosis in "multioperated" eyelids, i.e., eyelids that have undergone one or more prior surgical procedures, with scarred tissue planes. In a normal eyelid, levator aponeurosis and Müller's muscle are distensible, and the anatomic tissue layers slide upon themselves. In reoperation cases, tarsus and the full-thickness eyelid tissue encompassing scar along the superior tarsal margin are nondistensible. When this nonfluid tissue is resected in full-thickness fashion, a predictable millimeter-for-millimeter blepharoptosis correction is achieved.

Let us employ an analogy. If one purchases a pair of trousers and later realizes that the trouser legs are 3 in. too long, how is this problem fixed? An expert tailor would measure the excess length and cut 3 in. off the bottom of each

N.Shorr (✉)
Division of Oculoplastic Surgery,
Jules Stein eye Institute, UCLA School of Medicine,
LosA ngeles, CA, USA
e-mail:dr shorr@pacbell.net

A.J. Cohen and D.A. Weinberg (eds.), *Evaluation and Management of Blepharoptosis*,
DOI 10.1007/978-0-387-92855-5_22, © Springer Science+Business Media, LLC 2011

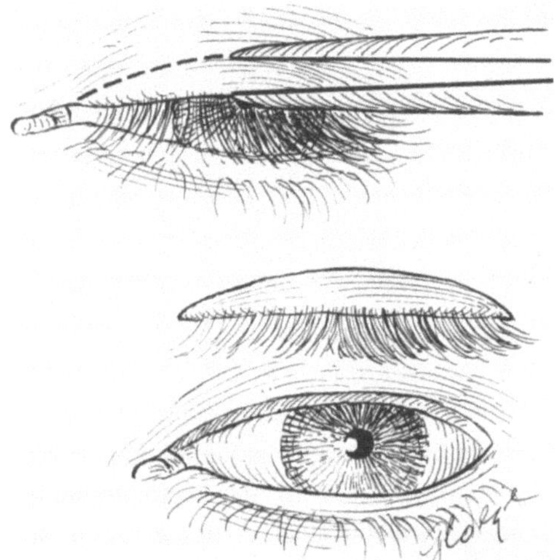

Fig. 22.1 Illustration of the theory behind full-thickness eyelid resection. If the desired amount of blepharoptosis correction is excised from the lid margin, an accurate and predictable amount of correction would be achieved. Reprintedw ithpe rmissionf romH enryB aylis,M D

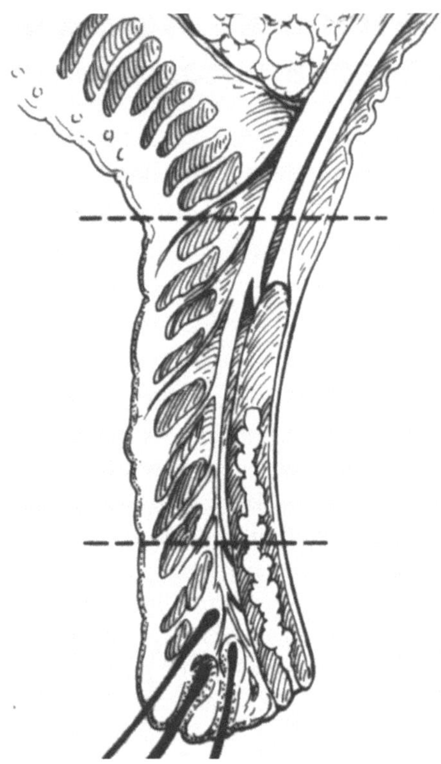

Fig. 22.2 Cross-section of normal upper eyelid. The *dotted lines* demarcate the segment of tissue recommended for full-thickness eyelid resection. The inferior incision should spare at least 4 mm of tissue at the eyelid margin. The superior incision should not be so high as to breach the orbital septum. Reprinted with permission fromH enryB aylis,M D

trouser leg. The trousers would then be the perfect length. Similarly, if an upper eyelid is 3 mm too low, resecting 3 mm of full-thickness eyelid from the margin would solve the length problem (Fig. 22.1). Of course, this is impractical because critical eyelid margin structures, such as lashes, blood vessels, and meibomian glands, need to be preserved for proper ocular surface function. We recommend sparing the inferior 4 mm of upper eyelid but performing full-thickness resection within the area superior to this demarcation and inferior to the level of the orbital septum (Fig. 22.2). In this area, tissue planes are less fluid, especially in multioperated scarred eyelids. Full-thickness eyelid resection in these cases can achieve a predictable amount of blepharoptosis correction. Additionally, eyelid margin contour abnormalities can be resolved reliably.

Two techniques for this surgery were previously published. In 1977, Baylis and Shorr described the lamellar dissection method and Baylis et al. subsequently described the en bloc dissection method [6, 7]. Both techniques are described in detail below.

Indications

Although full-thickness eyelid resection by either technique may be performed with satisfactory results in primary correction of blepharoptosis, we find ourselves utilizing full-thickness eyelid resection most frequently for especially challenging cases of secondary blepharoptosis repair. The underlying etiologies of the ptosis and procedures, which had been used for the primary repair, are irrelevant. Full-thickness eyelid resection has long been used successfully for secondary correction of residual upper eyelid blepharoptosis due to congenital, neurogenic, and myogenic causes. In congenital blepharoptosis, the levator muscle is relatively less distensible or nondistensible. Therefore, full-thickness blepharoptosis surgery is more predictable and efficacious.

Techniques

The preoperative preparation is identical whether using the lamellar or en bloc full-thickness eyelid resection technique. Pay detailed attention to MRD1, eyelid margin contour, and palpebral fissure height at various points along the horizontal axis of both upper eyelids. Additionally, record the margin-to-crease distance (MCD) as well as the margin-to-fold distance (MFD); the latter is the vertical distance between the eyelid margin and the skin draping over the eyelid crease in some patients. Compare these measurements between the two upper eyelids. Asymmetric MCD or MFD, which result in asymmetric tarsal platform show, is often more cosmetically bothersome to patients than true eyelid margin blepharoptosis. We believe that a crucial component of blepharoptosis correction is the attainment of symmetric tarsal platform show. It is our experience that the majority of patients who are candidates for full-thickness blepharoptosis correction surgery have a higher eyelid crease on the ptotic eyelid and that the vertical distance between the existing and desired crease positions equals the amount of needed blepharoptosis correction (Fig. 22.3a). Thus, the ensuing description of surgical techniques applies to this patient presentation. Management of asymmetric MCD is discussed in the challenges and solutions section of this chapter.

The amount of tarsus to be resected is the predetermined millimeter-for-millimeter difference between the preoperative eyelid margin level and the target eyelid margin level. Photographic documentation of both eyes is especially useful for preoperative planning and intraoperative comparison.

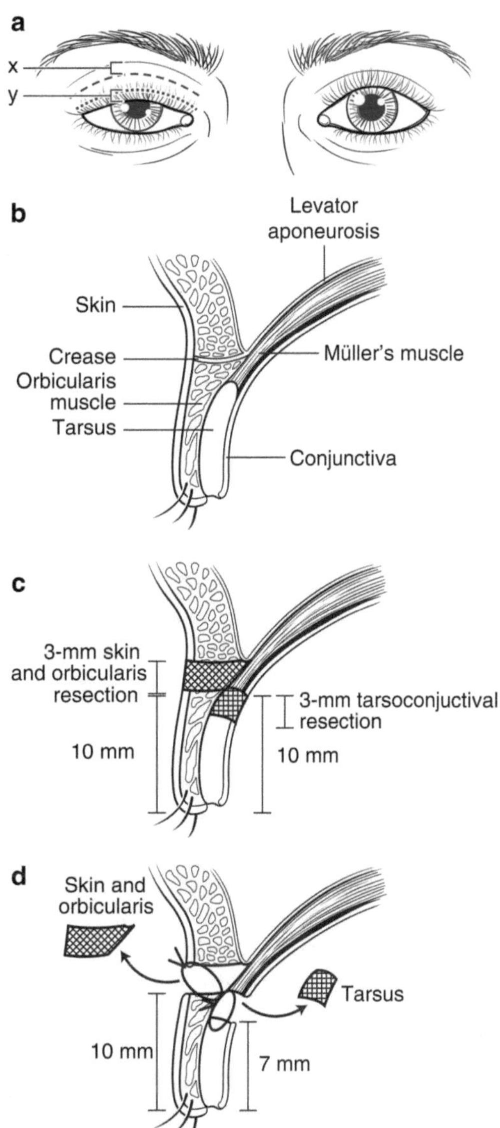

Fig. 22.3 Lamellar dissection technique. (**a**) The majority of patients have a higher crease on the ptotic eyelid, as shown here. On the ptotic right upper eyelid, *long dashed line* represents the desired crease position and *short dashed line* represents the desired eyelid margin position, both matching the fellow nonptotic eyelid. The vertical amount of eyelid crease asymmetry (x) is equal to the amount of blepharoptosis correction needed (y), thus $x=y$. The initial incision should be made at the existing eyelid crease and tissue excision should be performed inferior to the crease. (**b**) Cross-sectional view of this eyelid. (**c**) 3 mm of superior tarsoconjunctiva is to be excised, and 3 mm of skin orbicularis flap is to be excised. (**d**) Deep closure is achieved by suturing the cut edge of tarsus to the cut edge of levator aponeurosis. The anterior lamella cannot be closed at the same level as the deep sutures, however, because this will shorten the eyelid crease to 7 mm. The superficial closure should be performed at the level of the preexisting eyelid crease, incorporating levator aponeurosis if a harsh crease is desired, and preservingthe infe riorl0m mof M CD

Lamellar Technique

Use a marking pen to trace along the existing eyelid crease. Local anesthesia, usually consisting of 2% lidocaine with 1:100,000 epinephrine and hyaluronidase, is sparingly infiltrated into the upper eyelid along this marking. A protective corneal shield may be inserted at this point. Use a #15 blade to incise skin and orbicularis muscle along the marking. With Stevens scissors, carry the dissection inferiorly in a plane anterior to the levator aponeurosis, until the superior tarsal border is encountered.

Reflect the skin–orbicularis muscle flap such that the next step of surgery is performed beneath the flap. The #15 blade is now used to make a near full-thickness horizontal incision just superior to the superior tarsal border, cutting through all tissues anterior to the conjunctiva. Use scissors to expose the superior anterior surface of tarsus along the full horizontal length of the area to be operated, excising all pretarsal tissue including levator aponeurosis and intercalated scar tissues. On the bare anterior tarsal surface, use calipers and marking pen to delineate the segment of tarsus and underlying conjunctiva to be excised, from the superior tarsal border extending inferiorly toward the eyelid margin. The amount of tarsoconjunctival excision corresponds to the predetermined millimeter-for-millimeter difference between the preoperative and proposed eyelid margin positions. In the case of segmental upper eyelid contour deformity, divide the horizontal length of the tarsus into segments to facilitate accurate marking. For example, if the medial one-third of the eyelid is 2 mm low, the central one-third of the eyelid is 1 mm low, and the lateral one-third of the eyelid is 2 mm low, mark this amount of tarsus for excision from each segment respectively. Once satisfied with the markings, use either the #15 blade or a Stevens or Wescott scissor to excise the desired amount of tarsus and underlying conjunctiva.

Place three interrupted simple vertical sutures centrally, centromedially, and centrolaterally, using 6-0 resorbable material on a half-circle spatula needle. First, pass the suture through the cut edge of the tarsal plate in a very deep lamellar fashion, then through the cut edge of the levator aponeurosis. Care is taken to avoid penetration of the conjunctiva. In cases with scarring and cicatricial loss of defined tissue planes, the tarsus may be sutured to scarred tissues superiorly. Some surgeons may choose to tie these sutures in a slip knot, sit the patient upright, and inspect the eyelid contour and eyelid margin level. If a corneal protector was inserted during the case, it should be removed so that the pupil and corneal light reflex are visible while gauging eyelid position. After inspection, residual irregularities may be repaired by adjusting suture tension or excising additional tissue. The eyelid margin position should be reinspected after each manipulation.

At this point, the posterior lamella reconstruction has been completed, and satisfactory eyelid margin position and contour have been achieved. Attention is now turned to trimming the excess skin–orbicularis flap. In the typical patient described, this excision starts from the superior edge of the reflected pretarsal skin–orbicularis flap. Care must be taken to preserve the vertical anterior lamella distance from the eyelid margin superiorly that is equal to the desired MCD (Fig. 22.3b–d). If the fellow nonptotic eyelid has excess skin draping over the eyelid crease, then the surgeon may consider purposely leaving excess skin to match the MFD of the fellow nonptotic eyelid, or perform blepharoplasty on the fellow nonptotic eyelid. Again, the goal is to achieve symmetric tarsal platform show.

Prior to skin closure, the surgeon should decide whether a soft or harsh eyelid crease is desired. Recall that the anatomic definition of an eyelid crease is the superior-most insertions of levator muscle fibers to the skin [8]. To achieve a soft crease, use several interrupted or a continuous running suture to close the skin edges only. A harsh crease is formed by incorporating 1–2 mm of levator aponeurosis into the skin closure with every other stitch such that the skin is adherent to the levator aponeurosis and the eyelid crease is clearly visible with the eyelids closed.

En Bloc Technique

Use a caliper and marking pen to delineate an ellipse of skin representing the millimeter-for-millimeter difference between preoperative and proposed eyelid margin levels. The superior edge of the ellipse should correspond to the existing eyelid crease. Segmental eyelid margin contour deformities may be accounted for in the same manner as in the lamellar technique, with the only difference being that the segmental borders of excision are drawn on the skin surface (Fig. 22.4a,b).

After infiltrating the upper eyelid with local anesthetic, insert a bone plate or similar device beneath the eyelid to protect the globe during eyelid tissue excision (Fig. 22.5). Then, use a #15 blade to make a full-thickness incision along the premarked ellipse (Fig. 22.6a, b). Stevens scissors may be used to complete the excision (Fig. 22.7a,b).

With the en bloc full-thickness eyelid resection technique, tissue layers are not dissected free, making it somewhat more difficult to identify the cut edge of the tarsal plate inferiorly and the cut edge of the levator aponeurosis superiorly. In fact, the edges of the incision may not show any tarsus in cases where a prior tarsectomy was performed and only dense scar tissues remain. Thus, interrupted simple vertical sutures should be passed in very deep lamellar fashion to incorporate near full-thickness eyelid tissue on either cut edge (Fig. 22.8). Again, care is taken to avoid penetration of the conjunctiva. As described with the lamellar technique, sutures may be tied temporarily while intraoperative adjustments are made by sitting the patient upright. Use several interrupted or a continuous running suture to close the skin, incorporating levator aponeurosis to reestablish a harsh eyelid creasea sde sired(Fig. 22.9a,b).

ChallengesandSo lutions

The techniques described above apply to cases in which the MCD is greater in the ptotic eyelid when compared to the fellow nonptotic eyelid. In cases where the eyelid crease in the ptotic eyelid is symmetric with the fellow eyelid, lower than the fellow eyelid, or nonexistent, the initial incision should follow a line that is drawn superior to the eyelid margin at a vertical distance that is equal to the MCD of the fellow nonptotic eyelid plus the amount of desired blepharoptosis correction. Full-thickness eyelid resection is then carried inferior to this incision using either the lamellar or en bloc technique. At the completion of surgery, bilaterally symmetric tarsal platform show should be achieved.

In patients with a contour deformity isolated to one segment of the eyelid, full-thickness tissue resection may be performed in only that

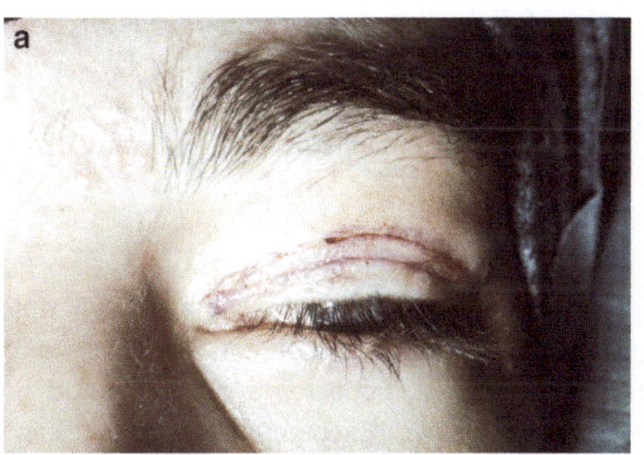

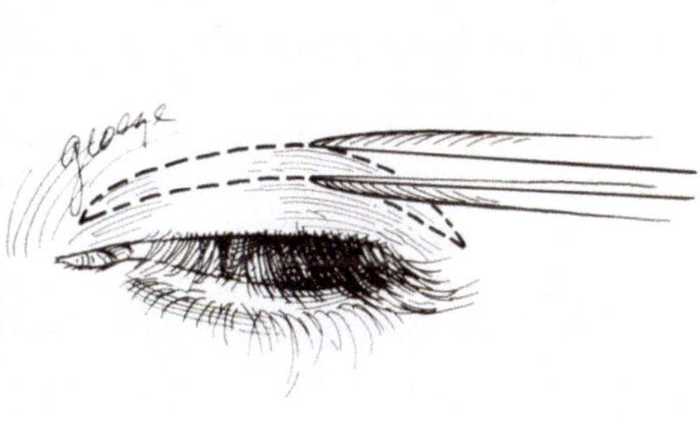

Fig. 22.4 (**a**) Skin marking delineating the ellipse of full-thickness tissue to be excised. (**b**) Artist schematic of intraoperative photograph. Reprinted with permission from Henry Baylis, MD

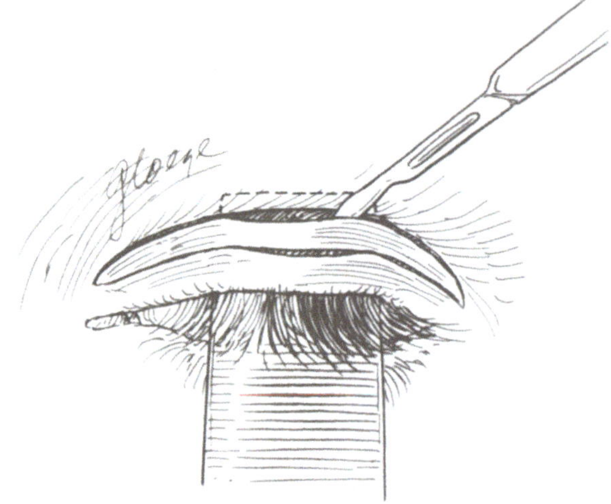

Fig. 22.5 A bone plate is inserted beneath the upper eyelid. This provides a hard surface against which the full-thickness incision is made, and protects the globe. Reprinted with permission from Henry Baylis, M D

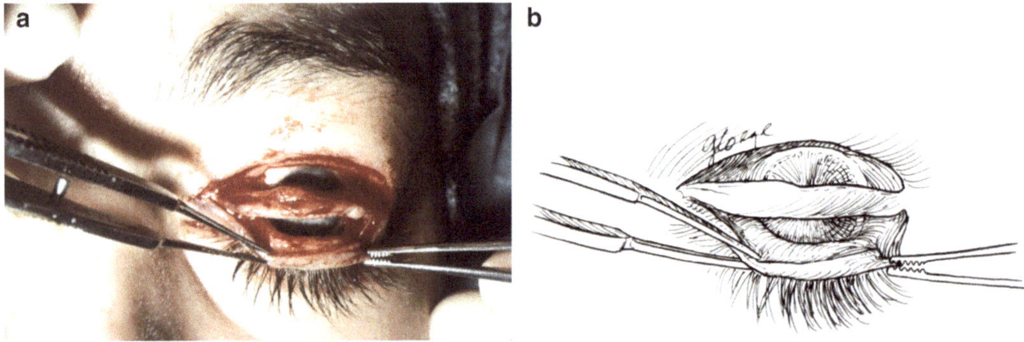

Fig. 22.6 (**a**) Full-thickness incision using the en bloc technique. (**b**) Artist schematic of intraoperative photograph. Reprinted with permission from Henry Baylis, MD

segment of the eyelid (Fig. 22.10a–c). If the area of tissue to be excised fits entirely within the head of a very large chalazion clamp, surgery may be performed with the aid of this clamp. To do so, place the clamp with the solid plate against the globe and the ring entirely encompassing the tissue marked for excision. The clamp now serves several purposes: to facilitate manipulation of the eyelid, to provide a firm surface against which the incision is made, and to protect the globe. The remainder of the surgery may be completed using either the lamellar or en bloc technique. If the area of tissue to be excised does not fit entirely within the head of the chalazion clamp, the clamp may be still be placed and the initial full thickness incision made centrally with the stability afforded by the clamp. The clamp can then be removed and the full thickness excisions extended medially and laterally with scissors.

In cases of severe eyelid margin contour deformities, the excised tarsus from one eyelid segment may be used to augment and thus lower another eyelid segment. This is a complicated eyelid reconstruction and should be reserved for use by surgeons with experience in full-thickness eyelid resection as well as eyelid reconstruction.

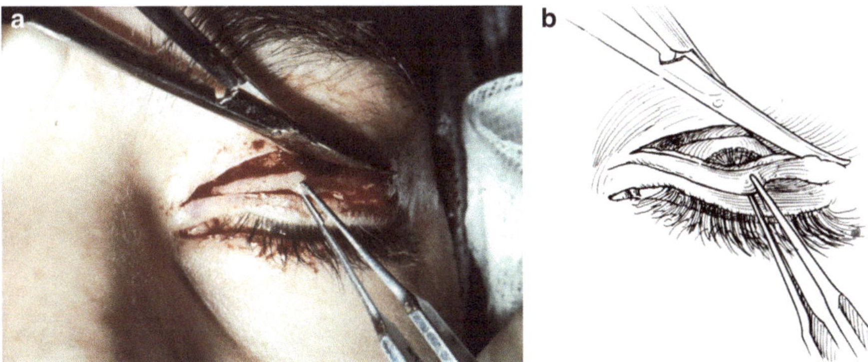

Fig. 22.7 (**a**) Scissors may be used to complete the full-thickness eyelid excision. (**b**) Artist schematic of intraoperative photograph. Reprinted with permission from Henry Baylis, MD

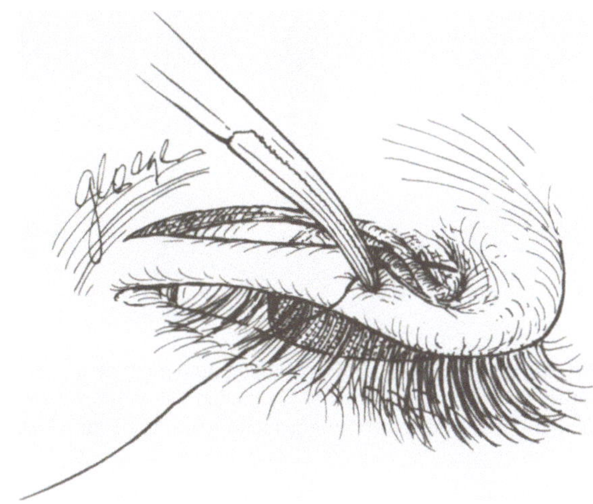

Fig. 22.8 The cut edges are reapproximated with interrupted simple vertical sutures in near full-thickness fashion. Reprinted with permission from Henry Baylis, MD

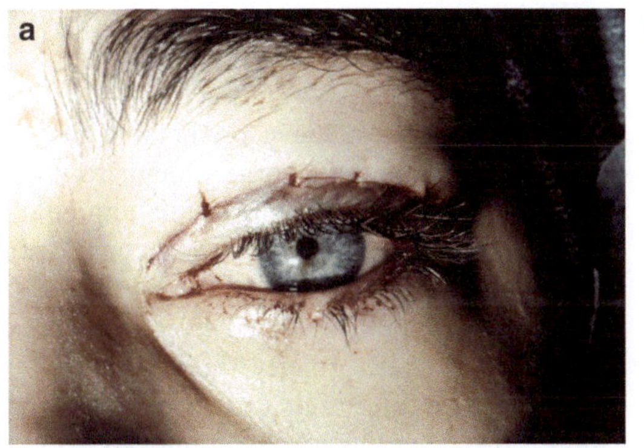

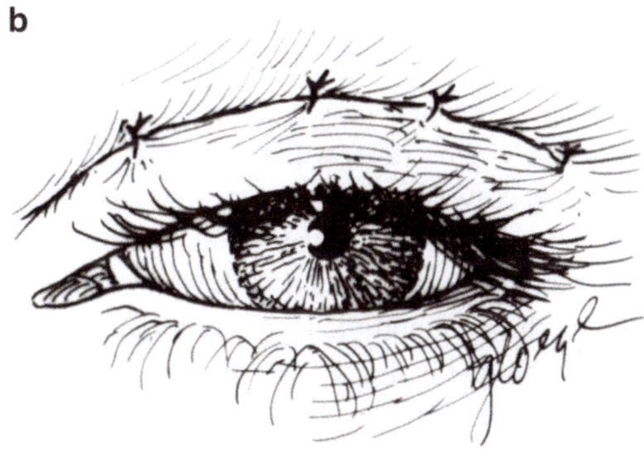

Fig. 22.9 (**a**) Skin closure is accomplished with interrupted sutures, incorporating underlying levator aponeurosis to create a harsh eyelid crease. (**b**) Artist schematic of intraoperative photograph. Reprinted with permission fromH enryB aylis,M D

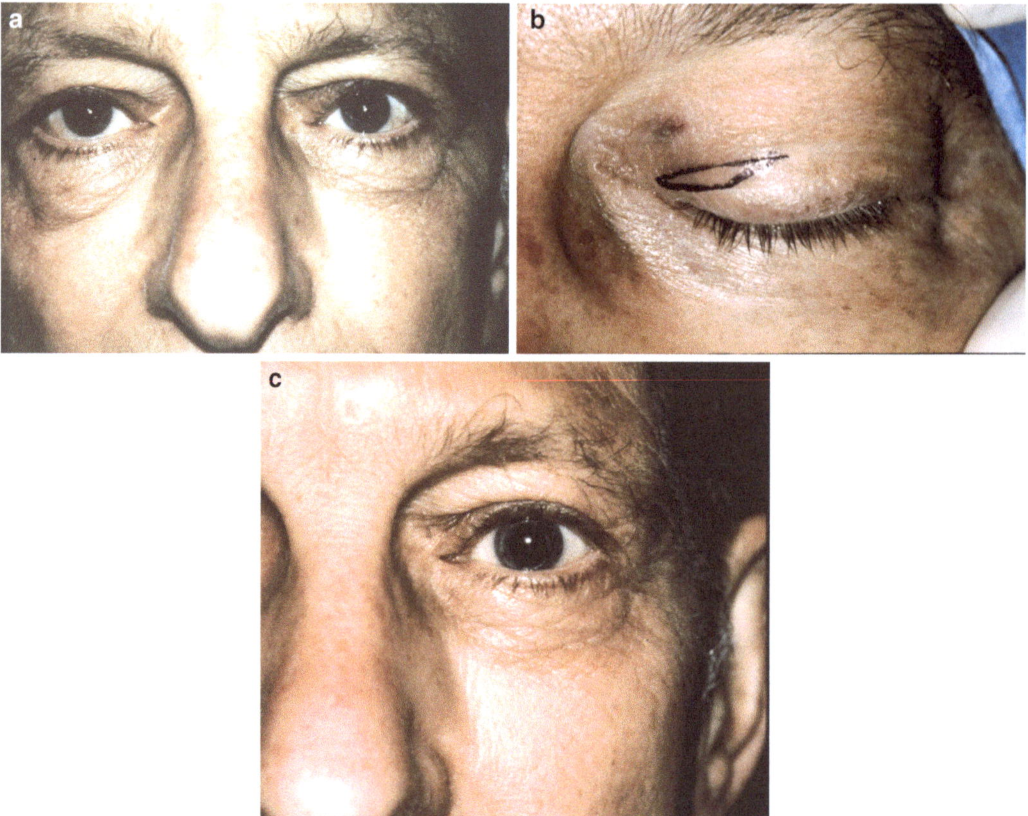

Fig. 22.10 (**a**) This is a preoperative photograph of a patient with segmental ptosis of the medial one-third of the left upper eyelid. (**b**) Intraoperative marking of the ellipse of full-thickness eyelid to be resected. (**c**) Postoperative photograph showing resolution of the medialbl epharoptosis

Pearls

It is the authors' suggestion to use the lamellar technique when teaching residents or in particularly challenging cases where added precision is required. Layer-by-layer dissection allows for direct visualization of tissues and avoids potential inaccuracies associated with simultaneously cutting through multiple layers of tissue. The en bloc technique is a good alternative in severely scarred eyelids or in eyelids that have undergone prior tarsectomy. In these cases, it may be impossible to separate tissue layers. Or, even if dissection is carried down to bare tarsus, vertical tarsus length may be insufficient to perform the necessary amount of millimeter-for-millimeter resection and still preserve the ideally desired 4 mm of vertical tarsal height at the eyelid margin.

The ability to achieve predictable results remains the elusive goal of any blepharoptosis surgery. One major reason for this unpredictability is the variable healing associated with surgery on thin, distensible, and fluid tissue layers. When multioperated eyelids become scarred such that formerly fluid tissue layers adhere into a single cicatricial mass continuum, this variability is removed. Full-thickness surgery then offers an opportunity to achieve predictable amounts of blepharoptosis correction.

References

1. Hervouet F, Tessier P. Technique chirurgicale du ptosis. Bull Mem Soc Fr Ophtalmol. 1956;239–42.
2. Beard C. Ptosis. St. Louis, MO: Mosby; 1969. p. 260.
3. McCord Jr CD. An external minimal ptosis procedure – external tarsoaponeurectomy. Trans Sect Ophthalmol Am Acad Ophthalmol Otolaryngol. 1975;79:683–6.
4. Mustarde JC. Correction of ptosis by split level resection. Clin Plast Surg. 1978;5:533–5.
5. Karesh JW. Multilevel full-thickness eyelid resection for the correction of severe acquired ptosis in the poorly functioning eyelid. Ophthalmic Surg. 1991;22(7):399–405.
6. Baylis HI, Shorr N. Anterior tarsectomy reoperation for upper eyelid blepharoptosis or contour deformities. Am J Ophthalmol. 1977;84:67–72.
7. Baylis HI, Axelrod RN, Rosen N. Full thickness eyelid resection for the treatment of undercorrected blepharoptosis and eyelid contour defects. Adv Ophthalmic Plast Reconstr Surg. 1982;1: 205–12.
8. Anderson RL, Beard C. The levator aponeurosis. Attachments and their clinical significance. Arch Ophthalmol.1977; 95(8):1437–41.

Chapter23
Frontalis Suspension for the Correction ofB lepharoptosis

Eve E. Moscato and Stuart R. Seiff

Abstract Frontalis suspension is the surgery of choice for congenital or acquired blepharoptosis with poor levator function (less than 5 mm). This procedure can be performed unilaterally or bilaterally in both children and adults. A variety of materials have been used with varying success. The ideal material is readily available, inert, adjustable, and has good, long-lasting tensile strength. Autologous materials frequently include fascia lata, temporalis fascia, and palmaris longus tendon. Allograft materials include mainly preserved fascia lata. Synthetic materials used for frontalis suspension include monofilament nylon, polypropylene, polybutylate-coated braided polyester, polyfilament cable-type suture, polyester fiber, expanded polytetrafluoroethylene (ePTFE), and silicone. Each of these materials has its own advantages and disadvantages. Adjustable sling materials may have specific advantages in patients with progressive ptosis or who are at risk for corneal decompensation. Excellent functional and aesthetic results can be obtained with frontalis slings when carefully placed with attention to surgical detail in all age groups.

S.R.Se iff(✉)
Department of Ophthalmology, University of California-San Francisco School of Medicine, SanFra ncisco, CA, USA
e-mail:s seiff@sfgh.ucsf.edu

Indications

Frontalis suspension is the surgery of choice for congenital or acquired blepharoptosis with poor levator function (less than 5 mm). The sling serves to raise the upper lid as the brow elevates. This procedure can be performed unilaterally or bilaterally. Traditionally, congenital ptosis repair has been delayed until 4 or 5 years of age unless there is a visual or general developmental delay that may be improved with earlier intervention. Frontalis suspension is also considered in adults with neurogenic or myogenic ptosis (e.g., chronic progressive external ophthalmoplegia, myasthenia gravis, or third nerve palsy) with poor levator function. In addition, frontalis suspension can be used effectively in Marcus Gunn jaw winking syndrome, congenital fibrosis syndrome, and double elevator palsy.

There are many materials that can be used in frontalis suspension surgery. The ideal material is readily available, inert, adjustable, and has good, long-lasting tensile strength. Numerous materials including autologous tissues, allografts, and synthetic materials can be used with varying success, each with its own advantages and disadvantages.

Autologous Tissue for Frontalis Suspension

Autogenous Fascia Lata

Autogenous fascia lata remains the gold standard for frontalis suspension. The fascia lata, or

A.J. Cohen and D.A. Weinberg (eds.), *Evaluation and Management of Blepharoptosis*, DOI 10.1007/978-0-387-92855-5_23, © Springer Science+Business Media, LLC 2011

iliotibial tract, is a thick band of tissue coursing from the lateral tibial condyle to the iliac crest. Fascia lata has excellent tensile strength, lack of significant inflammatory response in surrounding tissues, and minimal risk for rejection. Disadvantages include the need for a second operative site and increased surgical time. Complications of the donor site can include a hematoma, muscle herniation, infection, postoperative pain, and an unsightly scar. Because biointegration of fascia lata creates permanence, postoperative adjustment and removal is extremely difficult. Additionally, autogenous fascia lata may be difficult to harvest in children under 3 years of age since it is not yet adequately developed.

Harvesting Fascia Lata

Proper leg positioning is important for adequate tension on the fascia lata. Under general anesthesia, the leg is internally rotated and flexed at the knee. After prepping the outer thigh and knee and administration of local anesthesia for hemostasis, a 3-cm vertical incision is made 8–10 cm above the lateral condyle (Fig. 23.1a). Blunt dissection is carried out with Metzenbaum scissors through the superficial fascia until the glistening white fascia lata is exposed. Soft tissue is bluntly spread with long scissors off of the anterior surface of the fascia. A "U" shaped incision is made in the fascia, with the arms approximately 1 cm apart. A blade of the scissors is placed in the medial portion of the "U" incision, and the fascia is opened superiorly for a distance of approximately 10 cm. This step is repeated with the lateral incision. The flap of fascia lata is then placed in the fascia lata stripper. The stripper is guided superiorly and posteriorly toward the iliac crest to avoid transecting fibers (Fig. 23.1b) [1]. A 20-cm long strip should be obtained (Fig. 23.1c). The strip is then cut into narrower strips, each 3–4 mm in width. This will typically provide 3–4 strips, enough for two lids. However, if more fascia is needed, a second strip can be obtained in a similar fashion. Subcutaneous tissue is approximated with interrupted 3-0 Vicryl sutures, and skin is closed with a running 5-0 fast-absorbing plain gut suture. Antibiotic ointment and a Tegaderm dressing (3M, St. Paul, MN, USA) are placed over the wound, and a bandage is wrapped around the thigh.

Alternatively, a high leg incision can be used to minimize scar and muscle herniation [2]. Malhotra et al. have described an endoscopic approach to harvest fascia lata, using either a high thigh or low thigh incision and manual dissection under direct visualization without use of af asciatome [3].

Temporalis Fascia

Temporalis fascia is an alternative autologous material that is pliable and provides good tensile strength. Overlying the temporalis muscle, it originates in the temporalis fossa, and it is continuous with the galea. Temporalis fascia can be harvested with relative ease in the same operative field during ptosis surgery, and the scar is ultimately hidden by the hairline [4]. Disadvantages include a second operative site, prolonged surgical time, and difficulty in obtaining long strips. It is also more delicate than fascia lata.

Harvesting Deep Temporalis Fascia

After instillation of local anesthetic, a 3-cm incision is made 4 cm behind the hairline and approximately 2 cm above the ear. Blunt dissection is continued though superficial temporal fascia until temporalis fascia proper is identified. A 1-cm incision is made horizontally in the anteroposterior direction, and a strip of temporalis fascia proper is excised (Fig. 23.2) [4]. Subcutaneous tissue is closed with 3-0 Vicryl, and skin is approximated with skin staples.

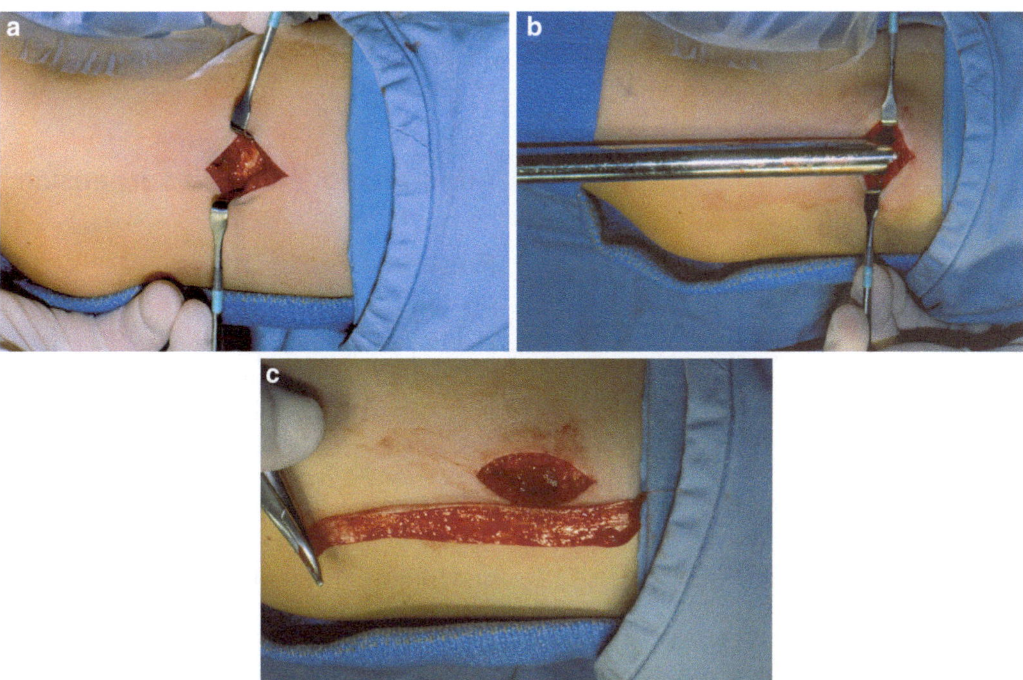

Fig. 23.1 Harvesting autogenous fascia lata. (**a**) Exposed fascia lata, demonstrating location of vertical incision that is made 8–10 cm above the lateral condyle. (**b**) A fascia lata stripper is guided superiorly and posteriorly toward the iliac crest. (**c**) Harvested strip of fascia lata, 20 cm in length. This strip can then be cut into strips 3–4 mm in width

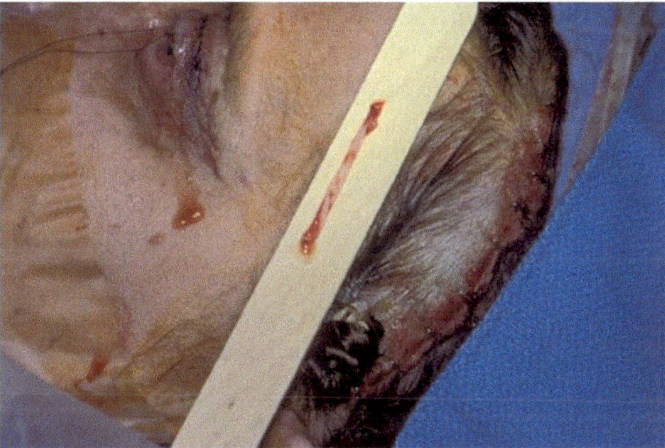

Fig. 23.2 Harvested strip of temporalis fascia, demonstrating location of vertical incision 4 cm behind the hairline and2c ma bovethe e ar

Palmaris Longus Tendon

The palmaris longus tendon can be used for frontalis suspension with good long-term success and can be performed under local anesthesia with minimal donor-site morbidity. The tendon is superficial in the forearm and is easily located. The loss of the tendon causes no functional deficit. The palmaris longus tendon is fully developed at birth, so it can be used in younger children as compared to autogenous fascia lata. Additionally, it provides greater tensile strength than fascia lata [5]. Preoperative evaluation of the palmaris longus tendon is a prerequisite, since only 80% of the population has a palmaris longus tendon. The patient should be asked to flex the wrist and touch the pad of the fifth digit to the thumb to confirm the presence of the tendon. The surgeon must know the anatomical landmarks and be careful not to harvest the median nerve in the absence of the palmaris longus tendon.

Harvesting Palmaris Longus Tendon

The forearm is placed in an elevated, supinated position. A pressure bandage is placed from the wrist to above the elbow, and a tourniquet is placed above the elbow for 1 min. A 1-cm incision is made transversely over the proximal wrist flexion crease (Fig. 23.3a) [6]. A second incision is made 10 cm from the initial incision (Fig. 23.3b). Mosquito forceps aid in separating the superficial fascia and deep fascia from the tendon. The tendon is identified at both incision sites. The presence of the tendon can be confirmed with gentle traction at one end. The tendon is then severed at the distal end and pulled gently through the proximal incision (Fig. 23.3c, d). It should be cut several times to create thinner strips. Skin is closed with interrupted 6-0 Nylon sutures.

Frontalis Muscle Flap Advancement

Direct frontalis muscle suspension has been used in the past as an alternative to frontalis suspension techniques. Through a lid crease incision, a frontalis flap is pulled inferiorly and secured to the anterior tarsus. Alternatively, the frontalis flap can be passed beneath a bipediculated levator aponeurosis flap for a more physiologic horizontal vector [7]. Although described in the literature, this technique has been inadequate in the authors' experience. The elasticity of the muscle flap does not provide sufficient support and allows recurrence of ptosiso vertime .

Allografts for Frontalis Suspension

Preserved Fascia Lata

Use of preserved fascia lata rather than autogenous fascia lata avoids comorbidities of a donor site and decreases surgical time. A major disadvantage includes a much higher recurrence rate of ptosis with higher reoperation rates. In fact, it has been reported to occur in up to 50% of patients at 8 years [8, 9]. Another disadvantage is the theoretic risk of disease transmission and rejection. Overall, irradiated fascia lata has had increased success, perhaps due to its more natural characteristics and higher tensile strength compared to lyophilized fascia lata [10]. Preserved fascia lata can be obtained from local tissue banks and may be of variable quality.

Other Processed Tissues

In the past, a variety of other processed tissues have been used with varying success, including collagen strips, pericardium, and human sclera [11]. These tend to dissolve and lead to high recurrence rates of ptosis. They also carry the theoretic risk of disease transmission.

Synthetic Materials for Frontalis Suspension

Synthetic materials used in frontalis suspension include: monofilament Nylon, polypropylene (Prolene; Ethicon, Inc., Somerville, NJ, USA), polybutylate-coated braided polyester (Ethibond 4-0; Ethicon, Inc., Somerville, NJ,

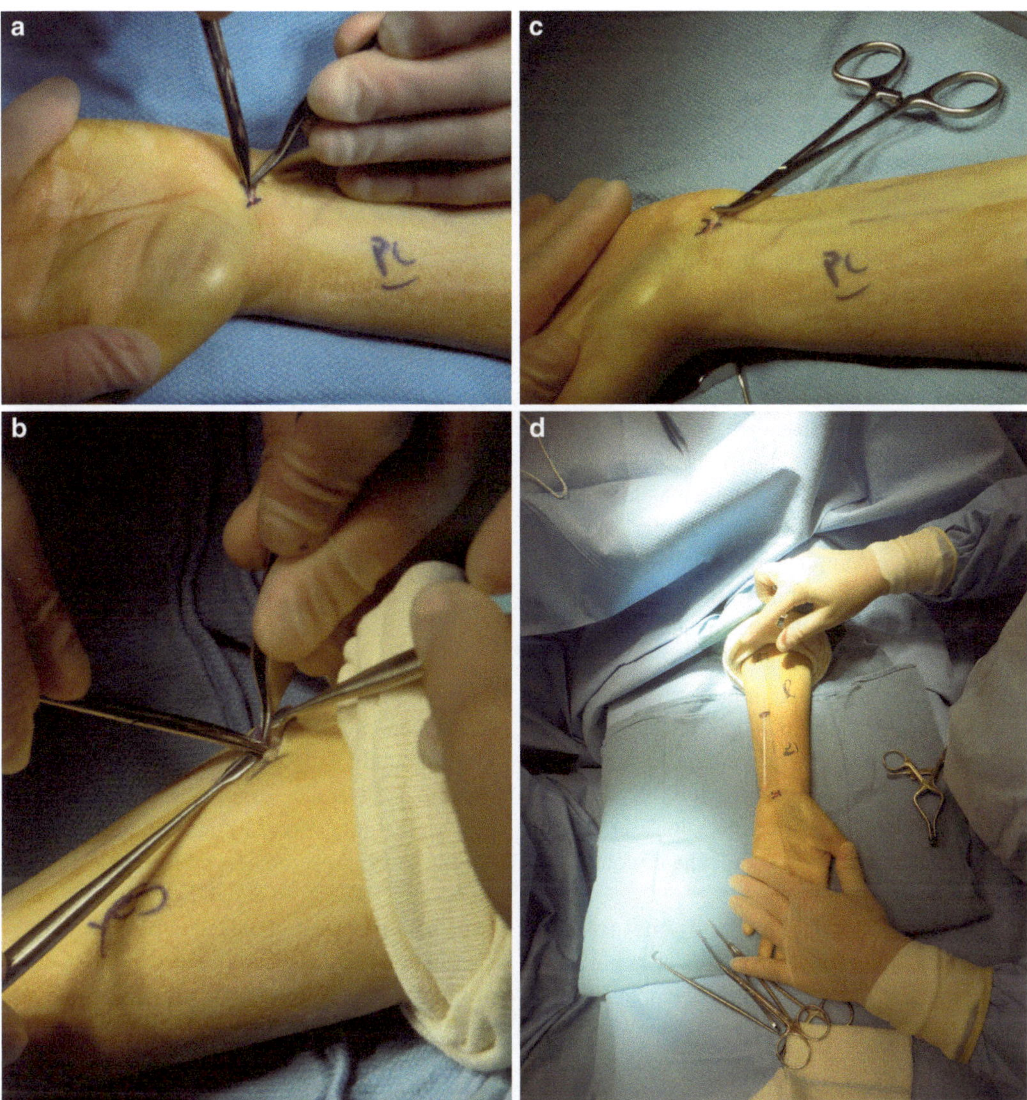

Fig. 23.3 Harvesting the palmaris longus tendon (Courtesy of Alan Harmatz, MD). (**a**) Transverse incision over the proximal wrist flexion crease and dissection to identify the palmaris longus tendon. (**b**) Second incision 10 cm from the initial incision. Once dissection has been performed, confirmation of palmaris longus tendon is obtained using gentle traction at one end. (**c**) After gentle traction to confirm the palmaris longus tendon, the tendon is cut at the distal end. (**d**) The palmaris longus tendon is pulled gently through the proximal incision

USA), polyfilament cable-type suture (Supramid Extra; S. Jackson, Inc., Alexandria, VA, USA), polyester fiber (Mersilene polyester fiber mesh; Ethicon, Inc., Somerville, NJ, USA), expanded polytetrafluoroethylene (ePTFE) (Gore-Tex; W.L. Gore & Associates, Inc., Flagstaff, AZ, USA), and silicone. The major advantages of synthetic materials are availability, avoidance of a donor site, and lack of disease transmission. Nylon, polypropylene, polyfilament cable-type suture, and silicone are easily adjustable due to lack of tissue integration.

Monofilament Nylon, polypropylene (Prolene), and polybutylate-coated braided polyester (Ethibond) have achieved variable success.

Disadvantages include granuloma formation, infection, and recurrent ptosis secondary to slippage. These narrow gauge materials are prone to cheesewiring through tissue. They may be considered a temporary measure. An alternative is polyfilament cable-type suture (Supramid Extra), which is inert, easily inserted, nonabsorbable, and reversible. Placing this material with a Wright fascia needle through the skin decreases the need for multiple skin incisions. Disadvantages include fragility with trauma, short-term effect, and infection.

The use of polyester fiber (Mersilene polyester fiber mesh or suture) has had variable success in the past. Although it has good tensile strength, it provides a scaffold for fibrovascular ingrowth, and soft tissue complication rates can be as high as 20%. Infection, granuloma formation, and extrusion may occur despite meticulous surgical technique [12]. Cutting thinner strips of Mersilene mesh and soaking the sling in antibiotic solution may help reduce infection. Ends should be sutured together rather than knotted to reduce bulkiness and decrease the risk of granuloma formation. Burying the suture ends in a deep frontalis pocket with adequate wound closure may reduce extrusion rates.

Expanded polytetrafluoroethylene (ePTFE) has led to successful outcomes, yet is not without complication. It is inert, biocompatible, and resistant to breakdown by tissue enzymes. Although it can be used as patches or strips, ePTFE suture provides superior results for frontalis slings. Stability is provided by biointegration through fibrovascular ingrowth, thereby enhancing longevity of ptosis correction. The authors note that this biointegration is a major disadvantage if the sling needs to be revised or removed. Additionally, the rates of infection and granuloma formation are up to fourfold higher with ePTFE compared with other synthetic materials. This may be due to the inherent porous fibrous matrix of the material with potential for bacterial sequestration [13]. Extrusion rates are also higher with this material. Soaking the implant in antibiotic solution and meticulous wound closure may decrease the risk of infection and extrusion of ePTFE.

The silicone rod frontalis sling has been used with good success. It is readily available and well tolerated. Infection and extrusion rates are low. Unlike autogenous fascia lata, it can be used in children before 3 years of age. No harvesting is necessary, and the sling can be easily adjusted since there is no tissue incorporation into the silicone. Major disadvantages include sling migration, cheesewiring, infection, and exposure. Although in the past, silicone was thought of as a temporizing measure until the child was old enough to undergo ptosis repair with autogenous fascia lata, the authors have had good, long-term success using silicone, with some slings remaining for over 30 years without revision.

Silicone rods are especially advantageous in those at risk for corneal exposure, such as those with chronic progressive external ophthalmoplegia, myasthenia gravis, myotonic muscular dystrophy, congenital fibrosis, third nerve palsy, and a poor Bell's phenomenon [14]. The elasticity of the silicone allows for better eyelid closure and less lagophthalmos compared to materials that are less flexible. The ease of adjustment through the original mid-forehead incision allows the lid height to be lowered if exposure keratopathy develops. The silicone rod is also particularly beneficial in those patients with progressive ptosis, such as chronic progressive external ophthalmoplegia, who may need adjustment as the disease process continues. Adjustment is critical in patients with variable ptosis, such as in myasthenia gravis. Because of lack of integration into surrounding tissues, the silicone sling is easily removed if no longer needed. In summary, silicone rods provide distinct advantages when compared with other surgical materials. The authors maintain that the silicone rod is an ideal suspensory material, suitable for all ages, and can be used in many conditions causing ptosis with poor levator function.

Techniques for Frontalis Suspension

The frontalis sling is placed in a similar fashion for all materials, with the exception of frontalis muscle flap advancement. There are various configurations of the sling, including original descriptions by Crawford [15] and Fox [16], as well as more recent modifications [17–19].

Double Triangle or Rhomboid Frontalis Sling

A double triangle or rhomboid, described by Crawford, uses a double-loop configuration with two strands. This technique has been used primarily for autogenous fascia lata suspension. It provides good contour and stability, yet is not easily adjustable postoperatively [15, 20]. The authors do not use this technique with synthetic materials due to excessive bulk and a possible increase in the risk of infection.

The authors use a modified Crawford technique for autogenous fascia lata frontalis suspension, consisting of the following six steps:

1. A 4-0 silk traction suture is placed in the central upper lid margin. Six incisions are made using a #15 blade. Three equidistant incisions are placed 3 mm above the lash line of the lid (medial, central, and lateral) and carried down to the anterior tarsal surface (Fig. 23.4a). Two incisions are made at the superior brow hairs, just above the medial and lateral lid incisions, and carried down to periosteum. A similar forehead incision is made 1.5 cm above the superior brow hairs between the lateral and medial brow incisions. Tenotomy scissors are used to create a pocket superiorly beneath the frontalis muscle through the forehead incision.
2. A bone plate coated with ophthalmic ointment is placed beneath the upper lid for corneal protection. An empty Wright needle (Storz; St. Louis, MO, USA) is passed from the medial lid incision to the central lid incision. The fascia is passed into the eye of the Wright needle and drawn across the lid.

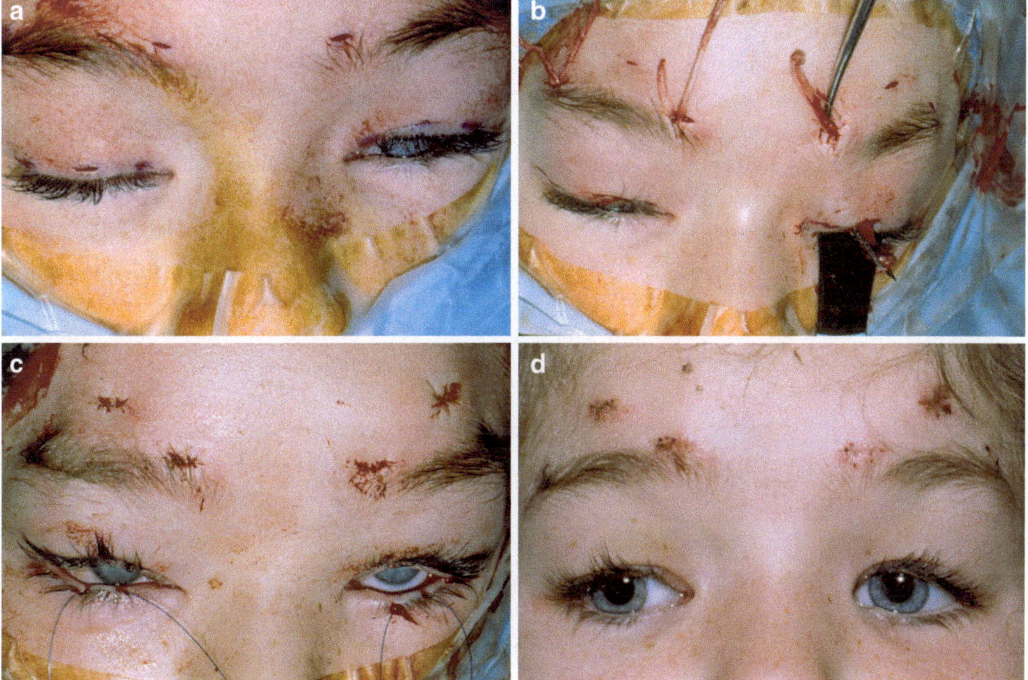

Fig. 23.4 Modified double triangle Crawford technique for frontalis suspension with fascia lata. (**a**) Demonstrates three lid incisions, two brow incisions, and a mid-forehead incision. (**b**) Two strips of fascia lata are passed, forming a medial and lateral triangle. The ends are pulled, thus tightening the slings, to adjust lid height and contour. (**c**) Closure of brow and mid-forehead incisions. (**d**) Postoperativea ppearanceonda y1

The empty Wright needle is then passed from the medial brow incision, posterior to the septum, and through the medial lid incision. Care is taken to avoid a full-thickness pass through the lid. One end of the sling is then threaded through the needle and pulled superiorly, bringing the end through the brow incision. The empty Wright needle is then passed from the same medial brow incision through the central lid incision, threaded, and pulled gently superiorly through the medial brow incision where the end is retrieved (Fig. 23.4b). This configuration forms a medial triangle.

3. Similarly, a second sling is used to create a lateral triangle. An empty Wright needle is passed from the lateral lid incision to the central lid incision. The fascia is passed into the eye of the Wright needle and drawn across the lid. The empty needle is then passed from the lateral brow incision, posterior to the septum, through the lateral lid incision, taking care to avoid a full thickness pass through the lid. One end of the sling is then threaded through the needle and pulled superiorly, bringing the end through the brow incision. The empty Wright needle is then passed from the same lateral brow incision through the central lid incision, threaded, and pulled superiorly through the lateral brow incision where the end is retrieved.
4. The tension on each triangle is adjusted for predetermined height and contour. A knot is tied, and the ends are left long. The empty Wright needle is then passed from the mid-forehead incision to the medial brow incision, threaded with the ends of the medial triangle, and pulled superiorly through the mid-forehead incision. This is also performed for the ends of the lateral triangle.
5. The ends of each sling are tied with a single square knot, reinforced with a 6-0 Nylon suture, and buried superiorly in the pocket beneath frontalis muscle.
6. The brow and forehead incisions are closed using interrupted 6-0 chromic suture for subcutaneous tissue and 6-0 fast absorbing plain gut suture for skin (Fig. 23.4c, d). Antibiotic ophthalmic ointment is placed over the incisions and in the eyes. The patient is given IV antibioticsintra operatively(Fig. 23.5a,b).

Single Pentagonal Frontalis Sling

Another technique is Fox's single pentagonal loop using one strand. This single-loop technique has the advantage of straightforward adjustment [16]. Additionally, less foreign body material is utilized compared to that of the Crawford technique.

Although there have been many deviations from original descriptions, the authors prefer a modified pentagonal loop [20]. They use a 0.8-mm silicone rod with swedged-on needles (BD Visitec frontalis suspension set (Seiff); Franklin Lakes, NJ, USA). The needles can be used or removed per surgeon preference. The authors' modified technique is outlined as follows:

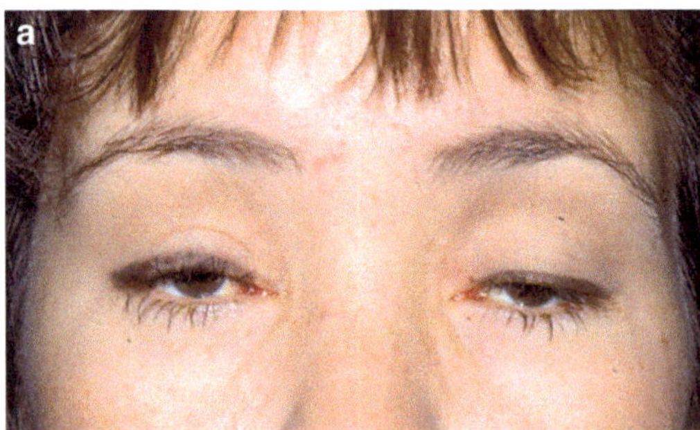

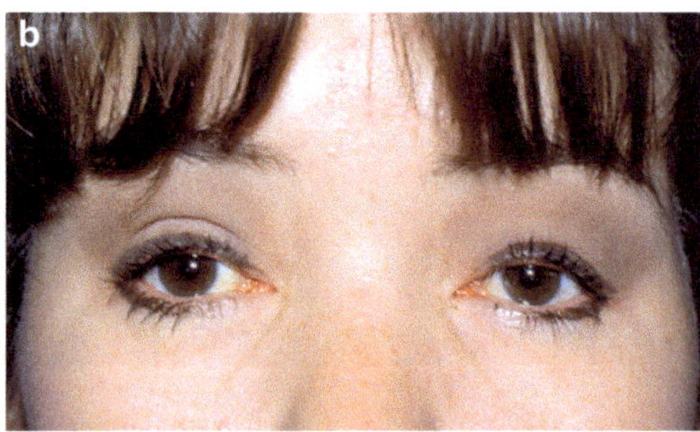

Fig. 23.5 (**a**) Preoperative appearance of a patient with congenital ptosis. (**b**) Postoperative appearance after autogenous fascia lata suspension demonstrating good lid height and contour

1. A 4-0 silk traction suture is placed in the central upper lid margin. Five incisions are made using a #15 blade. Two incisions are placed 3 mm above the lash line of the lid, corresponding to the medial and lateral edge of the corneal limbus, and carried down to the anterior tarsal surface. Two incisions are made at the superior brow hairs, just above the lid incisions, and carried down to periosteum. A similar forehead incision is made 1.5 cm above the superior brow hairs between the lateral and medial brow incisions. Tenotomy scissors are used to create a pocket superiorly beneath the frontalis muscle through the foreheadinc ision.
2. A bone plate coated with ophthalmic ointment is placed beneath the upper lid for corneal protection. An empty Wright needle is passed from the medial brow incision, posterior to the orbital septum, through the medial lid incision, taking care to avoid a full-thickness pass through the lid. The sling end is threaded through the needle, and pulled superiorly through the brow incision, where the end is retrieved. The opposite sling end is then brought from the medial lid incision to the lateral lid incision above the tarsus in a similarf ashion.
3. The empty Wright needle is passed from the lateral brow incision to the lateral lid incision, threaded, and pulled superiorly through the lateral brow incision (Fig. 23.6a). The empty Wright needle is then passed from the mid-forehead incision to the medial brow incision, threaded, and pulled superiorly through the mid-forehead incision where the end is retrieved. This is also performed to retrieve the end from lateral brow incision through the mid-foreheadinc ision(Fig. 23.6b).
4. When using silicone rods, a 3-mm silicone sleeve is placed over a hemostat, and the silicone ends are brought through the sleeve in a

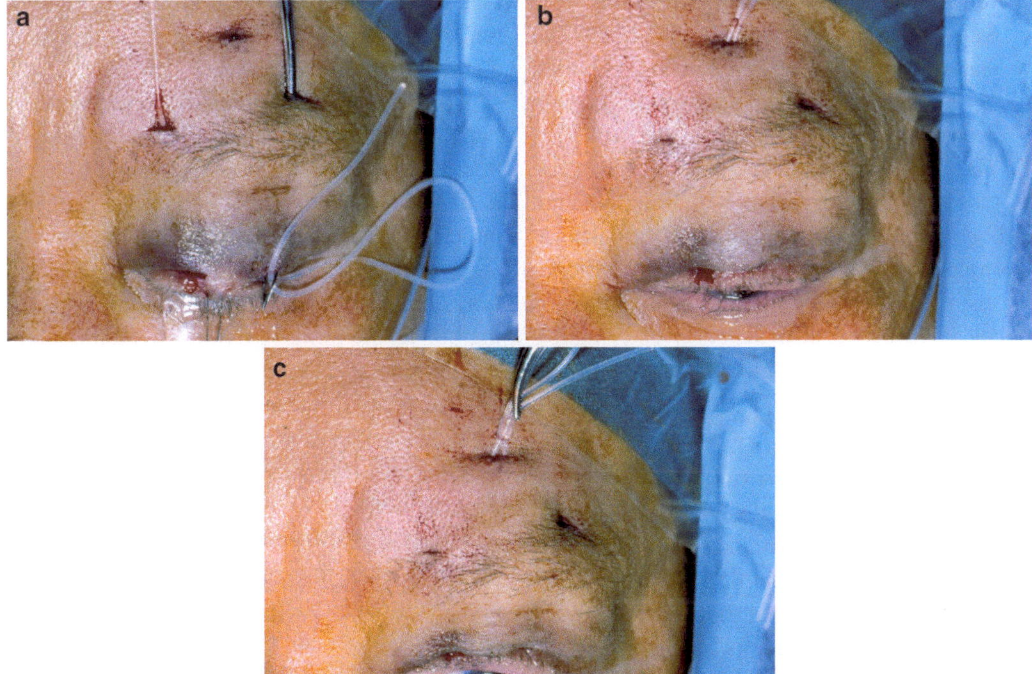

Fig. 23.6 Modified pentagonal Fox technique for frontalis suspension with silicone rod. (**a**) A silicone rod is threaded through the Wright needle before pulling the sling superiorly through the lateral brow incision. (**b**) Both ends of the silicone rod are brought through the mid-forehead incision. (**c**) The ends are brought through a 3-mm silicone sleeve. The sling tension is adjusted to achieve the desired lid height and contour before securing the sleeve into position with a 6-0 Nylon suture

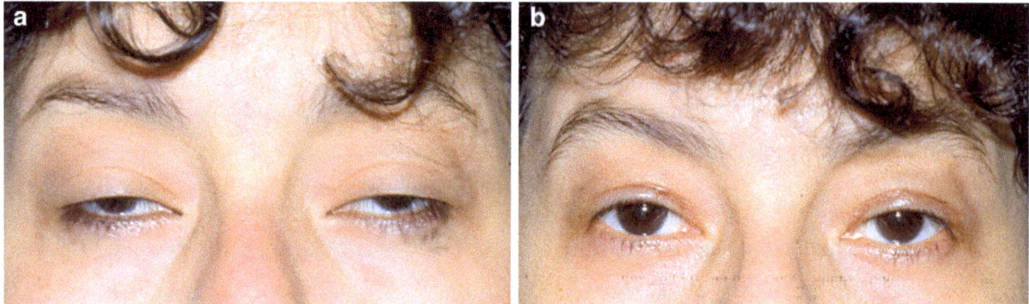

Fig. 23.7 (**a**) Preoperative appearance of a patient with chronic progressive external ophthalmoplegia. (**b**) Postoperative appearance after silicone rod frontalis suspension demonstrating good lid height and contour

parallel fashion (Fig. 23.6c). (Some surgeons prefer to pass the ends through the sleeve in opposite directions). The authors do not routinely fixate to the tarsus. The lid height is adjusted, and a 5-0 Nylon suture is passed through the sleeve and then wrapped around the silicone sling ends to prevent slippage of the loop. Care should be taken to not cut the sleeve or slings with the needle or suture. When using other synthetic materials, the ends are knotted together several times. All ends are left 10–15 mm in length and buried in the superior pocket previously created beneath the frontalis muscle.

5. The brow and mid-forehead incisions are closed using interrupted 6-0 chromic suture for subcutaneous tissue and 6-0 fast absorbing plain gut suture for skin. Antibiotic ophthalmic ointment is placed over the incisions and in the eyes. The patient is given IV antibioticsintra operatively(Fig. 23.7a,b).

Proper adjustment techniques vary for children and adults. When adjusting the lid height of a child intraoperatively, the surgeon should gently push the brow inferiorly to account for gravitational pull when the patient stands upright. With the brow in this position, the eyelid height should be set at the desired postoperative level. In the authors' experience, this produces excellent postoperative results with good predictability.

In adults, the height of the lid should be set slightly lower than in children, and lagophthalmos should be minimized. Avoidance of overcorrection is important, especially in adults with myasthenia gravis and third nerve palsy. Such adults carry increased risk for corneal exposure (due to weak eyelid closure and/or poor Bell's phenomenon) and diplopia secondary to impaired eye movement. Rather than positioning the lid for symmetry with the other side, the height should be set at an appropriate level above the pupil to prevent ocular surface issues. It is important to leave the silicone ends 10–15 mm in length from the sleeve to adjust the lid height in a graduated fashion, if needed.

Complications of frontalis sling placement include infection, granuloma formation, migration, and extrusion. The surgeon should be able to manage contour abnormalities, asymmetry, undercorrection, and overcorrection causing lagophthalmos. Passage of the sling too far inferiorly or anteriorly can cause eversion of the lid margin as the sling is tightened. Additionally, insufficient tarsus from prior surgery can lead to instability and unacceptable contour. Excess eyelid laxity can cause the sling to pull the eyelid away from the globe and create tear film abnormalities.

Frontalis suspension is the preferred method of ptosis repair in cases with poor levator function. Adjustable sling materials may have specific advantages in patients with progressive ptosis or who are at risk for corneal decompensation. In summary, excellent functional and aesthetic results can be obtained with frontalis slings when carefully placed with attention to surgical detail.

References

1. Jordan DR, Anderson RL. Obtaining fascia lata. Arch Ophthamol.1987; 105:1139–40.
2. Naugle Jr TC, Fry CL, Sabatier RE, Elliott LF. High leg incision fascia lata harvesting. Ophthalmology. 1997;104(9):1480–8.
3. Malhotra R, Selva D, Olver JM. Endoscopic harvesting of autogenous fascia lata. Ophthal Plast Reconstr Surg.2007;23(5):3 72–75.
4. Tellioglu AT, Saray A, Ergin A. Frontalis sling operation with deep temporal fascial graft in blepharoptosis repair. Plast Reconstr Surg. 2002;109(1):243–8.
5. Wong CY, Fan DSP, Ng JS, Goh TY, Lam DS. Long-term results of autogenous palmaris longus frontalis sling in children with congenital ptosis. Eye. 2005;19:546–8.
6. Lam DS, JS Ng, Cheng GP, Li RT. Autogenous palmaris longus tendon as frontalis suspension material for ptosis correction in children. Am J Ophthalmol. 1998;126:109–15.
7. Medel R, Alonso T, Giralt J, Torres J, González-Candial M, García-Arumí J. Frontalis muscle flap advancement with a pulley in the levator aponeurosis in patients with complete ptosis and deep-set eyes. Ophthal Plast Reconstr Surg. 2006;22(6):441–4.
8. Broughton WL, Matthews II JG, Harris Jr DJ. Congenital ptosis. Results of treatment using lyophilized fascia lata for frontalis suspensions. Ophthalmology.198 2;89(11):1261–6.
9. Wilson ME, Johnson RW. Congenital ptosis; long term results of treatment using lyophilized fascia lata for frontalis suspension. Ophthalmology. 1991;98:1234–37.
10. Esmaeli B, Chung H, Pashby RC. Long-term results of frontalis suspension using irradiated, banked fascia lata. Ophthal Plast Reconstr Surg. 1998;14(3):159–63.
11. Bodian M. Repair of ptosis using human sclera. Am J Ophthalmol.1968; 65:352–8.
12. Mehta P, Patel P, Olver JM. Functional results and complications of Mersilene mesh use for frontalis suspension ptosis surgery. Br J Ophthalmol. 2004;88:361–4.
13. Wasserman BN, Sprunger DT, Helveston EM. Comparison of materials used in frontalis suspension. Arch Ophthalmol. 2001;119:687–91.
14. Carter SR, Meecham WJ, Seiff SR. Silicone frontalis slings for the correction of blepharoptosis. Indications and efficacy. Ophthalmology. 1996;103(4):623–30.
15. Crawford JS. Repair of ptosis using frontalis muscle and fascia lata. Ophthalmology. 1956;60:672–8.
16. Fox SA. A new frontalis skin sling for ptosis. Am J Ophthalmol.1968; 65:359–62.
17. Friedenwald JS, Guyton JS. A simple ptosis operation: utilization of the frontalis by means of a single rhomboid-shaped suture. Am J Ophthalmol. 1948;31:411–4.
18. Tillet CW, Tillet GM. Silicone sling in the correction of ptosis. Am J Ophthalmol. 1966;62:521–3.
19. Rowan PJ, Hayes GS. Silicone sling for ptosis. South Med J. 1977;70:68–9.
20. Callahan MA, Beard C. Beard's ptosis. 4th ed. Burmingham, AL: Aesculapius Publishing Company; 1990.p.155–7,262–5.

PartV
OtherC onsiderations

Chapter 24
In-Office Surgery, Anesthesia, and Analgesia

C. Robert Bernardino

Abstract Ocular surface, refractive, cosmetic, plastic, and reconstructive surgery can now be performed safely and efficiently in the office setting without the aid of an anesthesiologist. To make the transition to office-based surgery, an ophthalmologist must minimize anxiety in the conscious patient, manage anesthesia during surgery, and prevent postoperative pain and nausea. Pearls on patient selection, conscious sedation, and pain and nausea prevention will be discussed.

The Transition to Office-Based Surgery

Ophthalmology is a specialty which embraces advances in technology in order to deliver better, and faster, eye care. This transition is evident where surgical services are offered. Intraocular surgery has transitioned from an inpatient endeavor to an outpatient, ambulatory affair. The next transition is to perform the surgery in the office; many surgical services can be offered safely and efficiently in the office setting.

C. R. Bernardino (✉)
Oculoplastics and Aesthetic Surgery,
Vantage Eye Center, 2 Upper Ragsdale
Drive, Suite B 130,
Monterey CA, 93940
e-mail: rbernardino@vantageeye.com

Reasons to Transition

Many of the reasons for transitioning from the inpatient setting to the ambulatory setting apply to this transition. The first reason is convenience for the surgeon and patients. Since the surgeon will operate out of the office, patient flow and scheduling of procedures are better controlled. Patients are familiar with the office, and they can typically just show up for surgery in the office without any specific preparation. Given the convenience of office surgery, patient satisfaction tends to be quite high.

Since the surgeon controls scheduling and patient flow, the patient processing is very efficient, leading to faster surgical turnover rates. In turn, the surgeon relies less on anesthesia and hospital staff to care for patients; this gives the surgeon additional control and higher satisfaction rates. A final consideration is financial. For most billing codes, the reimbursement is higher for surgery performed in the office when compared to an ambulatory surgery center or hospital setting. The higher reimbursement is to cover the cost of supplies and overhead. If the surgeon is careful with planning, in-office procedures can be more profitable than doing the surgery outside the office.

Surgical Space and Equipment

In order to successfully transition some procedures to the office, this requires a space to perform the surgical procedures. This can be as simple as a large

A.J. Cohen and D.A. Weinberg (eds.), *Evaluation and Management of Blepharoptosis*,
DOI 10.1007/978-0-387-92855-5_24, © Springer Science+Business Media, LLC 2011

eye lane or as involved as a dedicated minor procedure suite. Besides space, equipment is needed, including lighting (ceiling-mounted is ideal but not essential), microscope (if anterior segment procedures are performed), stool and surgical bed, surgical equipment, and supplies. The staff must be properly trained to assist and manage these office-based procedures including any postoperative and emergency situations that may arise.

StateR egulations

Prior to offering surgical procedures in the office, one has to ensure that they comply with any state regulations which might govern surgery performed in the office setting [1]. As of 2009, there are 21 states which have legislation on office-based surgery. These states include Alabama, California, Colorado, Florida, Illinois, Kansas, Louisiana, Massachusetts, Mississippi, New Jersey, New York, North Carolina, Ohio, Oklahoma, Oregon, Pennsylvania, Rhode Island, South Carolina, Tennessee, Texas, and Virginia. Although each state has nuances in the regulations, most have some common themes [2]. The first is based on level of sedation planned for a surgical procedure. Table 24.1 describes the level of sedation possible for a surgical procedure as originally defined by the American Society of Anesthesiology [3].

Surgery performed with minimal sedation is where oral medications are used for anxiolysis. At this level of sedation, patients have normal responsiveness and their breathing and cardiac function is unaffected.

At moderate levels of sedation, often called conscious sedation, responsiveness is further depressed. Whether intramuscular, intravenous, or inhaled medications are used, patients can still respond to purposeful verbal or tactile stimulus. Respiratory and cardiac function remains unaffected.

At deep levels of sedation, only painful or repeated stimulation causes a purposeful reaction from the patient. The patient's airway as well as spontaneous respiration can be affected, but cardiac function is intact.

General anesthesia, the deepest level of sedation, involves complete loss of patient responsiveness, even to painful stimuli. Respiratory and cardiac function can be compromised without direct intervention.

At a minimum, office-surgery regulations require that the surgeon and staff be prepared for emergency situations [4]. Therefore, the office must be equipped with a "crash cart" which should include an oral airway with positive pressure, and basic medications including epinephrine and atropine. The surgeon and staff should also be trained with the surgeon typically needing a minimum of Basic Cardiac Life Support certification. In some states, this is required even if one is only using local anesthetics or oral antianxiety medications; therefore, it is important to check local regulations. There should also be a dedicated transfer plan arranged with a local hospital in case of emergencies; the surgeon needs to have admitting/surgical privileges at that hospital. Documentation is also key when performing

Table24. 1 Levelsof s edation

	Minimals edation (anxiolysis)	Moderates edation/analgesia (conscious sedation)	Deep sedation/analgesia	General anesthesia
Responsiveness	Normalr esponse to verbal stimulation	Purposeful response to verbal or tactile stimulation	Purposeful response to repeated or painful stimulation	Unarousable,e ven to painful stimuli
Airway	Unaffected	Noi nterventionr equired	Interventionm aybe required	Interventionof ten required
Spontaneous ventilation	Unaffected	Adequate	Maybe i nadequate	Frequently inadequate
Cardiovascular function	Unaffected	Usuallym aintained	Usuallym aintained	Maybe i mpaired

surgical procedures in the office. Informed consent should be well documented in the medical record as well as a surgical procedure note. Finally, infection controls must be in place.

For many states, moderate sedation is defined as sedation which is delivered by intravenous, intramuscular, or inhaled medications. Regulations require the monitoring of vital signs (oxygen saturation, blood pressure, and level of sedation) preoperatively and during the procedure. For IV sedation, a running ECG strip and body temperature monitoring is also required. The surgeon should also be certified in Advanced Cardiac Life Support. Postoperatively, the patient needs to be evaluated by a dedicated staff member who documents O_2 saturation, blood pressure, pain control, and level of consciousness. Once a patient is stable for discharge, discharge instructions must be given and documented.

ProcedureS election

Many surgeries can be performed safely and efficiently in the office setting. However, certain surgeries may be better served in the ambulatory surgical center (ASC) or in the in-patient setting. Table 24.2 summarizes reasons why a surgery should be performed outside the office setting. In short, if you cannot provide a comfortable and safe environment for the patient's procedure in the office, then the surgery should be offered elsewhere. When considering appropriate surgical procedures for the office, the more complex the surgery, the less amenable it may be for the office; these issues of surgical complexity may include the presence of multiple surgical sites, the difficulty to anesthetize the surgical site, the risk of blood loss, and the risk of infection. Table 24.3 highlights some of the procedures that an ophthalmologist may consider performing in the offices etting.

Table 24.2 Reasons to operate in an ASC or in-patient setting

ASC	Unable to anesthetize surgical site in the office
	Unable to address anxiety issues in the office setting
	Lack of equipment or trained staff
	Need for higher sterility
In-patient	Complicated patient comorbidities requiring monitoring
	Patient needs hospital admission after surgery
	Need for special equipment or multiple surgeons

Table 24.3 Possible procedures performed in the office setting

Plastics	Eyelid, brow, forehead, midface, and lower face surgery (cosmetic and reconstructive), skin lasers, dermal fillers, abscess drainage including lacrimal, eyelid, periocular
Cornea/anterior segment	Pterygium excision, refractive surgery, simple corneal laceration or wound dehiscence repair, cryotherapy
Pediatrics/ strabismus	Lacrimal probing, extraocular muscle adjustments
Retina	Intravitreal injections, laser, and cryotherapy
Glaucoma	Bleb needling or revisions, laser, and cryotherapy

PatientSel ection

Like surgery selection, patient selection is important; the right patient can have surgery with minimal discomfort and risk of complication. Factors to be considered when offering surgery in the office include age and mental status of the patient, language barriers, comorbidities, ability to position the patient, and medications the patient is taking.

It is important to consider a patient's mental status when offering surgery in the office. The patient must be able to follow simple commands and be able to express pain or discomfort during the procedure. If there is any language barrier between the surgeon and the patient, this may limit the ability to successfully perform surgery on the patient in the office.

Comorbidities which make office-based surgery potentially unsafe include significant cardiovascular problems, sleep apnea, and latex allergies. Also, patients who cannot be comfortably positioned in the office including pregnant patients or those who cannot lie still for the procedure may not be optimal office surgery candidates. Furthermore, abnormal vital signs, and, in particular, uncontrolled hypertension can be a problem. Not only is hypertension a risk for bleeding during surgery, it is also a risk for cardiovascular events during surgery including stroke or myocardial infarction. Patient with systolic blood pressure ≥180 mm Hg and/or diastolic blood pressure ≥110 mm Hg should be rescheduled and referred to their medical doctor or emergency department for urgent evaluation.

Patient medications are the final piece of the puzzle when selecting the appropriate patients for office surgery. The main medications, which may alter the ability to offer safe surgery in the office, are those which inhibit coagulation. A surgeon needs to balance the risk of discontinuation of the medicine (stroke or heart attack) versus the risk of hemorrhage. The main medications which fall into this group are aspirin, nonsteroidal antiinflammatory drugs (NSAIDs), clopidogrel (Plavix, Bristol-Myers Squibb, New York, NY and sanofi-aventis US LLC, Bridgewater, NJ), and warfarin (Coumadin, Bristol-Myers Squibb, New York, NY) [5]. Table 24.4 lists these drugs and when they should be discontinued. Finally, herbal medications should be considered since many patients take these supplements without realizing that they can affect their risk for bleeding during surgery. Table 24.5 covers the most common herbal supplements that might affect surgery. In general, these should be stopped 7–10 days before surgery and may be resumed a day after surgery.

Table 24.4 Medications which inhibit coagulation

Medication	Discontinue (prior to surgery)	Resume (after surgery)
Aspirin	7–10 days	1 day
Clopidogrel (Plavix[a, b])	7–10 days (consult internist – beware of patients with cardiac stents)	1 day
NSAIDs	1 day for short-acting NSAID like ibuprofen/up to 3 days for long acting NSAID like naproxen	1 day
Warfarin (Coumadin[b])	3–14 days (consult internist)	1 day
Enoxaparin (Lovenox[a])	1 day	1 day

[a]Manufactured by Bristol-Myers Squibb, New York, NY
[b]Manufactured by Sanofi-Aventis U.S. LLC, Bridgewater, NJ

Table 24.5 Common herbal supplements and associated risks

Supplement	Hemorrhage	Hypertension
Ephedra		X
Feverfew	X	
Garlic	X	
Ginger	X	
Gingko Biloba	X	
Ginseng	X	
l-Tryptophan		X
Vitamin E	X	
Yohimbe		X

Evaluating Patients at Risk for Anxiety

The first task is recognizing that patients undergoing any invasive procedure can experience anxiety. Patients may not be able to completely describe what they are feeling, but often report a feeling of uneasiness or fear. This sensation is associated with an adrenergic response, leading to increased blood pressure and pulse, and dryness of the mouth. These symptoms can be exacerbated by pain or situations that are overstimulating.

When interviewing patients for a possible surgical procedure, it is important to prescreen them for anxiety. Factors that may be a sign of risk for anxiety around surgery include previous intolerance to surgical procedures or sitting still, history of pain intolerance, medical history of anxiety or other mental illness, or a medical condition leading to lability of blood pressure or heart rate. Patients who may be at risk for anxiety may benefit from techniques to reduce anxiety, or may be better candidates for surgery outside the office setting.

Nonmedical Prevention of Anxiety

Whether a patient is at risk for anxiety or not, all patients will benefit from techniques (medical and non-medical) to prevent anxiety during surgery. Nonmedical techniques are the easiest and should become a part of the standard operating procedure. The most important is probably the attitude of the surgeon and staff. If the surgeon exudes confidence, and talks with a calm and friendly voice before, during, and after the procedure, then it would help keep a patient calm and relaxed during surgery.

Likewise, if the environment of the office and staff is calm and relaxing, the patient will be more at ease. A distracting office environment and a hyperkinetic staff can add to patient anxiety. The surgical suite, whether an examination lane or dedicated procedure room, should be comfortable. Playing soft music, ensuring the ambient temperature is optimal, and putting the patient at ease can facilitate a comfortable procedure.

Medical Prevention of Anxiety

Pharmacologic intervention, when used properly, can make a case easily tolerable for the patient. In these instances, the ideal medication or "silver bullet" to treat anxiety around surgery would have a fast onset and resolution with no "hang-over," be an anxiolytic and a sedative, prevent pain, stabilize hemodynamic lability, and be amnestic. No single drug possesses these characteristics, but selection of certain medications can treat anxiety effectively and safely.

There are three main classes of drugs used to prevent anxiety in the office setting – opioids, benzodiazepines, and antiadrenergics. The classic opioid is morphine sulfate, acting as an analgesic and sedative. Diazepam (Valium, Roche Laboratories, Basel, Switzerland), a benzodiazepine works as an anxiolytic and sedative. Clonidine (Catapres, Boehringer Ingelheim Pharmaceuticals, Inc., Ridgefield, CT), known for its antihypertensive properties, also can provide analgesia and sedation. These are summarized in Table 24.6.

Table 24.6 Classesof s edatives

Class	Example	Effect	Side-effect
Opioids	Morphine sulfate	Analgesic	Respiratory depression
		Sedative	Nausea/ vomiting
Benzodiaz-epines	Diazepam (Valium[a])	Sedative	Respiratory depression
			Lowerspa in threshold
Antiadren-ergic	Clonidine	Analgesic	Longha lfl ife (8–12 h)
		Sedative	Vascular effects at high doses

[a]Manufactured by Roche Laboratories, Basel, Switzerland

Table 24.7 Clonidine dosing based on blood pressure

SystolicB P	Clonidinedos e
≤105	None
>105	0.1 µg
>160	0.2 µg

If patient >80 years old or <110 lbs, decrease dose by 50%
If BP >140 after 40 min, may augment with 0.1 µg

Clonidine deserves special mention because it has many of the characteristics of the ideal anxiolytic [6]. Clonidine works centrally, stimulating the alpha-adrenoreceptors in the brain stem. In turn, it reduces sympathetic outflow, decreasing peripheral vascular resistance, heart rate, and blood pressure. Clonidine has an onset of 30 min and must be dosed based on systolic blood pressure. Table 24.7 summarizes the clonidine dosing based on systolic blood pressure.

Once a medication is selected to pretreat anxiety, one needs to consider its onset of action. For patients who are particularly nervous about a procedure, dosing the night before surgery can be helpful in allowing for a restful night prior to surgery. It is also reasonable to administer the medication on the morning of surgery; but its effects may wear off before the time of surgery. Preprocedural use is also helpful; the patient is instructed to arrive about 30 min before surgery. Their vital signs are checked, and then the medication is given. The patient should be asked if they feel the effects of the medication, and, if so, surgery may begin. During surgery, if the patient needs more sedation, a sublingual tablet may be given. Table 24.8 is a summary of the common

Table24.8 Orals edation

Drug	Class	Dosage	Notes
Acetaminophen 325/Oxycodone 5 (Percocet[a])	O	1–2t ablets	Antiinflammatory
Acetaminophen 300/Codeine 30 (Tylenol #3[b])	O	1–2t ablets	Antiinflammatory
Meperidine(D emerol[c])	O	50–100m g	Analgesic
Morphines ulfate	O	10–30m g	Analgesic
Alprazolam(Xanax[d])	B	0.5–1m gi ncrements	Shorta cting
Midazolam(V ersed[e])	B	0.1–0.2m g/kg	Shorta cting
Lorazepam(A tivan[f])	B	2–4m g	Mediumdur ation
Diazepam(Valium[e])	B	5–10m g	Longa cting
Clonidine	A	1.5 μg/kg	Peak at 60 min

O opioid; *B* benzodiazepine; *A*a ntiadrenergic

[a]Manufactured by Endo Pharmaceuticals, Chadds Ford, PA

[b]Manufactured by Ortho-McNeil-Janssen Pharmaceuticals, Inc., Raritan, NJ

[c]Manufactured by sanofi-aventis U.S., LLC, Bridgewater, NJ

[d]Manufactured by Pfizer, Inc., New York, NY

[e]Manufactured by Roche Laboratories, Basel, Switzerland

[f]Manufactured by Biovail Pharmaceuticals, Inc., Bridgewater, NJ

Table24.9 Orals edationpr otocole xample

Length of case	Benzodiazepine	Type of case
<1 h	Xanax 0.5 mg or Valium 5 mg	Upper lid surgery
1–1.5h	Xanax1m g	Complicated eyelid surgery
>1.5 h	Xanax 1 mg+Triazolam (Halcion[a]) 0.25 mg	4 Lid surgery/face lift/brow coronal surgery

[a]Manufactured by Pfizer, Inc., New York, NY

medications used for office-based procedures. Note that short acting drugs have a faster onset; therefore alprazolam (Xanax, Pfizer, Inc., New York, NY) or midazolam (Versed, Roche Laboratories, Basel, Switzerland) are perfect for short office procedures. Table 24.9 is a sample protocol using multiple classes of sedatives for different surgical procedures.

If used appropriately, these drugs are unlikely to cause serious adverse reactions or over-sedation. However, the surgeon should always be prepared for those possibilities. To treat a benzodiazepine reaction, flumazenil (Romazicon, Roche Laboratories, Basel, Switzerland) can be given, 0.2 mg IV over 15 s, then 0.2 mg every minute for a total of 1 mg as needed. Naloxone (Narcan, Endo Pharmaceuticals, Chadds Ford, PA) is used for an opioid overdose, 0.4–2 mg IV/IM/SC and can be repeated every 2–3 min for a total dose of 10 mg.

During surgery, if the patient has any discomfort or anxiety, the cause of pain or discomfort should be determined and alleviated with local anesthesia, if possible. Assuring the patient during the surgery and having a staff member hold a hand are helpful. Increasing sedation should be considered, as needed.

Postoperative Nausea and Vomiting

Besides anxiety, postoperative nausea and vomiting (PONV) can turn a surgical experience into a miserable one. Besides retching and vomiting, a patient may experience the unpleasant sensation of nausea. Thirty percent of all procedures are associated with PONV. PONV can cause wound dehiscence, hematoma, and aspiration [7].

Like anxiety there are certain factors for which patients can be prescreened. These factors include a history of motion sickness, PONV, or low pain tolerance, and surgical issues such as extended surgical times and procedures around the eye or face.

Although there are many medications to prevent and/or treat PONV, many nonmedical interventions work well. The first is preoperative fasting at least 6 h for solid meals and 2 h for liquids. Furthermore, reducing anxiety during the surgery

Table24. 10 Medications for PONV prophylaxis and treatment

Drug	Class	Sedating	Dosage	Notes
Prochlorperazine maleate (Compazine[a])	Phenothiazine	Y	5–10m ge very3–4h	EPS
Promethazine(Phenergan[b])	Phenothiazine	Y	12.5–25m ge very4–8h	EPS
Trimethobenzamide(Tigan[c])	Benzamide	Y	250m ge very6–8h	EPS
Metoclopramide(Reglan[d])	Benzamide	Y	10–20m ge very3–4h	EPS
Ondansetron(Zofra n[e])	Serotonin5- HT3 antagonist	N	8–16 mg every 6–8 h	Sublingual

Extra-pyramidal symptoms (EPS): Involuntary muscle contractions or spasms can occur as a side effect of these medications. Patients with a history of this side effect should not be given these classes of medications

[a]Manufactured by GlaxoSmithKline, London, UK

[b]Manufactured by Baxter Healthcare Corp., Deerfield, IL

[c]Manufactured by JHP Pharmaceuticals, Parsippany, NJ

[d]Manufactured by Alaven Pharmaceuticals, LLC, Marietta, GA

[e]Manufactured by GlaxoSmithKline, London, UK

Table24 .11 Commont opicala nesthetic

Name	Tradena me	Strength	Notes
Cocainetopic als olution		1–4%	Controlleds ubstance
Lidocainetopic als olution		4%	
Proparacaine	Alcaine[a]	0.5%	
Tetracaine		0.5%	More painful initially than proparacaine
Benoxinate/fluorescein	Fluress[b]	0.4%/0.25%s ol	
Fluorescein/proparacaine	Fluoracaine[b]	0.25%/0.5%s ol	
Lidocainevi scousge l	Akten[b]	3.5%	Povadone iodine must be used first in surgery

Typical onset = 1 min, typical duration = 30 min for all topical anesthetics

[a]Manufactured by Alcon Laboratories, Inc., Fort Worth, TX

[b]Manufactured by Akorn, Inc., Lakeforest IL

may help prevent PONV. Controlling pain during and after surgery is important, although opioids may also contribute to PONV. Limiting position changes during surgery, that is, making the patient sit up and sit down, can help prevent PONV.

If PONV needs to be treated, many medications are available and are quite effective. These are summarized in Table 24.10. All of these drugs are quite effective at treating PONV. All except odansetron (Zofran, GlaxoSmithKline, London, UK) have the risk of extrapyramidal symptoms, in which patients develop involuntary muscle contractions. A history of this side effect may preclude use of these drugs.

Anesthesiaf orSur gery

The goals of perioperative anesthesia include minimizing pain and sensation during facilitation hemostasis via epinephrine injection (if desired) and preventing postoperative pain. Anesthetics for ocular and periocular surgery come in three varieties – topical, local injection, and regional block.

TopicalA nesthetics

Topical anesthetics have many advantages over injectables. These include fast onset, eliminating risk of globe injury/perforation; ocular motility and pupillary function are unaffected. They do not cause vasoconstriction, and some topical medications can block the bactericidal effects of povadone iodine (Betadine, Purdue Pharma LP, Stamford, CT). Table 24.11 is a list of common topical anesthetics used for ocular surgery. These topical anesthetics have an onset of 1 min and duration of action of 20–30 min. These topical anesthetics work only on mucous membranes, such as the ocular surface.

Ice and EMLA are two effective topical anesthetics [8]. Underutilized, ice can work as a quick anesthetic, particularly for small excisional biopsies or to dampen the pain from injections. It is quite helpful before botulinum toxin or filler injections. EMLA, or Eutetic Mixture of Local Anesthetic (APP Pharmaceuticals, LLC, Schaumburg, IL), is a 5% mixture of topical prilocaine and lidocaine [9]. It is commonly used prior to IV insertion, but is useful before injections and laser skin surgery. However, its onset is up to 90 min and requires an occlusive dressing to facilitate skin absorption. Common side effects from these topical anesthetics can include lightheadedness, local erythema and edema, and allergic reactions, while serious reactions including arrhythmias and seizures have been reported. Other topical anesthetics exist including topical lidocaine 3% in a lotion or cream (LidaMantle, PharmaDerm, Melville, NY), lidocaine 3.5% ophthalmic gel (Akten, Akorn, Inc., Lakeforest IL) as well as a generic 4% solution or 5% ointment; these all have similar efficacy.

InjectableA nesthetics

Injectable anesthetics can be used locally around the surgical site and regionally via a nerve block. Local injections work well because the anesthetic is placed directly at the surgical site. If vasoconstriction is desired, epinephrine may be employed. Disadvantages of local anesthetic injections include tissue distortion and muscle paresis, both of which may be problematic during external levator resection surgery, in which intraoperative titration of eyelid height and contour is critical for the optimal result. In such cases, the minimum amount of local anesthetic injection necessary should be used, that is, less than 1 cc per upper eyelid.

Regional blocks work by delivering anesthetic to a nerve supplying the surgical site. Examples include frontal, supraorbital, lacrimal, and infraorbital nerve blocks. The quantity of local anesthetic necessary is typically reduced with a regional block. Excellent intraoperative and postoperative pain control can be achieved, particularly if a long-acting anesthetic is used. However, the advantage of local vasoconstriction with epinephrine is lost, unless one combines a regional and local block.

When choosing an injectable anesthetic, time of onset and duration are factors to consider. Typically, fast-acting anesthetics have a shorter duration whereas long-lasting anesthetics have a longer time of onset, and therefore the surgeon has to plan appropriately. In order to take advantage of faster onset of one medication and longer duration of another, anesthetics can be mixed. Table 24.12 has a list of commonly used injectable anesthetics.

Injectables may be modified with the addition of epinephrine for vasoconstriction. All anesthetics cause vasodilatation, except cocaine, and can exacerbate bleeding. Therefore, epinephrine is compounded into many local anesthetics to

Table24 .12 Commoni njectablea nesthetics

Name	Maximumdos e	Onset	Duration
Bupivicaine 0.25–0.75% (Marcaine[a])	2 mg/kg or 175 mg/dose, 400 mg/24 h	2–10 min	3–6 h
Chloroprocaine 1–3% (Nesacaine[b])	11 mg/kg or 800 mg/dose	6–12 min	0.5–1 h
Lidocaine 1–2% (Xylocaine[b])	4 mg/kg or 280 mg/dose	4–6 min	0.75–1.5 h
Mepivacaine 1–2% (Carbocaine[a])	4 mg/kg or 400 mg/dose	3–5 min	0.75–1.5 h
Procaine 1–4% (Novocain[a])	10 mg/kg or 1,000 mg/dose	2–5 min	0.5 h
Ropivacaine 0.25–1% (Naropin[c])	2.5 mg/kg or 300 mg/dose	1–15 min	2–6 h

Note: Epinephrine can double the duration of an anesthetic and decrease the systemic toxicity

[a]Manufactured by Hospira, Inc., Lake Forest, IL

[b]Manufactured by APP Pharmaceuticals, Schaumburg, IL

[c]Manufactured by AstraZeneca Pharmaceuticals, LP, London, UK

Table24.13 Oralm edicationsf orm ildpa in

Drug	Dosing(mg)	Onset	Duration(h)
Aspirin	325–650	30m in	3–4
Acetaminophen	325–650	15–30m in	3–4
Ibuprofen	200–800	30m in	4–6
Naproxen(Naprosyn[a])	250–500	60m in	6–12
Indomethacin(Indocin[b])	25–75	30m in	4–12
Piroxicam(Feldene[c])	10–20	1–2h	24

[a]Manufactured by Roche Laboratories, Basel, Switzerland

[b]Manufactured by Iroko Pharmaceuticals LLC, Philadelphia, PA

[c]Manufactured by Pfizer Inc., New York, NY

improve hemostasis, prolong the anesthetic effect, and decrease systemic toxicity. Epinephrine should be used with caution when operating on a digit, that is, finger or toe, since tissue necrosis may occur. Furthermore, if pupil dilation is not desired, epinephrine should be avoided.

Anesthetics are acidic by nature, and therefore buffering an anesthetic with sodium bicarbonate can reduce the pain associated with injection [10]; 8.4% sodium bicarbonate is usually added to local anesthetic in a 1:5 ratio. Although it is believed that buffering an anesthetic may decrease the efficacy of the anesthetic, Davies [11] found no decrease in efficacy after buffering in a metaanalysis of 63 articles.

PostoperativePai nC ontrol

Proper intraoperative prevention of pain with appropriate anesthesia will help reduce postoperative pain. Nonetheless most patients will experience some discomfort after surgery. Educating the patient to anticipate some degree of pain and appropriate dosing of analgesia can minimize postoperative pain and anxiety [12]. Patients who are informed about the possibility of postoperative pain and the amount of discomfort they might experience are more accepting of it and are able to deal with it better, with potentially less anxiety about the pain. Therefore, telling the patient that there will be no discomfort after surgery is doing them a disservice and may reduce pain tolerance. Anticipating the amount of pain a patient may experience after a procedure is essential.

Treating postoperative pain should be performed in a staged approach [13]. The first level of analgesics is NSAIDs or acetaminophen. These are effective for mild postoperative discomfort. However, NSAIDs and aspirin may increase the risk for postoperative hemorrhage or hematoma. The drugs used for mild pain relief are listed in Table 24.13.

For patients with moderate pain, adding a narcotic to a NSAID or acetaminophen is appropriate. For convenience, many combination drugs are available. Table 24.14 lists the most common combination analgesics. When using any combination drug, one must be mindful that the maximum dose of acetaminophen is 4.0 g per day and 1,000 mg per dose based on average liver clearance; therefore if a patient is taking a combination medication with acetaminophen, such as acetaminophen 500 mg/oxycodone 5 mg (Roxicet, Boehringer Ingelheim Pharmaceuticals, Inc., Ridgefield, CT) two tablets every 4 h, s/he is taking a total of 6,000 mg of acetaminophen which exceeds the 4.0 g safety level. Following this scenario, two Roxicets every 4 h has an equivalent of 60 mg of oxycodone per day. Substituting oxycodone (OxyContin, Purdue Pharma LP, Stamford, CT) 30 mg every 12 h provides an equivalent narcotic dose, and one may supplement with Roxicet for breakthrough pain. In these cases, an analgesic for severe pain listed on Table 24.15 should be used, and the combination medication used for breakthrough pain. Of course, one must

Table24 .14 Oralme dicationsf orm oderatepa in

Trade	Generic	Dose
Darvocet N 100[a]	100 mg PNAP/650 mg APAP	1 tablet every 4 h maximum 6 tablets in 24 h
Darvon[a]	65 mg PHCL	1 tablet every 4 h maximum 6 tablets in 24 h
Lortab7.5/500 [b]	7.5 mg HCD/500 mg APAP	1 tablet every 4–6 h maximum 8 tablets in 24 h
Percocet5/325 [c]	5 mg Oxycodone/325 APAP	1–2 tablet every 6 h maximum 12 tablets in 24 h
Tylenol#3 [d]	30 mg codeine/300 mg APAP	1–2 tablet every 4 h maximum 12 tablets in 24 h
Vicodin[e]	5 mg HCD/500 mg APAP	1–2 tablet every 4–6 h maximum 8 tablets in 24 h

APAP acetaminophen; *HCD* hydrocodone; *PHCL* propoxyphene HCL; *PNAP* propoxyphene napsylate

[a] Manufactured by Xanodyne Pharmaceuticals, Inc., Newport, KY

[b] Manufactured by UCB Pharma, Inc., Brussels, Belgium

[c] Manufactured by Endo Pharmaceuticals, Chadds Ford, PA

[d] Manufactured by Ortho-McNeil-Janssen Pharmaceuticals, Inc., Raritan, NJ

[e] Manufactured by Abbott Laboratories, Abbott Park, IL

Table24.15 Oralme dicationsf ors everepa in

Trade	Generic	Dosing
Demerol[a]	Meperidine	5–10 mg every 3–4 h
Dilaudid[b]	Hydromorphone	2–4 mg every 4–6 h
MSC ontin[b]	Morphine sulfate extended release	30–60 mg every 12 h
OxyContin[b]	Oxycodone extended release	10–80 mg every 12 h
Percocet10/650 [c]	10 mg Oxycodone/650 mg APAP	1 tab every 6 h

[a]Manufactured by sanofi-aventis U.S. LLC, Bridgewater, NJ

[b]Manufactured by Purdue Pharma LP, Stamford, CT

[c]Manufactured by Endo Pharmaceuticals, Chadds Ford, PA

keep in mind that severe pain may herald the presence of a potentially serious complication, for example, hemorrhage, infection, or corneal abrasion.

Preventing pain with proper anesthesia during surgery, patient education, and postoperative analgesia will improve the patient experience and allow the surgeon to successfully perform many procedures in the office [14].

Conclusion

Offering surgical services in the office can give a surgeon better control of patient flow, may be financially advantageous, and can make the experience more tolerable for the patient. However, office-based surgery should be well thought out and should anticipate patients' issues including preventing and managing anxiety, intraoperative and postoperative pain, and postoperative nausea and vomiting. Furthermore, selecting the appropriate patients and types of procedures for the office will increase the chances of a successful outcome. Finally, a protocol for the day of surgery will allow for a seamless flow of patients and ensure that quality care and safety are provided. Table 24.16 is a sample office surgery protocol. This can be used as a guideline to create a customized protocol for thes urgeon'sne eds.

Table24.16 Offices urgerypr otocol

Patient arrives 30 min before procedure
Must be accompanied by family member or friend
Check vital signs (blood pressure and pulse; consider O_2 pulse oximetry if using significant oral sedation)
Obtain surgical consent
Preoperative medication
Xanax 1.0 mg (0.5 mg tabs × 2)
Clonidine according to protocol
Check for sedation
If adequate, administer anesthetic
Consider topical anesthetic or ice before injection
If inadequate, supplement with Xanax 0.25–0.5 mg
After surgery
Assess/addresspa in
Ice packs to surgical site (unless a skin graft was used)
Acetaminophen 650 mg
Lortab or Percocet for breakthrough pain
OxyContin for significant anticipated pain
Discharge patient when ambulatory
Evening/day after surgery
Contact patient to ensure patient satisfaction and pain control and to answer any questions and address all patient concerns
Confirm postoperative instructions – medications, dressing changes, etc.
Confirm follow-up appointment

References

1. Sutton JH. Office-based surgery regulation: improving patient safety and quality care. Bull Am Coll Surg. 2001;86(2):8–12.
2. Sutton JH. Patient safety update – office based surgery regulation expands. Bull Am Coll Surg. 2002;87(4):20–4.
3. American Society of Anesthesiology. Continuum of Depth of Sedation. Joint Commission on Accreditation of Hospitals, House of Deligates. Oct. 1999.
4. American Society of Anesthesiologists Task Force on Sedation and Analgesia by Non-Anesthesiologists. Practice guidelines for sedation and analgesia by non-anesthesiologists. Anesthesiology. 2002;96:1004–17.
5. Otley CC, Fewkes JL, Frank W, Olbricht SM. Complications of cutaneous surgery in patients who are taking warfarin, aspirin, or nonsteroidal anti-inflammatory drugs. Arch Dermatol. 1996;132:161–6.
6. Maze M, Segal IS, Bloor BC. Clonidine and other alpha2 adrenergic agonists: strategies for the rational use of these novel anesthetic agents. J Clin Anesth. 1988;1(2):146–57.
7. Kranke P, Schuster F, Eberhart LH. Recent advances, trends and economic considerations in the risk assessment, prevention and treatment of postoperative nausea and vomiting. Expert Opin Pharmacother. 2007;8(18):3217–35.
8. Chen BK, Eichenfield LF. Pediatric anesthesia in dermatology surgery: when hand-holding is not enough. Dermatol Surg. 2001;27:1010–8.
9. Friedman PM, Mafong EA, Friedman ES, Geronemus RG. Topical anesthetics update: EMLA and beyond. Dermatol Surg. 2001;27:1019–26.
10. Hanna MN, Elhassan A, Veloso PM, et al. Efficacy of bicarbonate in decreasing pain on intradermal injection of local anesthetics: a meta-analysis. Reg Anesth Pain Med. 2009;34(2):122–5.
11. Davies RJ. Buffering the pain of local anaesthetics: a systematic review. Emerg Med (Fremantle). 2003;15(1):81–8.
12. Crews JC. Multimodal pain management strategies for office-based and ambulatory procedures. JAMA. 2002;288(5):629–32.
13. Ducharme J. Acute pain and pain control: state of the art. Ann Emerg Med. 2000;35(6):592–603.
14. Schecter WP, Bongard FS, Gainor BJ, Weltz DL, Horn JK. Pain control in outpatient surgery. J Am CollS urg.2002; 195(1):95–104.

Chapter25
Ethnicand G enderC onsiderationsi nPt osisSur gery

Jed Poll and Michael T. Yen

Abstract All eyelids are not created equal. There are many anatomical and technical differences when evaluating and treating blepharoptosis in different genders and different ethnicities. This chapter reviews some of the ethnic and gender issues that a surgeon should consider when performingble pharoptosisre pair.

All ptotic eyelids are not created equal. This chapter addresses ethnic and gender differences in blepharoptosis. With regard to eyelid and facial surgery, much of what we aim to accomplish as surgeons is dictated by our patients' self-awareness and perception of how their eyelids and facial structures do and should appear. Ethnic and gender identification plays an important role in self perception and therefore serves as a useful framework in guiding assessment and surgical intervention. Ethnic and gender differences in eyelid shape, height, contour, and anatomy require an individualistic, rather than a "cookbook," approach to ptosis repair.

While there are certainly ethnic and gender differences in eyelid and facial anatomy, and the surgical techniques used may be directed towards these unique anatomical features [1–5], perhaps the most important element to successful eyelid surgery is understanding what the patient desires to achieve. While a single surgical technique could be used across all gender and ethnic lines, it would likely yield an unsatisfactory result and an unhappy patient. For example, many female patients desire to have a tight upper eyelid to serve as a flat platform for their cosmetic products (Fig. 25.1a, b). To give this appearance to a male patient is possible, and could technically be considered a surgical success, but is usually not the desired surgical outcome. Similarly, many Asian patients do not desire the deep superior sulcus and high eyelid crease that is often associated with the occidental eyelid. Yet, when some Asian patients present for surgical evaluation, they express their desire for the "double-eyelid" appearance to be synonymous with the occidental eyelid. Discordant expectations between surgeon and patient can often be avoided with a thorough and thoughtful preoperative discussion with the patient who identifies his/her unique anatomical features and desired postoperative appearance. This can be challenging if cultural or language barriers limit the preoperative discussion, but must be accomplished if a successful outcome is to be achieved.

GenderC onsiderations in Ptosis Surgery

To understand and appreciate how gender interplays with ptosis evaluation and repair, we must return to eyelid anatomy. Evaluating and at times manipulating the upper eyelid crease is very important. Careful attention to eyelid crease

M.T.Y en (✉)
Cullen Eye Institute, , Department of Ophthalmology
BaylorC ollegeof M edicine, Houston, TX, USA
e-mail:mye n@bcm.tmc.edu

A.J. Cohen and D.A. Weinberg (eds.), *Evaluation and Management of Blepharoptosis*,
DOI 10.1007/978-0-387-92855-5_25, © Springer Science+Business Media, LLC 2011

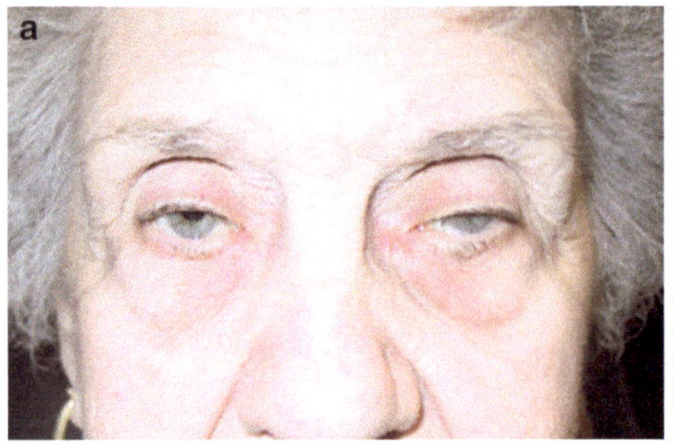
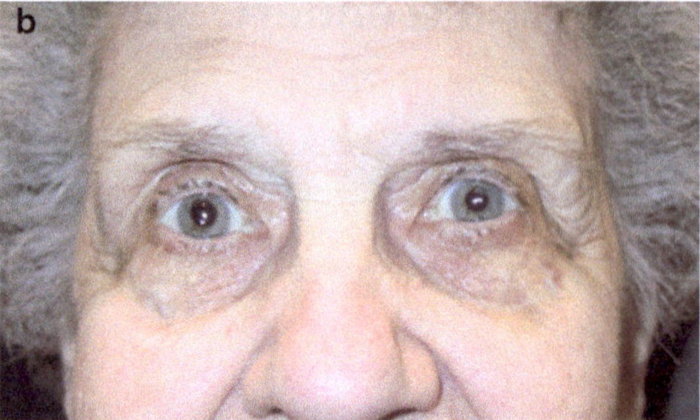

Fig. 25.1 (**a**) A 72-year-old female with the classical appearance of deep superior sulcus with high eyelid crease associated with aponeurotic disinsertion. (**b**) After ptosis repair, a flat pretarsal area is maintained to allow thea pplicationof e yelidc osmetics

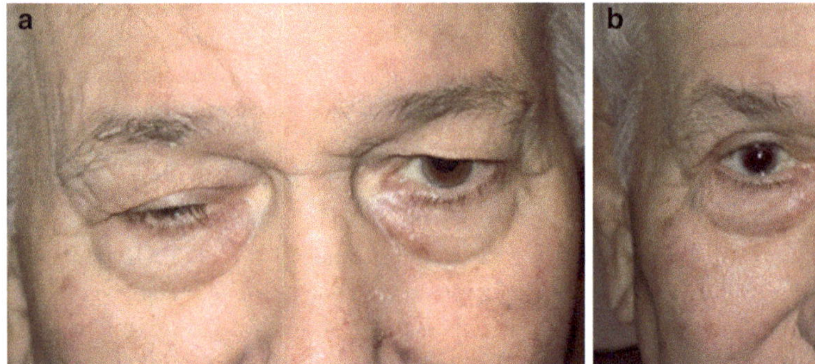
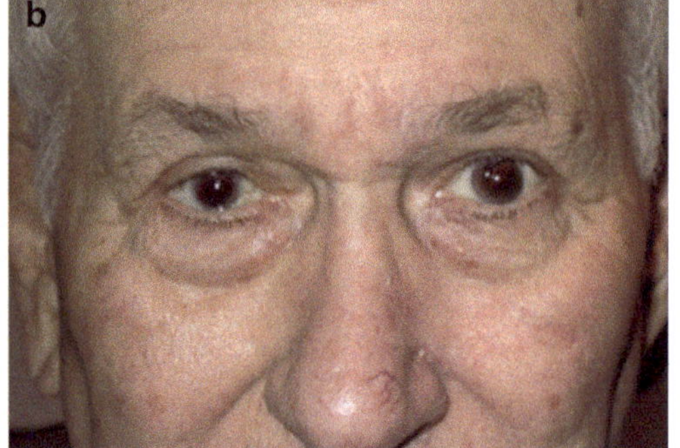

Fig. 25.2 (**a**) A 77-year-old man with significant asymmetry between the *right* and *left side*. (**b**) After eyelid surgery, improved symmetry draws less attention to the periorbital region

position and definition is crucial, particularly in female patients. Maintaining the proper height and symmetry of the eyelid crease is essential in patient satisfaction with ptosis surgery (Fig. 25.2a, b). Despite excellent eyelid height, asymmetry of the eyelid crease can produce an unhappy patient and a frustrated surgeon.

The normal eyelid crease in the male eyelid is about 8–9 mm above the lid margin. In contrast, the normal eyelid crease in a female counterpart is 9–11 mm above the lid margin, and usually more sharply defined [3, 5]. The more defined lid crease in female patients establishes a distinct, flat pretarsal platform to which cosmetics may be applied. Aponeurotic disinsertion or rarefaction often produces a higher, less defined lid crease. Such an appearance would likely be more noticeable and less tolerable by female patients. Using supratarsal fixation during skin closure, the surgeon can sharpen and/or alter the position of the lid crease.

The eyelids also cannot be adequately assessed in isolation. Upper eyelid position is intimately associated with eyebrow position and function. In males, the eyebrow usually rests along or slightly above the superior orbital rim. In females, brow position is slightly higher and generally more arching (Fig. 25.3a–d). In evaluating and treating patients with ptosis, it is important to consider eyebrow appearance, symmetry, and function. Repositioning of the eyebrows should be considered, if necessary, to maintain the appropriate eyelid–eyebrow relationships.

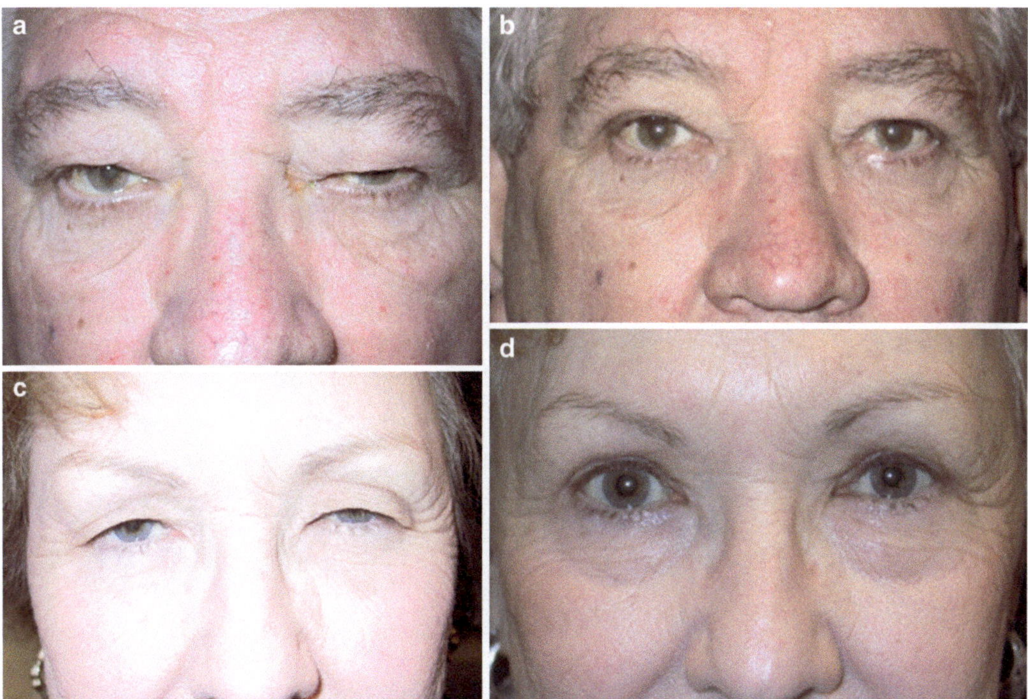

Fig. 25.3 (**a**) In a male patient, the brow is usually flat along the orbital rim. (**b**) After ptosis surgery, this brow configuration should be maintained. (**c**) In a female patient, the desired brow configuration is slightly arching towards the tail. (**d**) When considering ptosis surgery, eyebrow elevation may be necessary to achieve the desired brow configuration

Ethnic Considerations in Ptosis Surgery

When evaluating and treating a patient with blepharoptosis, identification of the patient's ethnic and cultural differences can be vitally important in guiding successful surgical intervention. Anatomical factors such as eyelid height, eyelid crease location, canthal anatomy, sulcus definition, and eyebrow positioning are all very important. However, perhaps the most important factor is the patient's cultural expectations. Oftentimes, the patient is not exactly sure what they expect from eyelid surgery. The surgeon and patient must be concordant with regard to surgery and anticipated outcome.

In terms of eyelid anatomy, perhaps the most striking differences are between the Asian and non-Asian eyelids. Even among Asian eyelids, there are distinct anatomical differences (Fig. 25.4a–f). Subtle anatomical differences can be indentified in other ethnicities as well. In our experience, many Hispanic patients have eyelid features akin to Asian eyelids; yet, other Hispanic patients have a more occidental appearance. Ptosis evaluation and repair is very similar in Caucasian and African-American patients. Eyelid anatomy and the relative position of the eyebrow and eyelid crease are comparable between the two ethnicities; however, preaponeurotic fat is generally less abundant in African-American patients (Fig. 25.5a–b) [1, 2]. While preaponeurotic fat is usually not sculpted in routine ptosis surgery, it does serve as an important landmark intraoperatively when identifying the levator. Probably, the most important factor to consider in ptosis repair in African-American patients is the tendency to form hypertrophic scars. Operating through a small incision can help minimize the effect of keloid formation, although hypertrophic scars

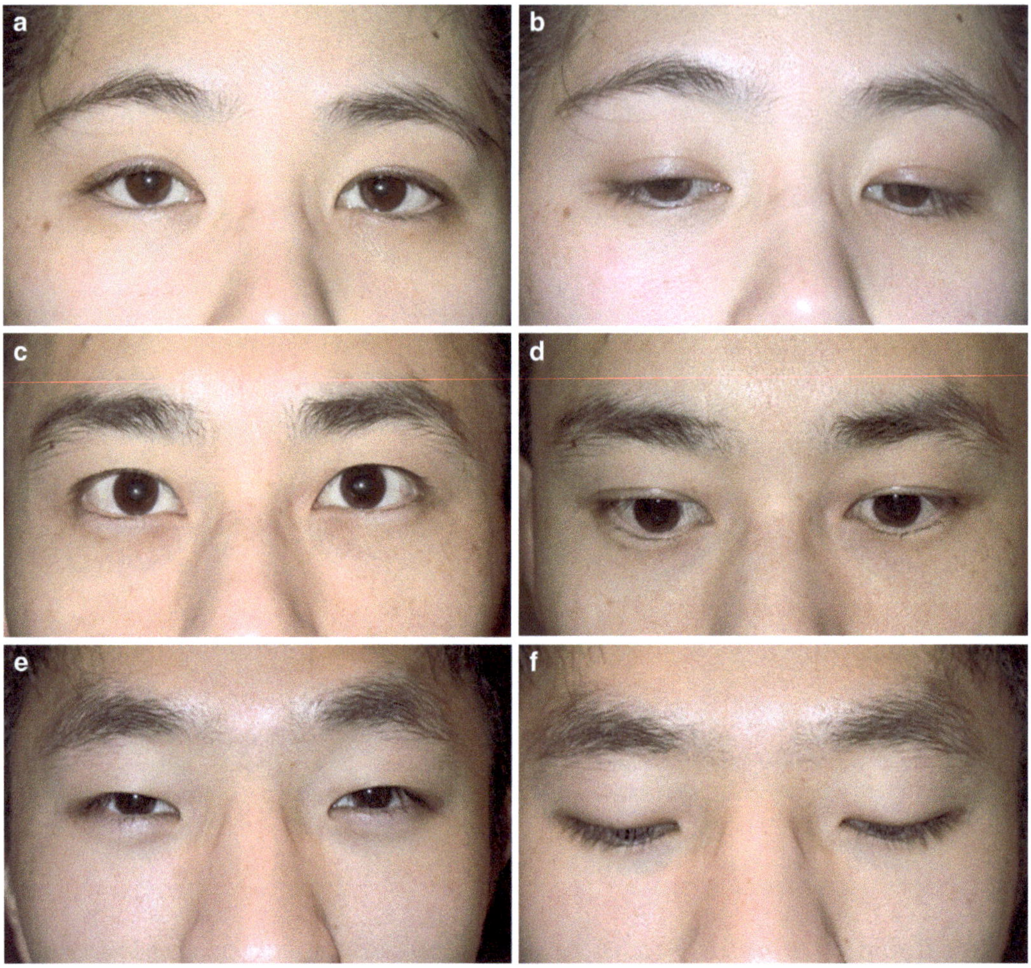

Fig. 25.4 Three anatomical configurations of the Asian eyelid. (**a**) The Asian double eyelid with the pretarsal eyelid distinctly visible. (**b**) In downgaze, the eyelid crease is visible in the Asian double eyelid. (**c**) The Asian single eyelid with crease. Note that the supratarsal fold extends down to the eyelid margin. (**d**) In downgaze, the eyelid crease is visible in the Asian single eyelid with crease. (**e**) The Asian single eyelid without crease. Note that there is no supratarsal fold as the eyelid crease is nonexistent or very low towards the eyelid margin. (**f**) In downgaze, no eyelid crease is identifiable in the Asian singlee yelidw ithoutc rease

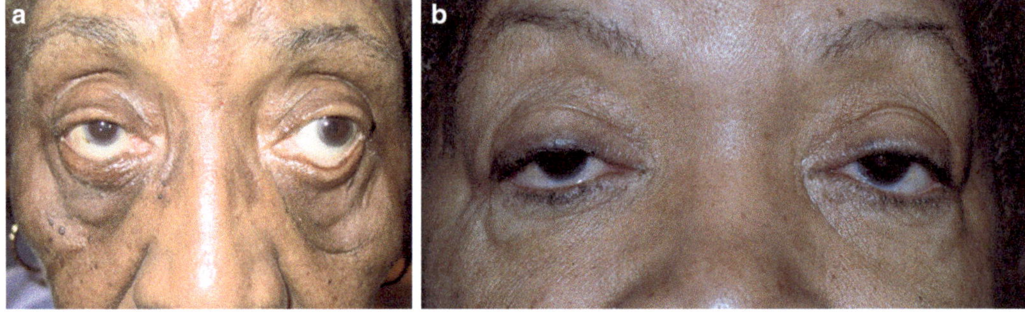

Fig. 25.5 Similar to the occidental eyelid, the African American eyelid is also characterized by a relatively high eyelid crease. (**a**) This patient has a deep superior sulcus with high eyelid crease typical of aponeurotic disinsertion. (**b**) This patient has a fuller appearing sulcus with dermatochalasis but still has a high eyelid crease

are uncommon and keloids are extremely rare on the thin skin of the eyelids.

Evaluation and surgery for ptosis in Asian patients can be very difficult. Understanding the anatomical differences in the Asian eyelid is the key to successful surgery. In the Asian upper eyelid, a notable difference is that the eyelid crease is lower, an average of 2–3 mm from the eyelid margin [4, 6]. In many cases, a defined lid crease cannot be appreciated, thus giving the appearance of a "single eyelid." Anatomically, this difference is due to a lower insertion of the septum and levator aponeurosis along the anterior surface of the tarsus. In non-Asian eyelids, the levator aponeurosis and septum fuse before inserting along the superior border of the tarsus. Another notable difference in the Asian eyelid is fat distribution. In the Asian lid, the preaponeurotic fat descends closer to the eyelid margin, giving a more full appearance to the upper eyelid. Relative lack of aponeurotic projections to the skin contributes to a less defined eyelid crease. In addition, there is more subcutaneous fat in the Asian eyelid, while in Caucasians and African-Americans there is essentially no subcutaneous fat.

A key determination in Asian ptosis surgery is whether to alter the eyelid crease height and definition. Many younger patients have eyelid surgery simply to elevate the eyelid crease position to achieve a "double-eyelid" appearance [5, 7, 8]. However, in our experience, most older patients seeking ptosis surgery desire to lift the eyelid but maintain the eyelid crease position. A detailed preoperative discussion is necessary to align the goals of both the patient and surgeon.

In addition to the unique eyelid anatomy and lower eyelid crease position, Asian patients also often have prominent epicanthal folds. The appearance of the epicanthal folds may need to be softened with adjunct surgery at the time of ptosis repair since skin excision and eyelid crease elevation can accentuate the appearance of the folds. Epicanthoplasty can be performed in a number of ways. Common procedures include various modifications of Z-plasty and Y-V advancement procedures [7]. Our preferred technique is the subcutaneous epicanthoplasty, which allows softening or elimination of the epicanthal fold with minimal risk of medial canthal scarring (Fig. 25.6) [8]. The tissue beneath the epicanthal folds is undermined, and the excess fibrofatty tissue is debulked. A dissolvable suture is then used to fixate the fold deep into the medial canthal tissues, flattening and softening the epicanthal fold. This is an effective technique that does not require the complexity of transposition flaps required with other techniques of epicanthoplasty.

In summary, the challenge of ethnic and gender considerations in blepharoptosis is primarily

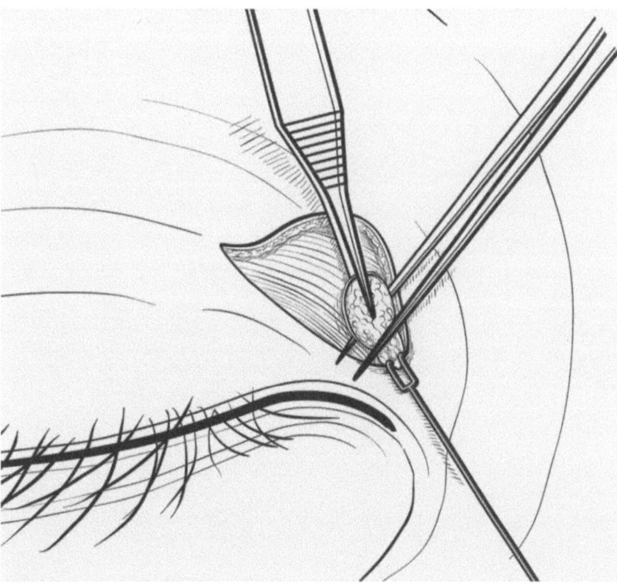

Fig.25.6 Line art of the subcutaneous epicanthoplasty. Through the medial portion of the eyelid crease incision, the subcutaneous tissues are dissected away from the overlying skin and excised

encountered in the preoperative assessment. Identifying and understanding the unique anatomical features of the specific gender and/or ethnicity is important. However, much more important is the communication between patient and surgeon to determine what the goals and expectationsofe yelids urgerya re.

References

1. Odunze M, Rosenberg DS, Few JW. Periorbital aging and ethnic considerations: a focus on the lateral canthal complex. Plast Reconstr Surg. 2008;121:1002–8.
2. Odunze M, Reid RR, Yu M, Few J. Periorbital rejuvenation and the African American patient: a survey approach. Plast Reconstr Surg. 2006;118:1011–8.
3. Stewart JM, Carter SR. Anatomy and examination of the eyelids. Int Ophthalmol Clin. 2002;42:1–13.
4. Doxanas MT, Anderson RL. Oriental eyelids – an anatomic study. Arch Ophthalmol. 1984;102:1232–5.
5. Flowers RS. The art of eyelid and orbital aesthetics: multiracial surgical considerations. Clin Plast Surg. 1987;14:703–21.
6. Kim MK, Rathbun JE, Aguilar GL, Seiff SR. Ptosis surgery in the Asian eyelid. Ophthal Plast Reconstr Surg.1989; 5:118–26.
7. Yi SK, Paik HW, Lee PK, et al. Simple epicanthoplasty with minimal scar. Aesthetic Plast Surg. 2007;31:350–3.
8. Yen MT, Jordan DR, Anderson RL. No-scar Asian Epicanthoplasty: a subcutaneous approach. Ophthal PlastR econstrS urg.2002; 18:40–4.

Chapter26
AestheticC onsiderationsf ort hePt osisSur geon

Adam J. Cohen and David A. Weinberg

Abstract Blepharoptosis is one of the most common age-related changes of the upper eyelids. It is frequently present in patients undergoing upper eyelid and facial rejuvenation. If the plan is to combine ptosis repair with other procedures, these additional procedures may impact which ptosisproc edureis s elected.

Blepharoptosis is one of the most common age-related changes of the upper eyelids. It is frequently present in patients undergoing upper eyelid and facial rejuvenation. If the plan is to combine ptosis repair with other procedures, these additional procedures may impact which ptosis procedure is selected.

Techniques for ptosis correction are well described elsewhere in this book, with each procedure having its own merits and drawbacks. Although under- or overcorrection of the ptotic lid is likely to be the most common complication, contour abnormalities of the eyelid margin may be even more disconcerting to the patient, particularly the cosmetic patient, and can be more difficult to correct. The Müller's muscle–conjunctival resection (MMCR) and Fasanella–Servat (FS) procedures described in previous chapters are reliable for eyelid elevation in suitable patients. MMCR and FS reportedly carry a lower incidence of postoperative eyelid margin contour abnormalities than levator advancement surgery since the attachments between levator aponeurosis and the anterior tarsal plate are left intact. However, the small incision, minimal dissection levator resection procedure (see chapter 19 on this procedure) may also accomplish the same goal of preserving many of the levator–tarsus attachments.

The external levator advancement technique is widely used. Some will argue that this approach is preferred when blepharoplasty or other procedures are concomitantly performed since only one incision is necessary. Furthermore, in patients with ptosis who desire ocular adnexal rejuvenation, external levator advancement allows for access to other periocular structures, including the upper eyelid skin and fat, lacrimal gland, subbrow fat pad, eyebrow, corrugator supercilii and procerus muscles, brow depressors, forehead, and midface. The ultimate decision regarding which ptosis surgery technique to use will be dictated by the surgeon preference, clinical findings (such as degree of ptosis, levator function, response to phenylephrine, status of the eyelid crease), need for access to periocular structures, and patient preference and expectations.

Regardless of which ptosis procedure is utilized, it is important to be aware that the following procedures may be performed via an upper eyelid crease incision:

1. Eyelid crease formation or repositioning in cases of crease asymmetry.
2. Lacrimal gland suspension for cases of lacrimal gland prolapse or prominence.

A.J.C ohen(✉)
PrivatePra ctice,The A rtof Eye s, Skokie, IL, USA
e-mail:a cohen@theartofeyes.com

A.J. Cohen and D.A. Weinberg (eds.), *Evaluation and Management of Blepharoptosis*,
DOI 10.1007/978-0-387-92855-5_26, © Springer Science+Business Media, LLC 2011

3. Removal of excess skin, orbicularis oculi muscle, and fat in the upper eyelid, i.e., upper blepharoplasty and orbicularis myectomy.
4. Lateral canthopexy or canthoplasty to tighten the eyelids and/or reposition the lateral canthus. One may attain satisfactory access to the lateral canthal tendon and lateral orbital rim through the lateral portion of the upper eyelid incision. Lateral canthopexy may be used to address horizontal eyelid laxity, lateral canthal dystopia, rounding of the lateral canthal angle, or involutional blepharophimosis. Disinsertion of the lateral canthal tendon allows for complete mobilization of the lateral retinaculum to achieve greater tightening of a very lax eyelid and a larger degree of freedom to move and refixate the tendon.
5. A weakening procedure of the corrugator supercilii and procerus muscles to alleviate glabellar frown lines. A superior dissection plane posterior to orbital portion of the orbicularis oculi muscle will expose the obliquely horizontal corrugator supercilii muscle. Care should be taken to avoid injury to the supraorbital neurovascular bundle when dividing and/or resecting the corrugator muscle. The vertical procerus muscle can be safely divided "blindly" in the midline.
6. Eyebrow fat pad sculpting. In certain patients, such as Asians, the subbrow fat extends down into the upper eyelid and contributes greatly to the fullness of the eyelid. This subbrow fat, which lies anterior to the orbital septum and has a prominent fibrous component, should not be confused with the preaponeurotic fat that flows freely behind the septum. Thyroid eye disease patients often display hypertrophy of the brow fat pad, which may benefit from debulking to restore a more aesthetically desirable upper eyelid appearance.
7. Internal eyebrowpexy with or without resorbable fixation devices. While browpexy has limited ability to elevate the brow position, it may be particularly useful in stabilizing brow position to prevent brow descent after ptosis repair or upper blepharoplasty.
8. Subperiosteal elevation of the central forehead via inferior release. A horizontal incision is made in the periosteum just above the superior orbital rim, allowing for subperiosteal release of the central portion of the forehead within the boundaries of the temporal lines of fusion.
9. Superior repositioning of the suborbital orbicularis oculi fat (SOOF) and malar fat pads, i.e., midface lift, may be performed to a limited degree through an upper eyelid crease incision. Through the lateral end of an extended upper eyelid incision, the lateral portion of the SOOF may be approached and mobilized by releasing the orbitomalar ligament. The SOOF is then suspended from the lateral orbital rim and the deep temporal fascia.

There is often confusion between ptosis and dermatochalasis by patients and inexperienced clinicians, and patients may assume that "too much skin" is the cause of their "droopy eyelids." If excess skin is overhanging the eyelashes, then it is necessary to gently raise the brows to lift the skin out of the way to assess the eyelid margin position and determine the true margin-reflex distance. If only upper blepharoplasty is performed, and concurrent ptosis is not addressed, there is an increased likelihood of ending up with an unhappy patient. It is essential that the clinician educate the patient how to achieve the goals that the patient has set forth, assuming those goals are realistic. In addition, in terms of managing patient expectations, it is important to forewarn the patient of the possible need for additional surgery to achieve the desired outcome. One should bear in mind that ptosis surgery may "produce" excess upper eyelid skin. This results from eyelid elevation and descent of the brows since there is no longer any need for compensatory brow elevation. The surgeon must take these issues into consideration when deciding whether or not to remove skin, and how much skin to resect, at the time of ptosis repair.

While the elderly patient with a functional eyelid malposition may be quite tolerant of certain expected postoperative issues such as bruising and swelling, younger and aesthetically oriented patients may react more strongly. In addition to withholding any drugs and herbal supplements that may promote bleeding for the appropriate amount of time preoperatively, certain patients opt to take oral homeopathic *Arnica montana*. Despite these measures and judicious intraoperative cautery, some patients may still develop significant periocular bruising. A cover-up makeup may be used to conceal this, as well as pulsed dye laser in cases of more severe ecchymosis [1]. It is important to avoid direct sunlight exposure to bruised and red areas since that may lead to hyperpigmentation that may gradually resolve over time or can be managed with bleaching agents, such as hydroquinone.

Compared with functional patients, there is even greater pressure on the surgeon for the aesthetic patient to have a positive surgical experience. That may be enhanced by the use of bicarbonate in the local anesthetic mixture and IV sedation. Intraoperative IV dexamethasone may have a beneficial effect on postoperative nausea and edema. It is helpful to elevate the head of the bed and initiate ice compresses as soon as possible after completion of the procedure, even in the operating room. In some patients who may be more prone to edema, one may also consider a short course of oral corticosteroids postoperatively.

Patients often ask whether vitamin E ointment applied following surgery will improve the ultimate cosmetic appearance of the wound. There is no consensus in this regard, and a significant incidence of contact dermatitis due to the ointment has been reported [2, 3]. It might be safest to just use an emollient, such as Aquaphor (Beiersdorflnc .,W ilton,C T).

References

1. DeFatta RJ. Pulsed-dye laser for treating ecchymoses after facial cosmetic procedures. Arch Facial Plast Surg.2009; 11:99–103.
2. Baumann LS, Spencer J. The effects of topical vitamin E on the cosmetic appearance of scars. Dermatol Surg. 1999;25:311–5.
3. Zampieri N et al. A prospective study in children: Pre- and post-surgery use of vitamin E in surgical incisions. JP lastR econstrA esthetS urg.2010; 63(9):1474–8.

Chapter 27
Challenging Ptosis Scenarios

John B. Holds, Adam G. Buchanan, Morris Hartstein, David A. Weinberg, and Adam J. Cohen

Abstract Ptosis is a common feature of both benign essential blepharospasm and hemifacial spasm. Mechanisms include excessive protractor muscle tone, levator aponeurosis dehiscence, apraxia, or response to botulinum toxin therapy. Treatment modalities include botulinum toxin injections, surgical ptosis repair, and myectomy.

Benign Essential Blepharospasm and Hemifacial Spasm

Etiology and Evaluation

Benign essential blepharospasm (BEB, Fig. 27.1) and hemifacial spasm (HFS, Fig. 27.2) share a common phenomenology with an overactive orbicularis oculi muscle and involuntary eyelid closure. The assessment of eyelid position is difficult in these patients, as the lid height is dynamic, and the lid height observed at any moment is related to a balance of retractor (levator) muscle and protractor (orbicularis and corrugator) muscles.

Ptosis is a common feature of both of these conditions. Excess orbicularis tone can completely overpower the levator muscle and close the eye (as in a wink). A variably ptotic eyelid is a common feature of BEB and HFS.

Ptosis can also result from the usual involutional mechanism. Involutional or aponeurotic ptosis commonly occurs with advancing age, but is also seen in a variety of other situations including after surgical or other trauma or with chronic rigid contact lens wear. It is hypothesized that the increased orbicularis muscle tone associated with BEB and HFS place increased stress on the levator aponeurosis and contribute to the development of ptosis by accelerating aponeurotic dehiscence.

In BEB, a form of dystonia, involuntary eyelid closure may occur due to apraxia of eyelid opening (Fig. 27.3). This is an additional movement disorder, commonly associated with BEB, characterized by an inability to voluntarily initiate eyelid opening. Patients with apraxia of eyelid opening may display an inability to voluntarily open the eyes while the BEB is inactive or relaxed.

A final mechanism of ptosis, which must be considered in these patients, is ptosis secondary to botulinum toxin injection. Botulinum therapy is considered in a majority of patients with BEB and HFS. Factors that predispose a patient to ptosis after botulinum therapy include high doses of toxin, deep injections, injection over the central eyelid, and preexisting ptosis. Botulinum therapy-associated ptosis typically develops within 1–2 weeks of treatment, and seldom lasts

J.B. Holds (✉)
Departments of Ophthalmology and Otolaryngology/Head and Neck Surgery, Saint Louis University, Ophthalmic Plastic and Cosmetic Surgery, Inc., 12990 Manchester Road #102, St. Louis, Des Peres, MO, USA
e-mail: jholds@sbcglobal.net

A.J. Cohen and D.A. Weinberg (eds.), *Evaluation and Management of Blepharoptosis*,
DOI 10.1007/978-0-387-92855-5_27, © Springer Science+Business Media, LLC 2011

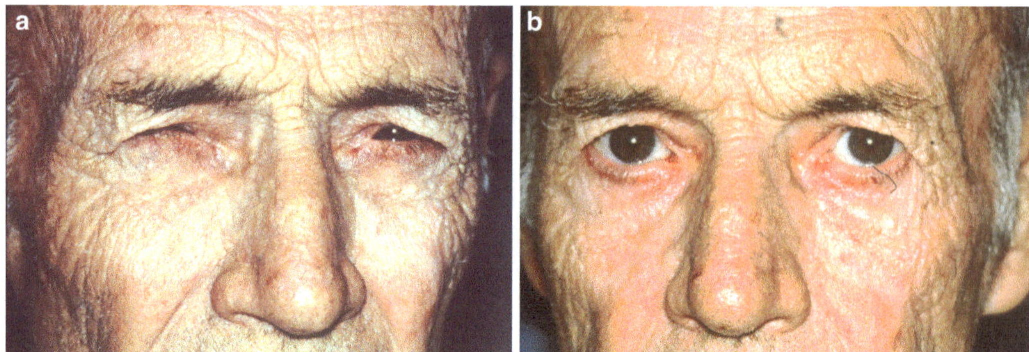

Fig. 27.1 Patient with benign essential blepharospasm (BEB) showing dystonic eyelid closure and associated ptosis: (**a**) pretreatment; (**b**)a fterbot ulinumt herapy

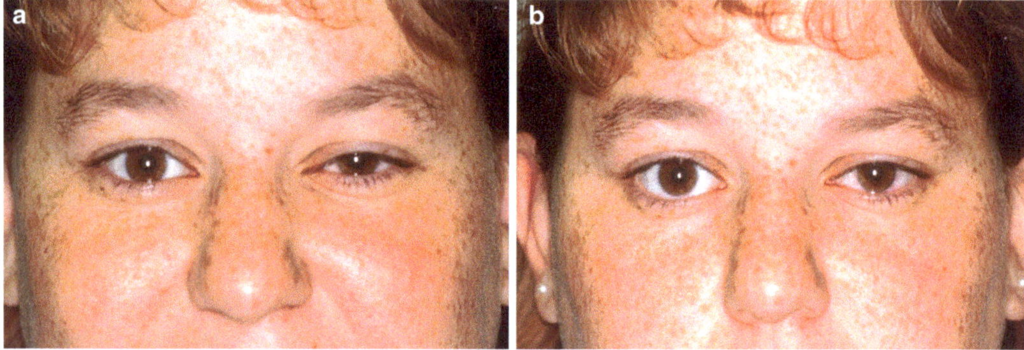

Fig. 27.2 Patient with hemifacial spasm (HFS) showing unilateral eyelid closure and associated ptosis: (**a**) pretreatment; (**b**)a fterbotulin umt herapy

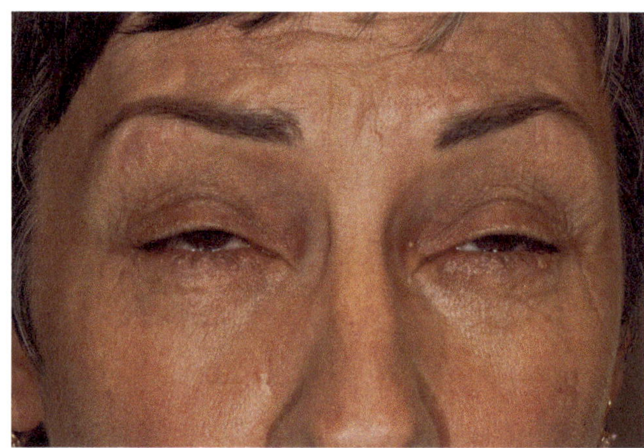

Fig.27.3 Patientw ithB EB and apraxia of eyelid opening. Orbicularis muscle spasm is relieved with botulinum therapy, but ptosis persists

more than a month. It is useful to evaluate patients with HFS and BEB 4–8 weeks after botulinum therapy. This aids in the assessment of the patients and their disease after botulinum therapy and before recurrent spasm and helps to guidefurthe rtre atment.

Treatment

In treating ptosis associated with BEB and HFS, one must first attempt to determine the relative contribution of excess orbicularis muscle tone versus true baseline ptosis in the eyelid height. As BEB and HFS are generally intermittent, careful observation during the preoperative interview may allow the surgeon to determine true ptosis versus closure secondary to orbicularis muscle activity.

As both BEB and HFS are customarily treated with botulinum toxin, it is important to ascertain what is the patient's predominant problem – ptosis (generally asymmetric and bilateral) or eyelid spasm. In patients whose eyelid spasm predominates, botulinum therapy is generally initiated first. It may be necessary to pass the patient through at least two cycles of botulinum therapy before considering ptosis surgery. If the ptosis is the predominant finding, it is reasonable to repair this before undertaking botulinum or other therapy.

If surgery is to be performed, it is helpful to schedule surgery in a window 4–8 weeks after botulinum therapy. This allows any preceding botulinum therapy to settle in and resolve temporary ptosis which may be due to botulinum toxin. After 3 months, spasm is often returning, and intra- and postoperative assessment of eyelid height may be a problem, if ptosis surgery is performed late in the treatment cycle.

Surgical repair is generally performed via a frontalis sling or external levator aponeurosis resection. External levator aponeurotic resection surgery is very adjustable. The external incision allows access to the orbicularis muscle, which is another object for treatment, via limited or radical myectomy surgery. In the setting of surgical myectomy, ptosis repair is virtually always bilateral. Even in surgical myectomy patients requiring no significant repositioning of upper eyelid position, the levator aponeurosis is generally reinforced at the time of myectomy surgery.

The completeness of myectomy surgery may be graded, and excision of several generous strips of orbicularis muscle at the time of ptosis repair often provides some improvement in the underlying eyelid spasm, lessening future botulinum toxin needs (both reduced total dose and increased duration of effect). Preoperative experience in observing the patient's response to botulinum therapy allows the surgeon to appropriately determine whether no myectomy, a limited myectomy, or a radical myectomy is required at the time of ptosis surgery (Fig. 27.4).

Frontalis sling surgery is effective in patients with severe apraxia of eyelid opening or otherwise recalcitrant ptosis. It is often appropriate to

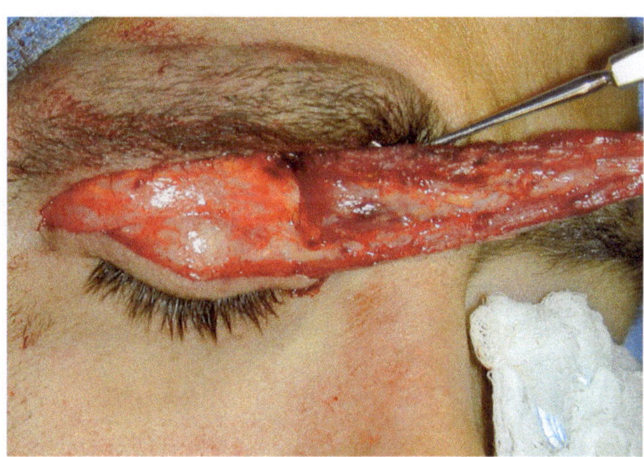

Fig.27.4 Intraoperative imageof m yectomys urgery

perform surgical myectomy and/or aponeurotic ptosis repair before considering frontalis sling surgery. Using a pentagon technique with a silicone rod, such as the Seiff frontalis suspension set (BD-Visitec, Inc.), a generally acceptable and functional ptosis result is achieved.

Surgical Technique

Aporneurotic Ptosis Repair

The surgical technique of aponeurotic ptosis repair is routine. Patients with HFS seldom require myectomy surgery and may undergo any sort of routine technique of aponeurotic repair. It is sensible to reinforce the aponeurosis with more sutures than are used in a small-incision technique.

Patients with BEB are a bit more difficult to repair, as apraxia of eyelid opening and dystonic spasm are bilateral and make intraoperative assessment of eyelid height more difficult and postoperative assessment of eyelid position more subjective. The addition of myectomy surgery requires the administration of local anesthetic over a broad area, with resultant intra- and postoperative edema (Fig. 27.5) and greater variability in eyelid position related to both edema and the possibility of anesthetic diffusion into the levator muscle. It is recommended that the ptosis repair in such patients be performed before anesthetizing more broadly for myectomy surgery.

Frontalis Sling

Frontalis sling surgery in patients with BEB may be performed with myectomy surgery, although it is generally better to perform an aponeurotic ptosis repair and myectomy initially, then reevaluate postoperatively. Even patients with severe apraxia of eyelid opening often will achieve a significant functional benefit from an aponeurotic ptosis repair and myectomy procedure and not require a frontalis sling. Frontalis sling performed with myectomy surgery will require suturing of the silicone rod to the tarsus. When performed at a later date, the silicone rod can generally be passed through supraciliary stab incisions, which is technically simpler and more predictable.

Complications

The common complications of ptosis surgery in patients with HFS and BEB are under and overcorrection, recurrence, and exposure keratitis. Patients' eyelid position is dynamic and varies significantly throughout the treatment cycle with botulinum toxin. The baseline increased tone of the orbicularis muscle with HFS causes a ptosis that frequently corrects with botulinum toxin alone (Fig. 27.2). The lid height in such patients after ptosis repair is thus dynamic and may vary significantly throughout the treatment cycle with botulinum toxin.

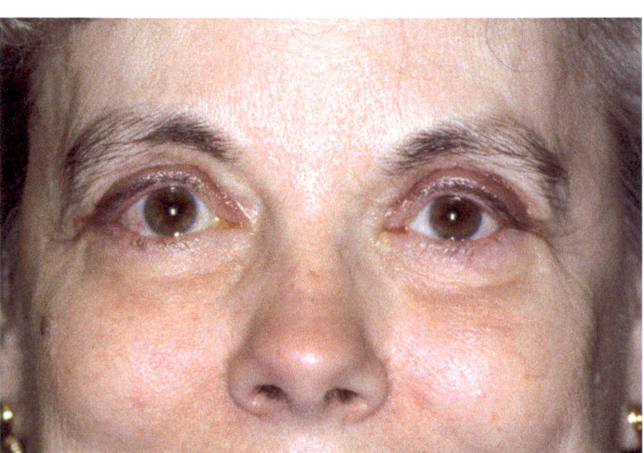

Fig. 27.5 Patient 1 month after myectomy surgery and ptosis repair showing significant edema

Recurrence of ptosis is more common in patients with HFS and BEB. These patients have a co-contraction of the levator and orbicularis muscle. Theoretically, this may create greater stress on the levator aponeurosis and the surgical repair. Prolonged postoperative edema may also play a role in this. Exposure keratitis is common and should be anticipated, with suggestions for significant ongoing lubrication after ptosis surgery in these patients. As most such patients will eventually undergo additional botulinum toxin therapy, it will be necessary to lubricate more aggressively at that time.

Botulinum toxin therapy is often altered after ptosis surgery in patients with BEB and HFS. The interval to the first treatment necessitated by symptoms is usually increased after ptosis repair. Myectomy surgery will further increase the interval to the next botulinum toxin therapy. The botulinum dose will be diminished in the area undergoing myectomy surgery in proportion to the amount of excised muscle. There is a lag to reinnervate any muscle left behind, so in limited efforts at myectomy, the necessary botulinum toxin dose will increase over the year after surgery. With myectomy the skin is generally anesthetic in the operated area for 6–12 months. Botulinum toxin treatment is relatively painless during this period. Following the return of sensation, the injections occur into a dense plane of scar tissue, and greater than normal amounts of pain are noted in the course of treatment. A marked permanent reduction in botulinum needs occurs only with aggressive removal of virtually all accessible orbicularis muscle.

Under- and overcorrection of ptosis may create difficult management decisions. If performed with little or no myectomy and a routine amount of postoperative edema, levator aponeurotic adjustments or adjustment of the frontalis sling is carried out in a routine fashion. Especially in the setting of myectomy surgery, postoperative edema may obscure the final eyelid height until the patient is well beyond the customary 2 week window of early ptosis adjustment. In such patients, it is appropriate to wait until the patient is 4–6 months out from surgery to reassess the eyelidhe ight.

Summary

Acquired ptosis is common in patients with BEB and HFS. The treatment is integrated into the patients botulinum toxin treatment regimen, and generally utilizes external aponeurotic resection and repair or an alloplastic frontalis sling. Despite a greater tendency to exposure and eyelid height issues, ptosis repair is a valuable component of the functional rehabilitation of the patient with BEB and HFS.

TarsalSw itch

In cases of chronic progressive external ophthalmoplegia, patients suffer from significant ptosis and poor eyelid closure and ocular motility limitation. These patients may adopt a chin-up head position in order to see better. Ptosis repair can be quite challenging. Often, these patients have a poor Bell's phenomenon, further contributing to risk of exposure keratopathy if there is any preoperative lagophthalmos. Frontalis suspension procedures are a reasonable option, especially when they can be adjusted in the case of corneal exposure. However, this requires good frontalis muscle function, which is not always the case with severe myopathies.

Another surgical option is the tarsal switch procedure. Since these patients' lids are already severely compromised, any additional elevation of their eyelid can potentially lead to corneal exposure and ulceration. In the tarsal switch procedure, the palpebral fissure height is not changed; rather, it is directed more superiorly so as not to obstruct the pupil, and therefore not increase the risk for exposure. That is, the upper lid is elevated while the lower lid is simultaneously raised. This procedure can be performed in patients with poor levator function, as is typically seen in CPEO.

The procedure is performed as follows: The lid crease is marked in standard fashion. A conservative amount of excess skin can be excised, if indicated. An incision is made and dissection is carried out to expose the tarsus and the levator muscle as described previously. The amount of resection can vary according to each patient's needs, but a general guideline can be to plan for a 6 mm vertical resection, including 3 mm of tarsus and 3 mm of levator. If additional elevation is needed and can be tolerated, further levator advancement can be performed. A corneal protector or lid plate should be placed before incising the tarsus full thickness. The incision is made with a #15 blade and then completed with Wescott scissors. The tarsal incision is angled superiorly medially and laterally with care taken not to injure the vascular arcades. Once removed, this graft should be placed in a saline-soaked sponge. The cut edge of levator is then sutured to the cut edge of the tarsus using interrupted 6-0 plain or chromic sutures, with care taken not to pass the sutures full thickness, which could abrade the cornea. This should elevate the upper eyelid into a more favorable position.

Attention is now directed toward the lower lid where an incision is made through conjunctiva and lower eyelid retractors along the inferior tarsal border. This can be performed with either Wescott scissors or needle-tip cutting cautery. Dissection is carried inferiorly in the subconjunctival plane to further release the lower lid retractors. At this point, if there is horizontal eyelid laxity, a lateral tarsal strip procedure can be performed. The free tarsal graft taken from the upper lid is now placed between the inferior tarsal border and the cut edge of conjunctiva (Fig. 27.6). The conjunctival side of the graft should be facing the globe. The graft is sutured using two running sutures of 6-0 plain gut. The tarsus acts as a spacer graft to support and elevate the lower lid, thereby leaving the palpebral fissure width unchanged but shifted superiorly into the primary field of gaze. By keeping the dimensions of the palpebral fissure unchanged (Fig. 27.7a, b), this procedure usually does not cause any worsening of the dry eye condition typically seen in these patients.

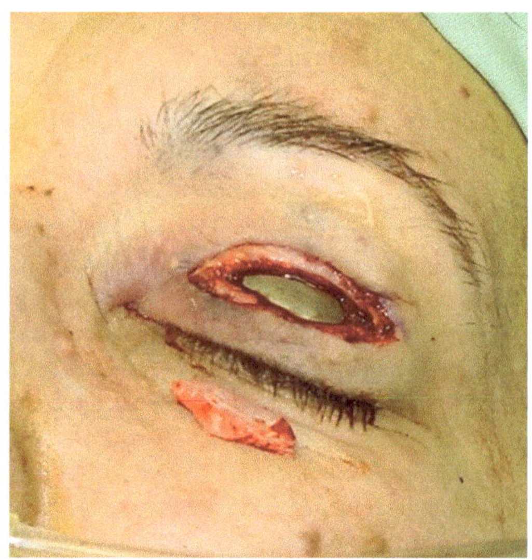

Fig. 27.6 Upper lid defect seen following full-thickness resection of tarsus and levator. Free tarsal graft is used as a spacer to elevate the lower lid

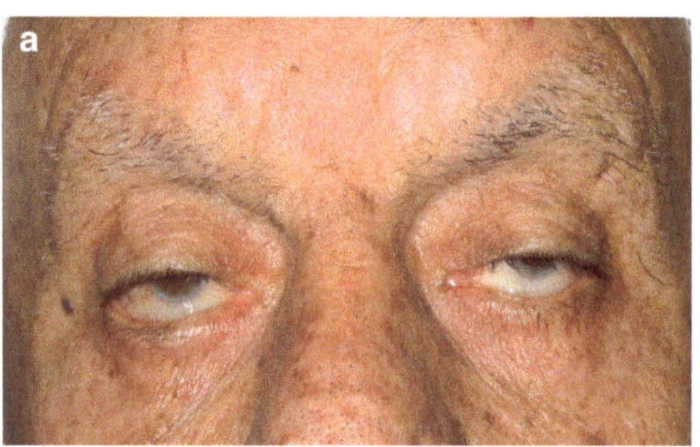

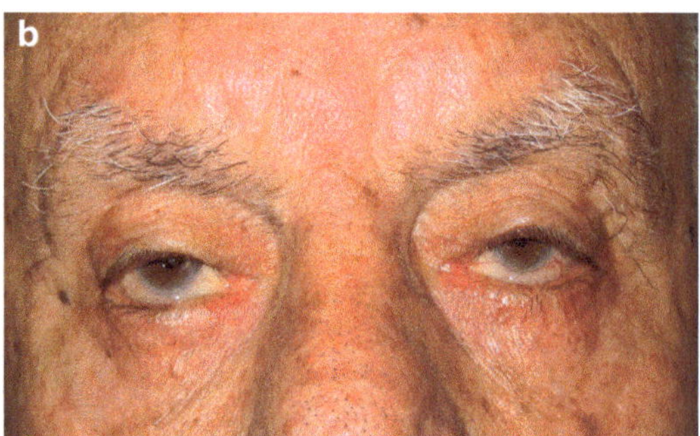

Fig. 27.7 (**a**) Preoperative photograph of severe myogenic ptosis, occluding pupil, with lower lid retraction. (**b**) Postoperative photograph following tarsal switch with papillary axis cleared, correction of lower lid retractionw hilel eavingP Func hanged

Eyelid Laxity and Tarsal Insufficiency

Severe Horizontal Eyelid Laxity

Severe horizontal eyelid laxity can pose a variety of challenges during ptosis surgery. Such laxity could result from floppy eyelid syndrome or may be acquired. In a setting of eyelid laxity, MMCR or limited levator advancement may be performed without encountering problems. However, if the laxity is severe enough, ptosis surgery may be complicated by:

1. Eyelidma rginc ontourde formity
2. Lateral tarsal shift due to medial canthal tendonla xity
3. Ectropion
4. Eyelash ptosis (especially with floppy eyelid syndrome).

Horizontal eyelid tightening may address some or all of these issues and may be accomplished by medial or lateral canthal tendon tightening or by full-thickness eyelid wedge resection. The latter is often employed in severe floppy eyelid syndrome, although the lateral tarsal strip procedure has also been described for upper eyelid tightening. Each surgical approach carries its own limitations. Full-thickness resection carries the risk of producing an eyelid margin notch, as well as greater chance of corneal abrasion from the sutures. Upper eyelid lateral tarsal strip procedures may endanger the lacrimal gland ductules, while medial canthal tendon tightening may disrupt the canaliculus and lacrimal sac, and potentially cause canthal dystopia.

Medial tightening is often reserved for cases of significant lateral tarsal shift; this shift may increase the likelihood of suboptimal upper eyelid contour, with the high point displaced laterally. With lateral tarsal shift, if one tries to move the eyelid margin high point more centrally by placing the levator sutures more medially, a medial peak may occur, usually at the medial end of the tarsal plate. This medial peak may be even less desirable than a lateral high point that is rounded. If optimal eyelid margin contour is important, as in an esthetically oriented patient, then medial canthal tendon tightening is a reasonable option to move the tarsal plate back to its proper anatomic position. Medial tightening can be accomplished either via resection or tendon plication. Resection requires canalicular reconstruction, generally over a silicone stent, unless the patient already has an occluded canaliculus or severe dry eye syndrome that would benefit from sacrifice of the superior canaliculus. While it is much easier to plicate the anterior limb of the medial canthal tendon than the posterior limb, anterior limb tightening carries a high risk of distracting the medial canthus anteriorly, away from the globe, unless the globe is very prominent or minimal tightening of the tendon is performed. A more favorable result is usually obtained with tightening of the posterior limb of the tendon, which may be accomplished through a transcaruncular approach. Care needs to be taken to avoid injury to the lacrimal sac.

Ectropion that develops during external levator advancement surgery may often be addressed by moving the tarsal sutures further superiorly so there is less everting effect at the eyelid margin. This will tend to shift the anterior vector of pull on the eyelid margin toward a more favorable superior vector. However, if a large levator advancement is being performed and the eyelid is very lax, then horizontal eyelid tightening is the best solution. Eyelash ptosis does not generally result from horizontal laxity, but often accompanies it. A variety of methods for the correction of eyelid laxity are covered elsewhere in thiste xt.

Inadequate Tarsus

Tarsus may be deficient in its vertical or horizontal dimension or in its thickness. Vertical, superior tarsal deficiency (see Fig. 27.8) may result from prior Fasanella–Servat or other superior tarsectomy ptosis repair, lower eyelid reconstruction utilizing a Hughes or Hewes tarsoconjunctival flap, tumor resection, or trauma. A vertically short tarsal plate forces one to anchor

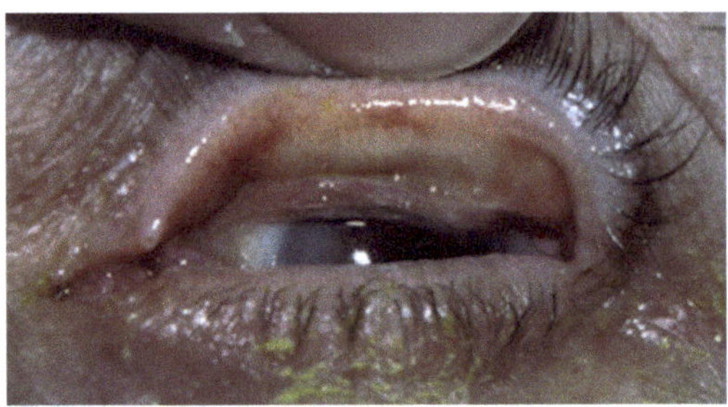

Fig. 27.8 Narrow vertical dimension of the upper tarsal plate due to an aggressive Fasanella–Servat ptosis repair years ago. This patient required repeat ptosis surgery, which was somewhat challenging due to the tarsal deficiency

the eyelid retractors along tarsus near the eyelid margin. This has a greater everting effect and carries a much higher risk of causing ectropion. Additionally, anchoring sutures closer to the eyelid margin often produces a contour deformity, i.e., a "peak," at the site of the suture. Ectropion and contour deformity may be at least partially alleviated by horizontally tightening the eyelid. Of course, excessive horizontal tightening of the eyelid may add a restrictive component to the ptosis, which would be counterproductive. One could certainly vertically lengthen the tarsal plate with a superiorly positioned spacer graft, but that is seldom necessary.

A horizontally short or absent tarsal plate may result from tumor resection or trauma. If tarsus is horizontally, but not vertically, deficient, a sliding tarsonconjunctival flap to "borrow" the superior portion of tarsus and transplant it to an area of absent or inadequate tarsus medial or lateral to the intact segment may be used. If a large or complete upper eyelid full-thickness defect was repaired with a Cutler-Beard flap, that provides no tarsal replacement in the upper eyelid, although a tarsal substitute, such as ear cartilage, is often added at the time that the eyelid-sharing flap is divided. A reverse Hughes flap will provide a narrow strip of tarsus to the upper eyelid.

Since tarsus provides structural support to the eyelid, absence or deficiency of tarsus predisposes to eyelid margin contour deformity and ectropion.

A thin tarsal plate, an anatomic variant in some patients, poses a different set of challenges. When levator is anchored to anterior tarsus with sutures, the goals is to place the sutures so that they are deep enough to hold securely, but to avoid suture exposure on the conjunctival surface; internally exposed sutures run a high risk of producing a corneal abrasion. With a thin tarsal plate, one may use a long, shallow suture bite, as is often utilized when suturing extraocular muscles to sclera. Such thin tarsal plates often lack structural rigidity, and one may compensate by horizontally tightening the eyelid, when necessary, to address contour problems or ectropion. If tarsus is too thin to achieve a satisfactory result, then one could potentially reinforce tarsus by placing some form of rigid onlay graft along the anterior surface, which would provide a more robust anchoring platform for the levator sutures.

Neurofibromatosis

Ocular adnexal neurofibromatosis may either be a component of generalized, peripheral neurofibromatosis (NF1) or isolated, localized orbitotemporal neurofibromatosis. NF1, an autosomal dominant disorder, has an incidence of 1:3,000 [1]. This subtype rarely involves the skull and face.

Orbitotemporal neurofibromatosis [2] occurs without systemic findings seen in NF1. The orbitotemporal variant may disrupt the greater and lesser sphenoid wings with resultant enlargement of the superior orbital fissure [3]. Temporal lobe herniation and pulsatile proptosis may ensue [2]. On the other hand, these patients may also develop enophthalmos due to prolapse of the intraorbital contents into the middle cranial fossa [2]. Both proptosis and enophthalmos may result in a pseudoptosis, with enophthalmos producing ipsilateral "ptosis," while exophthalmos widens the palpebral fissure and creates an illusion of contralateral ptosis. Widening of the inferior orbital fissure [3], orbital bone, and zygomatic hypoplasia [2] can manifest as hypoglobus, enophthalmos, and pseudoptosis. Canthal deformity may occur as a result of soft tissue infiltration or orbital dysplasia and increased bony orbital volume.

Arising from the peripheral nerve sheath, neurofibromas involving the eyelids may produce mechanical ptosis, eyelid deformity (often an S-shaped upper eyelid deformity), and potentially amblyopia in young children [4]. Patients may experience tearing, pain, and diplopia, among others ymptoms [4].

Diffuse soft tissue infiltration by plexiform neurofibromas makes their complete resection all but impossible, since it would require the sacrifice of significant amount of normal tissue. The infiltrative nature and high rate of recurrence of plexiform neurofibromas may result in persistent or recurrent deformity and the need for multiple surgeries when the tumor reaches a significant size.

Staged reconstruction and ptosis repair of a patient with isolated, right upper eyelid neurofibromas yielded a satisfactory result (see Figs. 27.9–27.11). The patient had been operated on previously with resultant eyelid scarring and persistent mechanical ptosis and contour abnormality.

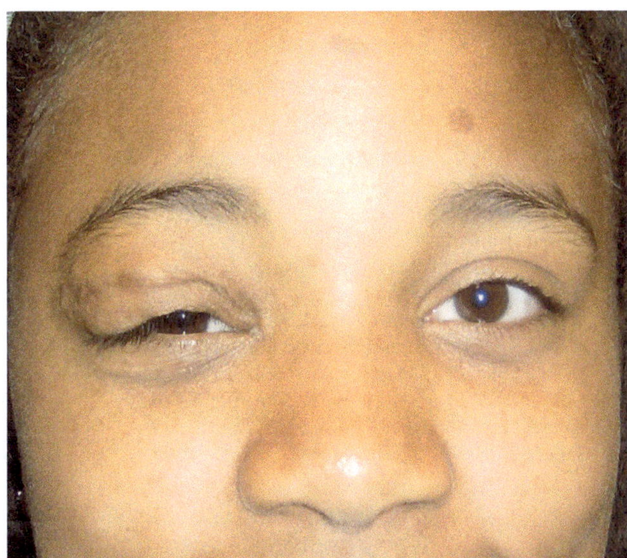

Fig.27.9 The patient at the time of initial evaluation with right upper eyelid mechanical blepharoptosis, neurofibromas with result eyelid laxity, anddi stortiona nds carring

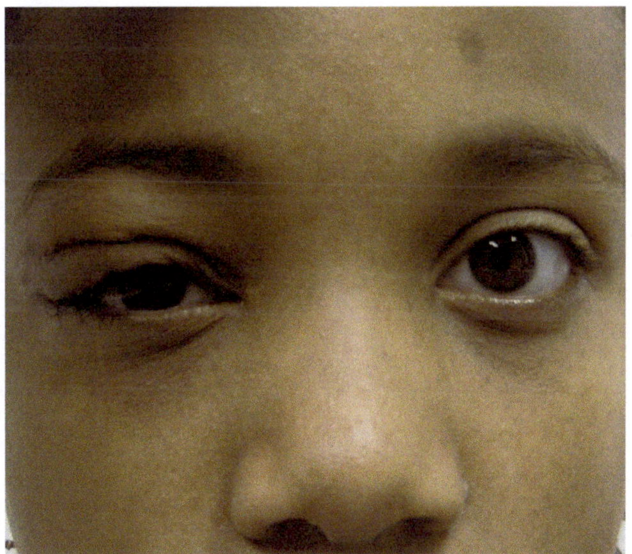

Fig.27.10 Thepa tienta fter the first surgery that included neurofibroma resection and scarre vision

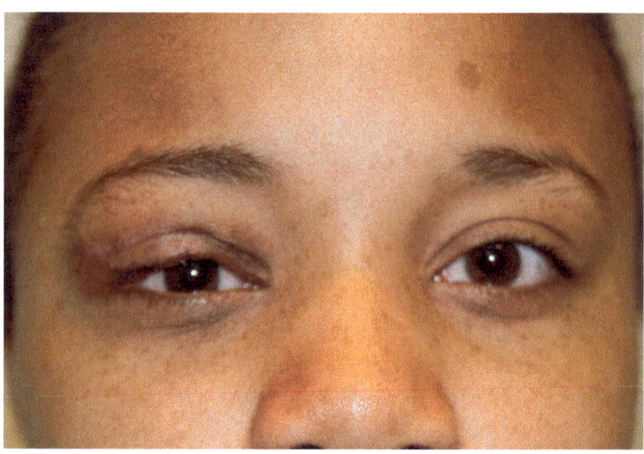

Fig. 27.11 Thepa tienta fter the second surgery that included repeat neurofibroma resection and Whitnall's sling procedureforptos isre pair

References

1. Fang LJ, Vidaud D, Vidaud M, Thirion JP. Identification and characterization of four novel large deletions in the human neurofibromatosis type 1 (NF 1) gene. Hum Mutat. 2001;18(6):549–50.
2. Jackson IT, Carbonnel A, Potparic Z, Shaw K. Orbitotemporal neurofibromatosis: classification and treatment. Plast Reconstr Surg. 1993;92(1):1–11.
3. Fukuta K, Jackson IT. Orbital neurofibromatosis with enophthalmos. Br J Plast Surg. 1993;46:36–8.
4. Jackson IT, Laws ER, Martin R. The surgical management of orbital neurofibromatosis. Plast Reconstr Surg.1983;71(6):7 51–8.

SuggestedR eading

5. Holds JB, White GL, Thiese SM, Anderson RL. Facial dystonia, essential blepharospasm and hemifacial spasm. Am Fam Physician. 1991;43(6):2113–20.
6. Anderson RL, Patel BCK, Holds JB, Jordan DR. Blepharospasm: past, present and future. Ophthal Plast Reconstr Surg. 1998;14:305–17.
7. Esteban A, Traba A, Prieto J. Eyelid movements in health and disease. The supranuclear impairment of the palpebral motility. Neurophysiol Clin. 2004;34(1):3–15.
8. Patrinely JR, Whiting AS, Anderson RL. Local side effects of botulinum toxin injections. Adv Neurol. 1988;49:493–500.
9. Lucci LM, Yen MT, Anderson RL, Hwang IP, Black RE. Orbicularis myectomy with levator advancement in Schwartz-Jampel syndrome. Am J Ophthalmol.2001; 132(5):799–801.
10. Anderson RL, Beard C. The levator aponeurosis. Attachments and their clinical significance. Arch Ophthalmol.1977; 95:1437–41.
11. Gillum WN, Anderson RL. Blepharospasm surgery. An anatomical approach. Arch Ophthalmol. 1981; 99(6):1056–62.
12. Anderson RL, Patrinely JR. Surgical management of blepharospasm. Adv Neurol. 1988;49:501–20.
13. Garland PE, Patrinely JR, Anderson RL. Hemifacial spasm. Results of unilateral myectomy. Ophthalmology. 1987;94(3):288–94.
14. Holds JB. Ptosis (Ch. 79). In: Albert DM, editor-in-chief. Ophthalmic surgery: Principles and techniques. malden, MA: Blackwell Science; 1999. pp. 1307–26.
15. Holds JB, Anderson RL. Blepharoptosis (Ch. 12). In: Tse DT, editor. Color atlas of ophthalmic surgery, Vol. 6– Oculoplastic Surgery. Philadelphia, PA: J.B. Lippincott Co.; 1992. pp. 151–74.
16. Baroody M, Holds JB, Vick VL. Advances in the diagnosis and treatment of ptosis. Curr Opin Ophthalmol.2005; 16(6):351–5.
17. Wabbels B, Roggenkämper P. Long-term follow-up of patients with frontalis sling operation in the treatment of essential blepharospasm unresponsive to botulinum toxin therapy. Graefes Arch Clin Exp Ophthalmol.2007; 245(1):45–50.
18. Leone CR, Shore JW, Van Gemert JV. Silicone rod frontalis sling for the correction of blepharoptosis. Ophthalmic Surg. 1981;12:881–7.
19. Demartelaere SL, Blaydon SM, Shore JW. Tarsal switch levator resection for the treatment of blepharoptosis in patients with poor eye protective mechanisms.O phthalmology.2006; 113:2357–63.

Chapter28
Ptosis Surgery: Comparing Different SurgicalT echniques

Alon Skaat and Guy Jonathan Ben Simon

Abstract Surgical techniques for the treatment of ptosis are varied, presenting the surgeon with a complex repertoire of options. The treatment plan should be best matched to each individual case, based on the etiology, severity of the ptosis, levator function, and surgeon's experience. Therefore familiarity with the different surgical techniques, their indications, advantages, and disadvantages may help the surgeon in making the best clinical decision. This chapter reviews the clinical outcome data in ptosis surgery based on comparative studies, comparing different surgical techniques, such as levator resection vs. Müller's muscle resection vs. Fasanella–Servat for involutional ptosis, frontalis suspension via autogenous fascia vs. banked fascia vs. an alloplastic material (silicone, Gortex, and Supramyd) for poor levator function ptosis, and levator resection vs. frontalis suspension for congenital ptosis.

Surgical treatment of ptosis dates as far back as 200 years, when one simple skin excision technique was performed; making the surgical decision very straightforward. Currently, various types of blepharoptosis surgeries exist, and the surgeon is faced with a more complex repertoire of options. In order to choose a treatment plan best matched to each individual case, the surgeon must be familiar with the range of available surgical options. To some degree, the treatment plan is based on the underlying condition, and therefore identifying the etiology of the ptosis is important. That being said, the particular surgical procedure is usually primarily dependent upon the severity of the ptosis and the levator function. Hering's effect should be checked in every case of ptosis, and if there is a strong dependency, the surgeon may wish to repair one eye at a time for a more reliable outcome. When comparing different surgical techniques, it is important to note that levator function has been defined in various ways by different authors (in terms of what they consider poor, fair, or good function), and it may vary with age and race [1]. So, one should be cautious in comparing surgical outcome in different studies, which may involve very different patient populations.

Involutional/Aponeuroticp tosis

Levator Advancement/Plication

Levator advancement or plication is one of the most common methods used in the management of ptosis. This technique enables direct visualization of the entire anatomy during the dissection, with precise results and intraoperative adjustment of eyelid height and contour [2]. Recurrence rate is reported to be between 9 and 12% [3], which may be due, in part, to the local anesthetic injections transiently weakening levator function, stimulating Müller muscle via

G.J.B enSimon (✉)
The Goldschleger Eye Institute, Sheba Medical Center, TelH ashomer, Israel
e-mail:guybe nsimon@gmail.com

A.J. Cohen and D.A. Weinberg (eds.), *Evaluation and Management of Blepharoptosis*, DOI 10.1007/978-0-387-92855-5_28, © Springer Science+Business Media, LLC 2011

the epinephrine, and distorting eyelid anatomy and altering eyelid mechanics by inducing swelling. These issues make it more difficult to accurately position the eyelid and may result in under- or overcorrection. Some surgeons use adrenaline-free local anesthetic solution to avoid activating Müller muscle, as well as injecting the smallest volume of local anesthetic solution necessary.

Müller Muscle Conjunctival Resection

The internal (transconjunctival) approaches, including conjunctivo-Müllerectomy (Müller muscle conjunctival resection – MMCR) and tarso-conjunctivo-Müllerectomy (Fasanella–Servat procedure) are best suited for minimal-to-moderate ptosis with good levator function. Most surgeons consider a positive response to phenylephrine a requirement for performing MMCR.

MMCR, first described in 1975, is reported to reproducibly result in a more predictable eyelid height with a better contour compared to levator aponeurosis surgery in cases with less than 3 mm ptosis with good levator function and a positive response to phenylephrine [4]. Major benefits of this method are lack of a skin incision/scar, less surgical tissue invasion, and avoidance of tarsal instability. It may be used for any type of ptosis, but tends to be employed in cases with minimal ptosis with good levator function and a positive phenylephrine test [2].

External levator advancement and MMCR, alone or with concurrent blepharoplasty, are both effective in correcting involutional upper eyelid ptosis. Reoperation rate for residual ptosis is low in MMCR (<3%) and can be as high as 17% in external ptosis repair. Overcorrection and eyelid retraction is not common (1.4%) but may be more prevalent with MMCR [4]. Cosmetic outcome, based on eyelid contour, eyelid crease, and eyelid symmetry, may be better in MMCR, especially when performed with upper blepharoplasty. However, it is important to realize that the degree of ptosis present preoperatively differs, on average, between these two techniques since patients who undergo MMCR tend to have milder ptosis compared to patients who undergo external levator advancement based on selection bias. The authors find MMCR to be more predictable, with lower reoperation rate and better cosmetic outcome in their hands.

While external levator resection enables intraoperative adjustment of the eyelid position and eyelid contour, MMCR requires careful preoperative planning of the desired tissue to be excised. This is aided by the instillation of phenylephrine (10 or 2.5%), which stimulates the sympathetically innervated Müller's muscle, causing it to contract, shorten, and elevate the eyelid. It is believed that if the eyelid fails to respond to the phenylephrine test, an alternative procedure such as external levator resection should be performed, albeit few surgeons perform MMCR in phenylephrine-negative cases.

Tarsoconjunctival resection (Fasanella–Servat procedure), first described in 1961, is best for the correction of mild ptosis with good levator function (preferably greater than 8 mm in acquired cases or 12 mm in congenital cases) in young patients with minimal asymmetry who do not want any visible scars. The technique may cause a peaked appearance and postoperative eyelid instability, if too much central tarsus is removed. This is a rare complication in experienced hands, and the resection of 3 mm of tarsus generally leaves sufficient tarsal plate remaining to maintain eyelid stability [5]. Symptomatic dry eye syndrome due to the resection of meibomian glands and accessory glands of Wolfring is also uncommon [5]. Surgical outcomes of Fasanella–Servat and MMCR cases have shown both procedures to be equally effective in ptosis correction [6].

CongenitalM yogenicPt osis

Frontalis Suspension

Frontalis suspension is used to manage myogenic ptosis, neuromuscular diseases, and cases in which linkage between the muscle and the eyelid is abnormal, such as Marcus Gunn jaw-winking phenomenon or third nerve palsy with aberrant regeneration. Autogenous fascia has been shown to result in lower ptosis recurrence and complication rate compared with banked fascia and therefore is considered the material of choice [7]. Historically, fascia lata from the thigh has been the gold standard for fixation. Recurrence rates after frontalis suspension vary and are reported to be between 0 and 100%.

Polytetrafluoroethylene (PTFE) and autogenous fascia have demonstrated the lowest recurrence rate [8], which is reported to be between 4 and 20%, while nylon or silicone has reported recurrence rates between 40 and 100%.

It is believed that the suture material serves only as a temporary skeleton for scar formation, and therefore no difference is anticipated between different suture materials as long as they remain in good position during the inflammation and scarring process. However, better cosmetic outcome was noted in cases in which a nylon sling was used [8]. Several suture designs such as single loop or double pentagon configurations are used for frontalis suspension surgery with no clinically significant difference between them [8].

Many investigators believe that eventually all cases of congenital ptosis that are treated with frontalis suspension will recur. This is evident from the higher recurrence rate (ranging from 4 to 100%) published in studies with longer follow-up periods (Table 28.1), regardless of the type of sling used. Success of frontalis suspension with lyophilized human fascia lata decreases from 90% at 2–3 years after surgery to 50% at 8 and 9 years [9]. In cases of congenital ptosis, parents and children should realize that the ptosis recurrence rate is high after surgery and that the patient is likely to need additional surgeries.

Despite the fact that autogenous fascia has better biocompatibility than alloplastic materials, similar functional and cosmetic outcomes and incidence of ptosis recurrence may be achieved with alloplastic materials [9]. Rates of common complications associated with frontalis suspension including early postoperative exposure keratopathy, inflammation or pyogenic granuloma, eyebrow scars, suture infection with preseptal cellulitis, and suture exposure vary with different sling materials. Higher rates of complications are associated with nylon monofilament and PTFE.

Frontalis suspension is the preferred option for poor levator function cases, although levator resection is often employed [18]. Both methods were found to be effective [19] in cases of poor levator function (2–4 mm). Levator function was reported to be the best predictor of surgical outcomeinthe sec ases [18].

A relatively new procedure termed "Incisionless frontalis suspension" utilizes a nylon monofilament suture for frontalis suspension [20]. The nylon suture is passed in a circling fashion via puncture wounds without making eyebrow incisions. Two puncture sites, approximately 10 mm apart, are marked 3 mm above the lash line centered over the area of desired maximal eyelid elevation. Another two puncture sites are marked above the eyebrow approximately in line with the lateral and medial canthi. This minimally invasive surgery is scarless and can be performed with little trauma to the orbicularis oculi muscle. In comparison to the results of frontalis suspension using allogenic (banked) material, which is not permanent and may be associated with late failures, this technique is a simple, safe, and temporary measure in elevating the eyelid for visual development until the child is old enough for definitive surgery using autologous tissues.

Levator Resection

More aggressive lifts are achievable with levator resection compared to levator advancement, so it is preferred in cases with decreased levator function [2].

Table 28.1 Comparison of previously published data of ptosis recurrence after frontalis suspension surgery with different sling materials

	Study										
Variable	Wasserman et al. [7]	Ben Simon et al. [8]	Wilson and Johnson [9]	Yoon and Lee [10]	Bajaj et al. [11]	Liu [12]	Hersh et al. [13]	Esmaeli et al. [14]	Carter et al. [15]	Wagner et al. [16]	Metha et al. [17]
Eyes (n)	102	164	112	239	60	112	72	132	61	145	32
Follow-up time (months)	24	20	86	6–144	16	84	46	120	22	31[a], 21[b]	29
Material: ptosis recurrence/failure (%)											
Autogenous fascia	4	22		31						8.3	
Banked fascia	51		43				35.3	28			
Silastic							13				
Nylon/nylon monofilament	69	25				100				40.5	
Polyester	27	36			7						23–25
Polytetrafluoro-ethylene (Gortex), Gore Medical, Inc., Flagstaff, AZ, USA	0	15									
Polypropylene	12										
Ethibond (modified polyester suture), Ethicon, Inc., Somerville, NJ, USA					17						
Silicone		44							7		

[a] 31 months for the synthetic group

[b] 21 months for the fascia group

The main disadvantage of this technique is the high rate of lagophthalmos causing exposure keratopathy. Plication of distal orbicularis fibers to the proximal fibers via a skin flap [21] was described in order to overcome the lagophthalmos issues and achieved good results irrespective of the disorder, showing few complications and no lagophthalmos.

Maximal Levator Resection

Maximal levator resection is a better surgical alternative to frontalis suspension in the treatment of severe congenital ptosis whether unilateral or bilateral. It provides a better cosmetic result and the recurrence rate is less than with frontalis suspension [22]. Complete transsection of the medial and lateral horns of the levator aponeurosis with preservation of the Whitnall's ligament is the most important surgical step in mobilizing the levator muscle. Satisfactory eyelid elevation (generally considered to be a difference of less than 1 mm between both eyelid fissures) can be achieved with this technique [23]. Possible complications of sacrificing the medial and lateral horns of the levator aponeurosis include: damage to the superior oblique tendon, severing the lacrimal gland or lacrimal gland ductules, sacrifice of accessory lacrimal glands, goblet cells, meibomian glands, conjunctiva, and loss of support to the lacrimal glad and temporal eyelid. These could be avoided by incising the medial horn slightly temporally and the lateral horn slightly medially. Maintenance of normal tear film is especially important in congenital ptosis surgery where postoperative eyelid lag and lagophthalmos are expected [22, 23].

Whitnall's Sling

In "Whitnall's sling" technique, only the levator aponeurosis is resected, preserving Whitnall's ligament and its attachments. This surgery preserves levator muscle, Müller's muscle, and Whitnall's ligament without altering the structures that produce the three-layer tear film. It is best suited for severe unilateral ptosis in which the opposite fissure height is 9 mm or less and levator function of the ptotic eyelid is 3–5 mm [24]. This technique is believed to be anatomically and physiologically superior to "maximal levator resection" with similar long-term results. More recent results have shown that the addition of a 5-mm superior tarsectomy provides an additional elevation of 1–1.5 mm.

Summary

The traditional approach for correcting ptosis is the use of frontalis suspension procedures for cases with poor levator function, and any of the other methods, depending on margin to reflex distance (MRD), for cases with good levator functions.

Minimal ptosis is best corrected using MMCR, but Fasanella–Servat and levator surgery are also viable options.

With moderate ptosis, levator aponeurosis surgery is usually applied. Levator muscle surgery may be preferred for moderate ptosis with fair levator function. For severe ptosis, levator function and the surgeon's personal preference dictate the choice of surgical procedure, where levator resection and frontalis suspension surgery are the most recommended options.

In general, the success of the procedure depends on the skill and experience of the surgeon; however, even in the most experienced hands, under or overcorrection, asymmetry, and contour deformity are not so uncommon.

References

1. Park DH, Jung JM, Song CH. Anthropometric analysis of levator muscle function. Plast Reconstr Surg. 2008;121:1181–7.
2. Cetinkaya A, Brannan PA. Ptosis repair options and algorithm. Curr Opin Ophthalmol. 2008;19:428–34.

3. McCulley TJ, Kersten RC, Kulwin DR, Feuer WJ. Outcome and influencing factors of external levator palpebrae superioris aponeurosis advancement for blepharoptosis. Ophthal Plast Reconstr Surg. 2003;19:388–93.
4. Ben Simon GJ, Lee S, Schwarcz RM, McCann JD, Goldberg RA. External levator advancement vs Müller's muscle-conjunctival resection for correction of upper eyelid involutional ptosis. Am J Ophthalmol. 2005;140:426–32.
5. Pang NK, Newsom RW, Oestreicher JH, Chung HT, Harvey JT. Fasanella-Servat procedure: indications, efficacy, and complications. Can J Ophthalmol. 2008; 43:84–8.
6. Skibell BC, Harvey JH, Oestreicher JH, Howarth D, Gibbs A, Wegrynowski T, et al. Adrenergic receptors in the ptotic human eyelid: correlation with phenylephrine testing and surgical success in ptosis repair. Ophthal Plast Reconstr Surg. 2007;23:367–71.
7. Wasserman BN, Sprunger DT, Helveston EM. Comparison of materials used in frontalis suspension. Arch Ophthalmol. 2001;119:687–91.
8. Ben Simon GJ, Macedo AA, Schwarcz RM, Wang DY, McCann JD, Goldberg RA. Frontalis suspension for upper eyelid ptosis: evaluation of different surgical designs and suture material. Am J Ophthalmol. 2005;140:877–85.
9. Wilson ME, Johnson RW. Congenital ptosis. Long-term results of treatment using lyophilized fascia lata for frontalis suspensions. Ophthalmology. 1991;98:1234–7.
10. Yoon JS, Lee SY. Long-term functional and cosmetic outcomes after frontalis suspension using autogenous fascia lata for pediatric congenital ptosis. Ophthalmology.200 9;116:1405–14.
11. Bajaj MS, Sastry SS, Ghose S, Betharia SM, Pushker N. Evaluation of polytetrafluoroethylene suture for frontalis suspension as compared to polybutrylate-coated braided polyester. Clin Exp Ophthalmol. 2004;32:415–9.
12. Liu D. Blepharoptosis correction with frontalis suspension using a nylon monofilament sling: duration of effect. Am J Ophthalmol. 1999;128:772–3.
13. Hersh D, Martin FJ, Rowe NJ. Comparison of silastic and banked fascia lata in pediatric frontalis suspension. J Pediatr Ophthalmol Strabismus. 2006;43:212–8.
14. Esmaeli B, Chung H, Pashby RC. Long-term results of frontalis suspension using irradiated, banked fascia lata. Ophthal Plast Reconstr Surg. 1998;14:159–63.
15. Carter S, Meecham WJ, Steiff SR. Silicone frontalis slings for the correction of blepharoptosis: indications and efficacy. Ophthalmology. 1996;103:623–30.
16. Wagner RS, Mauriello Jr JA, Nelson LB, Calhoun JH, Flanagan JC, Harley RD. Treatment of congenital ptosis with frontalis suspension: a comparison of suspensory materials. Ophthalmology. 1984;91:245–8.
17. Metha P, Patel P, Olver JM. Functional results and complications of polyester mesh use for frontalis suspension ptosis surgery. Br J Ophthalmol. 2004;88:361–4.
18. Cates CA, Tyers AG. Outcomes of anterior levator resection in congenital blepharoptosis. Eye. 2001; 15:770–3.
19. Park DH, Choi WS, Yoon SH, Shim JS. Comparison of levator resection and frontalis muscle transfer in the treatment of severe blepharoptosis. Ann Plast Surg.2007; 59:388–92.
20. Yip CC, Goldberg RA, Cook TL, McCann JD. Incision-less frontalis suspension. Br J Ophthalmol. 2004;88:585–6.
21. Singh D. Orbicularis plication for ptosis: a third alternative. Ann Ophthalmol. 2006;38:185–93.
22. Mauriello JA, Wagner RS, Caputo AR, Natale B, Lister M. Treatment of congenital ptosis by maximal levator resection. Ophthalmology. 1986;93:466–9.
23. Press UP, Hubner H. Maximal levator resection in the treatment of unilateral congenital ptosis with poor levator function. Orbit. 2001;20:125–9.
24. Anderson RL, Jordan DR, Dutton JJ. Whitnall's sling for poor function ptosis. Arch Ophthalmol. 1990;108: 1628–32.

Chapter 29
Ptosis Surgery Failure and Reoperation

Jill Melicher and Jefferey A. Nerad

Abstract The purpose of this chapter is to discuss the risk factors for ptosis surgery failure. Preoperative assessment to identify patients with marginal reflex distance < 0 mm, poor levator excursion, and preoperative eyelid laxity should be performed. Treatment of eyelid laxity with lateral canthoplasty or full-thickness wedge resection should be performed prior to ptosis surgery. Intraoperative swelling, bleeding, and excessive sedation may negatively influence revision outcome and should be recognized. If significant corneal exposure and lagophthalmos exist postoperatively, early intervention is necessary. If undercorrection exists, surgical revision should be delayed to allow complete resolution of postoperative swelling.

Introduction

Ptosis surgery is among the most common procedures performed by oculoplastic surgeons. Acquired ptosis may be corrected by an external or internal approach. Severe ptosis of greater than 3 mm, in patients with moderate to good levator excursion (LE, defined as the distance the upper eyelid travels from extreme downgaze to extreme upgaze, measured in millimeters), requires an external approach with levator aponeurosis advancement. Müllers muscle-conjunctival resection is traditionally used to treat mild to moderate ptosis of 2 mm or less, although it has successfully been employed with 3 mm or greater ptosis. Frontalis suspension is required for patients with poor levator excursion. Most patients undergoing eyelid ptosis repair have satisfactory results. However, even the most experienced eyelid surgeon will have a few patients with unsatisfactory results. Honest, critical eyelid surgeons will agree that very few ptosis repairs have "perfect" height and contour.

The reoperation rates for ptosis repair in the literature vary. A recent study performed by Simon et al. reports a reoperation rate of 18% for external levator advancement and 3% for Müllers muscle-conjunctival resection surgery [1]. The overall success rates of external levator aponeurosis advancement surgery reported in the literature vary from 70% to more than 95% [2–4]. The largest study to date evaluating approximately 1,000 patients who underwent external levator advancement surgery for acquired ptosis with good levator excursion had a reoperation rate of 8.7% [3].

Both eyelid height and contour are important considerations. A patient with satisfactory eyelid height may complain about irregularities in the eyelid shape. Careful contour adjustments should be performed at the time of ptosis correction to decrease the likelihood of reoperation. Even with careful intraoperative adjustments, eyelid abnormalities in height and contour (nasal or temporal flare or droop and areas of peaking) may require

J. Melicher (✉)
Department of Ophthalmology, Cincinnati Eye Institute, Cincinnati, OH, USA
e-mail: jmelicher@cincinnatieye.com

A.J. Cohen and D.A. Weinberg (eds.), *Evaluation and Management of Blepharoptosis*,
DOI 10.1007/978-0-387-92855-5_29, © Springer Science+Business Media, LLC 2011

revision surgery. This chapter identifies factors increasing the likelihood of ptosis surgery failure and surgical approaches to ptosis reoperation.

Factors Increasing Ptosis Surgery Failure

Understanding our patient's goals for surgery is very important in achieving success with ptosis correction. Educating patients on the difference between dermatochalasis and eyelid margin height and illustrating to the patient how the presence of brow ptosis worsens upper eyelid dermatochalasis are very important. Many patients do not recognize eyelid or brow ptosis, but notice the presence of dermatochalasis. It is important to educate the patient regarding how the eyebrow, the skin fold, and the eyelid margin may contribute to a "droopy eyelid." Equally important is understanding the patient's cosmetic concerns, any functional difficulties, and the overall postoperative expectation.

Preoperative Factors

Several preoperative measurable eyelid characteristics have been noted in the literature to be risk factors for increased likelihood of reoperation following ptosis surgery. Marginal reflex distance (MRD_1, defined as the distance between the corneal light reflex and the upper eyelid margin, measured in millimeters) of less than 0 mm, decreased levator excursion, and the presence of Hering's law dependency are all predictors of over or undercorrection with ptosis surgery [3]. All three factors should be taken into consideration with preoperative surgical planning and in the informed consent process.

Hering's law dependency can be identified by instilling 10% phenylephrine in the superior fornix of the ptotic eye, in the case of unilateral ptosis, or the more ptotic eye, in the case of bilateral ptosis. The presence of a decrease in the contralateral MRD_1 indicates that Hering's effect is present. If Hering's effect is suspected, the phenylephrine test should be performed. If prominent Hering's dependency is found, bilateral ptosis surgery should be performed.

Additionally, the presence of eyelid laxity or floppy eyelid syndrome should be noted at the time of preoperative evaluation. Significant laxity can result in problems with contour adjustment intraoperatively. Surgeons may consider treating eyelid laxity with full-thickness wedge resection or lateral canthopexy prior to surgery to improve the overall success of ptosis correction. Wedge resection can result in some elevation of the eyelid margin and should be performed at least 3–6 months prior to ptosis repair.

Intraoperative Factors

Intraoperative factors influencing the success of ptosis surgery include bleeding, swelling, impaired levator function due to local anesthetic effect, unrecognized eyelid laxity, an excessively sedated patient, and scarring from injury or previous eyelid procedures. Shorter operative time tends to make ptosis correction easier. Careful use of intravenous sedation can make the patient comfortable, facilitating eyelid surgery, while too much sedation can interfere with intraoperative eyelid height. Severe intraoperative lagophthalmos may limit the amount of advancement possible.

Excessive bleeding or ecchymosis at the time of surgical correction may result in significant eyelid swelling that make adjustments difficult, or less accurate, during external levator aponeurosis advancement surgery. Slow injection of local anesthesia with epinephrine with a 30-gauge needle just under the skin should be used to minimize any bruising that may occur even before the skin incision. In most cases 1.0 cc of local anesthetic per eyelid is all that is necessary. Excessive injection contributes to eyelid swelling and potential weakening of the levator. Allow 5–10 min for the epinephrine effect to provide hemostasis prior to the skin incision. Cutting tools including the Colorado microdissection needle, thermal cautery, Ellman radiofrequency, or the CO_2 laser are useful to minimize bleeding during the skin incision and deeper dissection. Careful dissection of the aponeurosis from the underlying vascular Müller's muscle should be performed to minimize bleeding and bruising within Müller's muscle. Performing this dissection with high temperature battery cautery is helpful to decrease the risk of Müller's muscle hemorrhage. If bleeding occurs, immediate tamponade with a cotton tip applicator or digital pressure followed by bipolar cauterization of the bleeding vessel will minimize the swelling induced by the hemorrhage. If significant hemorrhage and swelling occur intraoperatively, the surgeon may need to make adjustments based on the amount of levator aponeurosis resected on the contralateral side or consider the degree of swelling in unilateral surgery and adjust the suture placement accordingly. If significant intraoperative hemorrhage is encountered, surgery may need to be aborted and the eyelid position adjusted a week later in the office, once swelling has deminished.

In unilateral ptosis and asymmetric bilateral ptosis cases, Hering's law dependency may result in contralateral eyelid drooping that makes reliable intraoperative adjustment more difficult. A study published by Wladis and Gausas in 2008 illustrated in a small number of patients that Hering's law dependency, although not demonstrated preoperatively, was present at the time of surgery, resulting in a mean intraoperative droop of greater than 2 mm in the contralateral eyelid height. They suggest raising the operated eyelid to the preoperative height (MRD_1) of the contralateral side to achieve postoperative symmetry. The Hering's effect resolved postoperatively in all the 12 patients studied [5]. Preoperative testing for Hering's law dependency does not reliably predict postoperative contralateral eyelid height according to Erb et al. [6]. Their study states that approximately 5% of patients undergoing unilateral ptosis repair require contralateral ptosis correction within 1 year.

Although infrequently encountered in our practice, cases of bilateral, asymmetric ptosis may present an intraoperative surgical challenge. These patients must be carefully evaluated for Hering's law dependency preoperatively and the levator function should be carefully assessed. This unique subgroup of patients may be best treated with the most ptotic lid being surgically corrected first, postoperative assessment of the height of the contralateral lid, and if necessary surgical intervention for the contralateral lid 2–3 months after the first surgery.

Unrecognized upper lid laxity may be encountered at the time of surgery and is exacerbated by the absence of orbicularis muscle tone following the injection of local anesthesia. Patients with eyelid laxity may require more than one suture to secure the aponeurosis to the tarsal plate to avoid contour abnormalities or eyelid margin peaking postoperatively. Severe eyelid laxity also predisposes to eversion of the tarsus, which can be alleviated by moving the sutures higher on the tarsal plate. Ideally, excessive laxity should be corrected with a separate surgical procedure prior to ptosis correction. Simultaneous wedge resection and ptosis repair should be avoided in these patients. Wedge resection requires additional local anesthesia, resulting in a decrease in levator tone and excursion and can make adjustment of eyelid height and contour more difficult intraoperatively. Horizontal lid tightening surgery should be performed at least 6–8 weeks prior to ptosis correction to allow appropriate time for healing and re-evaluation of eyelid position as wedge resection surgery often will lift the lid slightly, resulting in some ptosis correction.

Intraoperative qualitative assessment of lagophthalmos is challenging for eyelid surgeons. We typically ask ourselves: How much intraoperative lagophthalmos is too much at the time of ptosis surgery? Several preoperative factors should be considered to minimize exposure issues postoperatively. If the patient has robust orbicularis function, a good Bell's phenomenon and a healthy tear film, more aggressive lid elevation and greater intraoperative lagophthalmos can be tolerated. Once orbicularis tone improves following surgery, lagophthalmos should resolve, or at least improve, in most patients.

Patient goals and expectations should be considered during the informed consent process.

It is important to remember that not all patients require an MRD_1 of 4–5 mm postoperatively. Ptosis surgeons may consider a conservative postoperative lid height (MRD_1 of 2 mm) in elderly patients and those with previous corneal surface disease, prior corneal or glaucoma surgery, orbicularis muscle weakness, or poor levator excursion. Aggressive postoperative lubrication is recommended in all patients to minimize surface dryness. In patients at risk for exposure, minimal skin and muscle or skin only should be resected at the time of ptosis surgery.

Careful use of intravenous sedation is important to make the patient comfortable, but excessive sedation can make adjustment difficult or impossible. Ideally, the patient should receive propofol just prior to local anesthetic injection and then be allowed to awaken fully. Small amounts of additional sedation or narcotic pain medication can be used to keep the patient comfortable but awake enough for accurate eyelid adjustment. A discussion preoperatively with the anesthesia service is helpful to avoid over- or under-sedation.

Postoperative Factors

Severe and prolonged swelling may result in residual postoperative eyelid ptosis. Complete resolution of the swelling is necessary to assess the surgical outcome, in terms of eyelid height and contour. Severe postoperative edema may also result in suture loosening (cheese-wiring) or breakage. Early postoperative adjustment in height or contour should not be considered if significant eyelid swelling is present [7].

Lagophthalmos, or lid retraction with lagophthalmos, may result from septal scarring or excessive shortening of the levator aponeurosis and muscle. Minimal handling of the orbital septum is encouraged. One should avoid placing any sutures through the septum, i.e., closing the septum or suturing it to the tarsal plate. In patients with eyebrow ptosis, the novice surgeon may mistake the eyebrow (sub-brow) fat pad for the preaponeurotic fat, or confuse the septum with the levator aponeurosis. One should remember that the eyebrow fat contains fibrous septae, whereas the preaponeurotic fat does not. The orbital septum attaches to the orbital rim so that manual tugging on this layer will demonstrate firm resistance. On the other hand, one can appreciate some stretching when pulling on the aponeurosis. If there is any uncertainty, one can ask the patient to look up and down to identify levator movement or to feel a "tug" with upgaze.

Patients with postoperative lagophthalmos and lid lag on downgaze should be evaluated for septal scarring that will require surgical release if there is significant or symptomatic corneal exposure. If reduced upper eyelid excursion is noted preoperatively, significant resection of the levator may be required to achieve a "normal" eyelid height. Remember it is much better to have the eyelid remain a bit low, i.e., undercorrected, and the patient comfortable, rather than "normal" height and an uncomfortable patient.

Postoperative asymmetry in the eyelid skin crease or fold may give the appearance of residual postoperative ptosis. Careful preoperative eyelid skin crease measurements and marking may prevent this complication postoperatively. Lid crease reformation, with anchoring of the skin to the underlying levator, is necessary in some patients, especially those with reduced levatore xcursion.

Surgical Approach to Ptosis Reoperation

Reoperation rates following both external levator aponeurosis advancement and Müller's muscle-conjunctival resection are relatively low. The timing of revision surgery is typically determined by surgeon preference when treating both under- and overcorrection of ptosis. A study published by Shore et al. indicates that both early and late revisions were successful in correcting unacceptable results following external levator advancement surgery [4]. Although early and late revision surgery was equally successful, benefits of early intervention included minimizing time to final surgical result and ease of reoperation surgery due to minimal scarring. We typically perform all revision operations as an external approach through the lid crease, regardless of the initial surgical technique employed.

Several studies have suggested that resting eyelid position 1 week postoperatively in patients with minimal to moderate swelling is a good predictor of final eyelid height and outcome [8, 9]. Mild asymmetry may be observed for 4–6 weeks until all swelling resolves. Mild eyelid height asymmetry of less than 1 mm may resolve without surgical intervention or may be considered an acceptable surgical outcome.

If minimal overcorrection exists following levator aponeurosis advancement surgery, conservative management with eyelid "massage" can result in some improvement in eyelid height. Ask the patient to close the eye. While placing inferior traction on the closed upper eyelid, the patient looks upward, thus stretching the levator aponeurosis and muscle. Eyelid massage can be started as early as the second postoperative week, when the risk of wound dehiscence is greatly reduced.

If significant eyelid retraction and prominent lagophthalmos with significant corneal exposure are present at 1 week postoperatively, early surgical revision is indicated. At 1 week, the majority of postoperative eyelid edema has resolved, tissue planes are easily identified, and scar tissue formation is minimal, making revision surgery at this time relatively easy. The levator suture(s) may be cut from either an external or a transconjunctival approach to drop the upper eyelid. We prefer reopening the wound, identifying the suture resulting in the abnormality, and cutting the suture. Using an external approach allows additional suture placement if contour is disrupted when suture lysis is performed.

Postoperative abnormalities in contour (i.e., peaking and temporal flare) may be addressed from an external approach by moving or adding a suture to change the eyelid shape. If significant contour abnormality exists in patients with minimal to moderate swelling, early intervention is indicated [10]. The natural "peak" (high point) of the upper eyelid margin typically corresponds to the medial aspect of the pupil; however, some patients have relatively flat eyelid contour, and in unilateral ptosis surgery cases, contour symmetry should be the goal.

Residual ptosis following levator advancement or Müller's muscle-conjunctival resection requiring reoperation can be performed through a "mini" external approach through a small incision in the lid crease or previous incision. Inspecting for a broken or cheese-wire suture and repeating the aponeurosis advancement can be performed as early as 4–6 weeks following the initial surgery, giving ample time for residual edema to resolve. Some surgeons opt for reoperation following levator advancement using posterior approach repairs. This has not been our approach, however.

Patients with persistent lagophthalmos that exhibit signs of septal scarring on clinical exam require reoperation. If there is no evidence of corneal compromise, revision surgery should not be performed prior to 4–6 months following the initial operation, allowing scar tissue remodeling to complete. The lid crease should be opened, exposing the entire septum. Septal scarring should be released along the entire length of the levator and excised. Occasionally, we place Kenalog in the dissection planes at the time of revision surgery to decrease the inflammatory response and minimize scar tissue formation followingre operation.

Summary

Recognizing preoperative, intraoperative, and postoperative factors increasing the likelihood of surgical failure is essential to improve the success of ptosis operation. As always, patient education and reasonable goals and expectations are important to achieve a good postoperative result and a satisfied patient. Careful preoperative measurements (MRD_1 and levator excursion) and preoperative recognition of preexisting ocular conditions (such as lagophthalmos) and eyelid disorders (such as floppy eyelid syndrome) help to avoid potential problems. Meticulous hemostasis and careful dissection of surgical planes minimize intraoperative adjustment difficulties and postoperative scarring. In the best of hands, occasional cases that require reoperation are expected. Timing and technique for reoperation vary among ptosis surgeons, without a definitive consensus.

References

1. Ben Simon GJ, Lee S, Schwarcz RM, McCann JD, Goldberg RA. External levator advancement vs. Muller's muscle-conjunctival resection for correction of upper eyelid involutional ptosis. Am J Ophthalmol. 2005;140(3):426–32.
2. Anderson RL, Dixon RS. Aponeurotic ptosis surgery. Arch Ophthalmol. 1979;97:1123–8.
3. Berlin AJ, Vestal KP. Levatory aponeurosis surgery: a retrospective review. Ophthalmology. 1989;96: 1033–6.
4. McCulley T, Kersten RC, Kulwin DR, Feuer WJ. Outcome and influencing factors of external levator palpebrae superioris aponeurosis advancement for blepharoptosis. Ophthal Plast Reconstr Surg. 2003;19:388–93.
5. Shore JW, Bergin DJ, Garrett SN. Results of blepharoptosis surgery with early postoperative adjustment. Ophthalmology. 1990;97:1502–11.
6. Erb MH, Kersten RC, Yip CC, Hudak D, Kulwin DR, McCulley TJ. Effect of unilateral blepharoptosis repair on contralateral eyelid position. Ophthal Plast Reconstr Surg. 2004;20(6):418–22.
7. Tucker SM, Verhulst SJ. Stabilization of eyelid height after aponeurotic ptosis repair. Ophthalmology. 1999; 106(3):517–22.
8. Wladis EJ, Gausas RE. Transient descent of the contralateral eyelid in unilateral ptosis surgery. Ophthal Plast Reconstr Surg. 2008;24(5):348–51.
9. Linberg JV, Vasquez RJ, Chao GM. Aponeurotic ptosis repair under local anesthesia: prediction of results from operative lid height. Ophthalmology. 1988;95:1046.
10. Park DH, Jung JM, Choi WS, Song CH. Early postoperative adjustment of blepharoptosis. Ann Plast Surg.2006; 57(4):376–80.

Chapter30
Complications of Ptosis Repair: Prevention andManag ement

Milad Hakimbashi, Don O. Kikkawa, and Bobby S. Korn

Abstract Ptosis repair is one of the most common operations in oculofacial plastic surgery. In mild cases, eyelid ptosis can be purely cosmetic, but in severe cases, it can cause significant visual field compromise, hindering vision and resulting in amblyopia in children. Because a variety of mechanisms can cause ptosis, it is essential that the surgeon make the proper diagnosis and implement the right surgical plan to achieve the best result. Even in expert hands, however, a less than ideal result can occur. Variables exist beyond the surgeon's control, but it is the proper recognition and management of these problems that allow for optimized outcomes even in the face of complications.

This chapter details the most frequent complications associated with the different approaches to ptosis surgery. These include: under/overcorrection, lid contour abnormalities, lid malposition, and lagophthalmos. Recommended medical and surgical solutions to deal with each specific postoperative complication are also covered.

Ptosis repair is one of the most frequent operations in ophthalmic plastic surgery. Even in the best of hands, ptosis surgery can be challenging, and results may not be perfect. Although the vast majority of procedures achieve the desired outcome with patient and surgeon satisfaction, educating the patient and family about potential side effects and complications can decrease the element of surprise postoperatively. One of the most fundamental ways to decrease complications is the selection of the proper operation for the patient; simply performing an operation that the surgeon feels most comfortable with will likely lead to suboptimal outcomes [1–3].

Due to the unpredictable nature of ptosis surgery, even the most experienced and skilled surgeon will likely face complications at some point. This chapter highlights common complications and their management.

Under-andO vercorrection

Under- and overcorrection constitute the majority of complications depending on the type of operation, in some studies, the frequency is as high as 20% [4]. Some colleagues feel that sitting the patient up, often several times, during surgery to assess upper lid height and symmetry will improve the likelihood of a successful outcome.

Overcorrection typically occurs after levator advancement for acquired ptosis and in patients with good levator function. It is more rare in congenital ptosis, particularly in cases with poor levator function where undercorrection is more common. Although over or under correction is not

D.O.K ikkawa(✉)
Department of Ophthalmology, Division of Ophthalmic Plastic and Reconstructive Surgery,
Shiley Eye Center, University of California,
SanD iego,La J olla, CA, USA
e-mail:ki kkawa@eyecenter.ucsd.edu

A.J. Cohen and D.A. Weinberg (eds.), *Evaluation and Management of Blepharoptosis*,
DOI 10.1007/978-0-387-92855-5_30, © Springer Science+Business Media, LLC 2011

entirely avoidable, one can reduce the incidence with careful measurement of levator function, preoperative planning, and intraoperative lid adjustments based on patient cooperation during surgery, if done under local anesthesia [5]. Many intraoperative variables exist during levator advancement surgery. These include: amount of anesthetic infiltrated, degree of patient consciousness, and amount of swelling and hemorrhage (see chapter on levator advancement surgery for more details on surgical technique). We commonly use epinephrine (1:200,000) in our local anesthetic and infiltrate more anteriorly and for hemostasis. In theory, epinephrine can stimulate Müller's muscle causing contraction resulting in undercorrection in levator advancement and overcorrection in conjunctival Müllerectomy in conjunctival Müllerectomy, however, we keep the injection superficial and limit the amount to avoid diffusion posteriorly.

If possible, it is best to follow the patient for a minimum of 2 weeks prior to attempting repair of overcorrection. Patients can use frequent lubricants and tape their lid closed at bedtime to lessen exposure keratopathy. Conservative measures include downward massage, stretching, and asking the patient to squeeze his/her eyelids multiple times a day. If conservative measures fail and surgical repair is imminent, a frank discussion with the patient is necessary with the surgical goal of lowering the eyelid but preferably not returning the patient back to the preoperative ptotic state.

In adults undergoing levator surgery with either over- or undercorrection, an early office revision (Fig. 30.1a–d) has been recommended [6]. This technique involves an office visit as early as 3–4 days postoperatively. Minimal to no local anesthetic is used, and under sterile conditions, the wound is opened. Blunt dissection easily separates the wound edge, and the levator is identified. The levator sutures are removed, replaced (advanced in the case of undercorrection and recessed in the case of overcorrection), and tied with a temporary knot. The lid height is then examined until satisfactory height of the upper eyelid is established. Once the desired height has been determined, the suture is tied permanently. Skin closure is then performed.

Overcorrection can also occur after frontalis suspension. Depending on the type of material used, adjustment can range from simple to complex [7, 8]. If silicone is used, the central brow incision can be opened and the two ends loosened from the within the sleeve. If fascia or another synthetic material is used, two options exist. If early (within 1–2 months after surgery), an attempt can be made to loosen the knots at the brow attachment. If greater than 3 months after the initial surgery, the fascia becomes incorporated and it becomes very difficult to isolate the knots. Thus, in these cases, the eyelid wound can be opened and the fascia recessed from its tarsal attachment.

If overcorrection occurs with the posterior approach ptosis repairs, release of the suture and gentle downward stretch will usually help to resolve the overcorrection. However, one must be careful to avoid converting an overcorrection to an undercorrection by fully separating the internal wound during this maneuver.

In most cases of undercorrection, observation should be the initial approach. Postoperative swelling, which may restrict elevation of the eyelid, can take up to several months to resolve in certain cases. Once edema and hemorrhage subside, the lid is likely to get elevated to some degree. When considering a surgical repair of undercorrection, a fundamental decision must be made to either revise the same surgery or perform a different surgical technique. The early office-based revision can be applied to adults with mild to moderate undercorrection. However, if time has elapsed and the tissues have healed well, a complete reoperation is more likely.

Undercorrection occurs most commonly in congenital or acquired ptosis where levator function is poor or when the inappropriate type of ptosis procedure has been performed. In cases of levator resection, inadequate levator resection or postoperative loosening of the sutures (sometimes due to "cheesewiring" through a very attenuated aponeurosis) are the likely culprits. When operating on a patient with a very thin levator aponeurosis, sutures should be passed through a more robust portion of the aponeurosis more superiorly, or through Whitnall's ligament, and one can use a hang-back suture position if

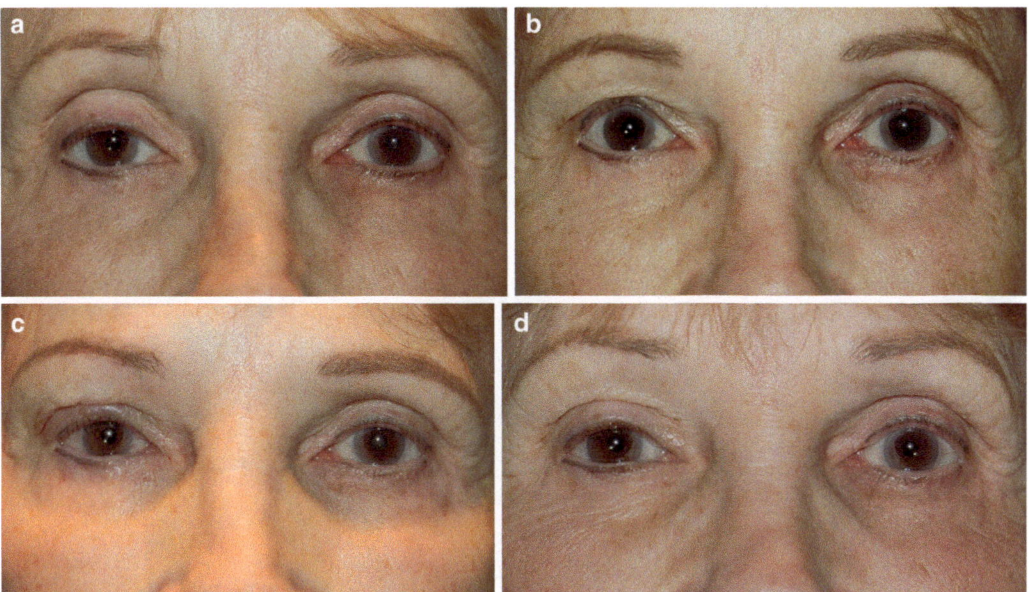

Fig. 30.1 (**a**) A 66-year-old female with right upper lid ptosis. (**b**) Patient 1 week after surgery with right upper lid symptomatic overcorrection. (**c**) Immediately after right upper lid in-office levator recession. (**d**) Final lid levels 3 months after officer evision

this results in excessive levator advancement, i.e., if overcorrection is noted intraoperatively. If there is persistent, significant undercorrection, then reoperation with additional levator resection should be considered, provided the ocular surface can tolerate it. In the case of poor levator function, if a maximal levator resection has already been performed and the patient has recurrent or persistent ptosis, then further levator resection is not an option, and either superior tarsectomy or frontalis suspension may be required. In cases of undercorrection with good levator function, readvancement of the levator is typically all that is necessary; in addition, a posterior lamellar procedure (Müller's muscle-conjunctival resection or Fasanella–Servat [9]) could be considered as a secondary procedure.

Treatment for unilateral ptosis with poor levator function has been controversial, with some surgeons electing a bilateral procedure with levator weakening on the normal side, and others preferring a unilateral surgical approach. A unilateral procedure will likely have associated lid lag (with greater eyelid asymmetry noted on down-gaze on the operated side). If undercorrection occurs following a unilateral frontalis suspension procedure, which may result from amblyopia in the ptotic eye or simply ocular dominance in the contralateral eye (such that the patient is not motivated to elevate the brow), then a bilateral frontalis suspension procedure should be considered.

In cases of undercorrection after a frontalis suspension procedure, a similar approach can be used as in the case of overcorrection. With a silicone sling the brow incision can be opened and the ends tightened within the sleeve (Fig. 30.2a–c). In the case of fascia or other materials, if the material cannot be found and tightened, advancing the sling further inferiorly on the tarsus and reanchoring the sling with additional sutures can provide additional lift. Finally, if the suspension material is inadequate and its tensile strength has weakened, a complete revision is recommended.

In the case of posterior lamellar approaches (Müller's muscle-conjunctival resection or the Fasanella–Servat procedure), repair of undercorrection typically involves using a different surgical approach. Some surgeons will perform a

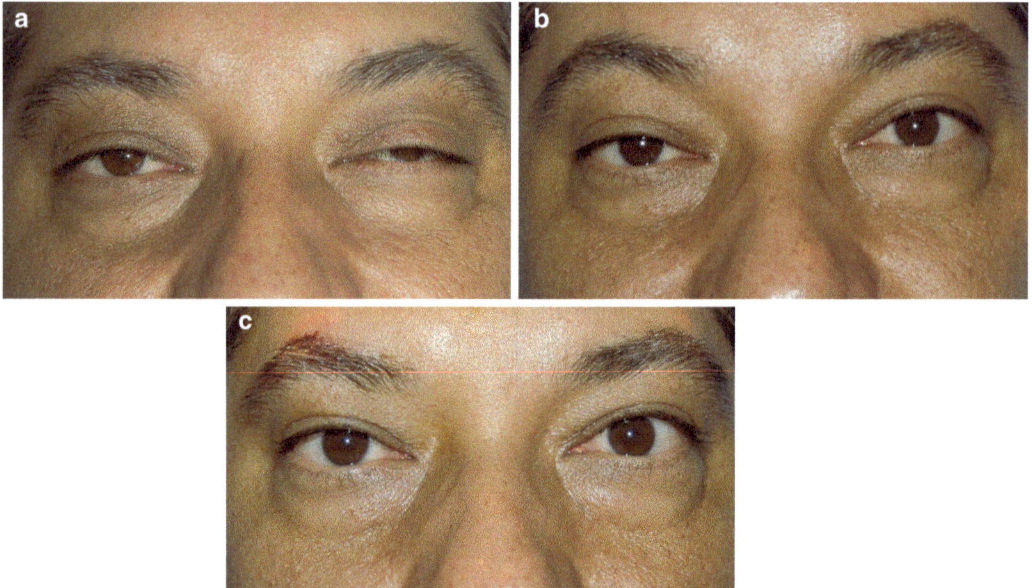

Fig. 30.2 (**a**) A 43-year-old male with myasthenia gravis and stable bilateral ptosis on maximally tolerated medical therapy. (**b**) After bilateral upper lid frontalis suspension with silicone band. Right upper lid is undercorrected. (**c**) Immediately after office revision with tightening of thes iliconeba ndt hroughc entralbr owi ncision

Fasanella–Servat procedure following a failed Müller's muscle-conjunctival resection with good results; however, there is a limit as to the amount of conjunctiva and tarsus that can be safely resected, and excessive resection can lead to symblepharon (see below) and tarsal instability. Patients with a failed posterior approach will likely benefit the most from levator advancement surgery (Fig. 30.3a–d).

Entropion

Entropion typically results when the posterior lamella of the eyelid has been shortened out of proportion to the anterior lamella. This can occur with almost every type of ptosis surgery. The posterior lamella is elevated superiorly, and the anterior lamella shifts inferiorly. It is the lack of everting forces that causes the lid margin to rotate inward. In addition to its cosmetic impact, entropion may result in inward eyelashes that abrade the cornea, a potentially disastrous complication that can cause severe keratopathy and corneal ulceration and requires prompt attention. However, if the entropion is mild and well tolerated, it is reasonable to carefully observe the patient to see if improvement occurs spontaneously.

Avoidance of entropion is best addressed at the time of the initial operation. A large levator resection with sutures placed too high on the tarsus may promote the development of entropion (Fig. 30.4), so it is best to lower the tarsal fixation points of the sutures. If the tarsus is divided vertically into thirds, the tarsal fixation points should be located between the junction of the middle and upper thirds for the best stability and contour of the lid postoperatively (Fig. 30.5).

Anterior lamellar repositioning is another useful approach when managing postoperative upper lid entropion and preventing its occurrence. This involves dissecting skin and muscle in the pretarsal space until the lash bulbs are visible. The anterior lamella is then elevated and secured by placing multiple 7-0 absorbable sutures from the pretarsal orbicularis to a higher

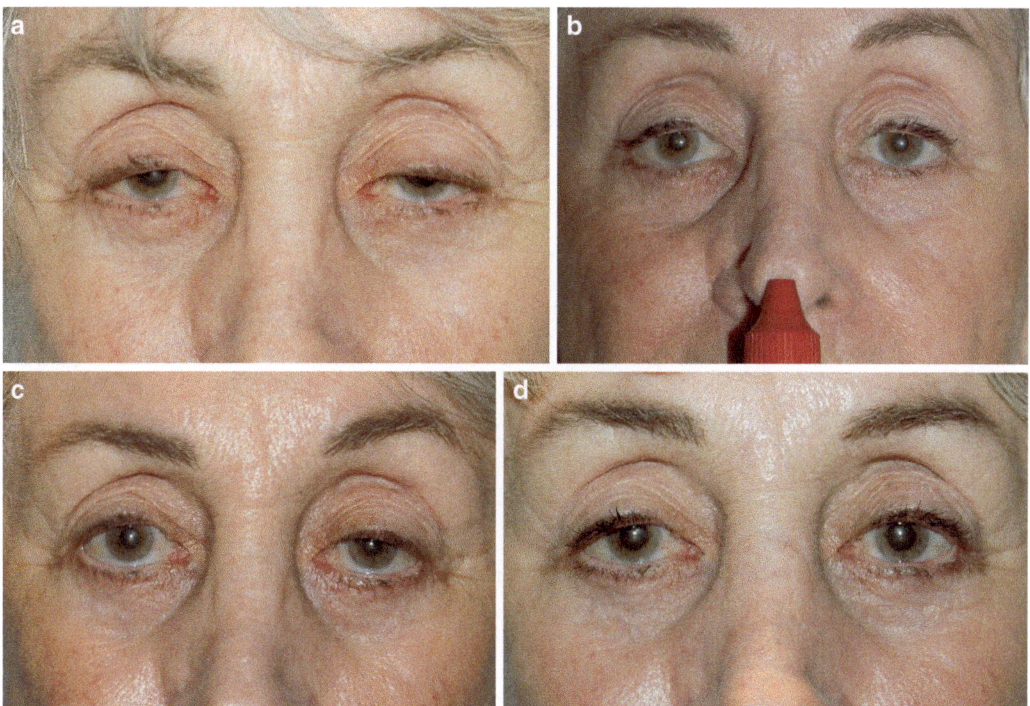

Fig. 30.3 (**a**) A 76-year-old female with bilateral acquired ptosis. (**b**) After instillation of 2.5% phenylephrine showing good response. (**c**) Same patient after undergoing bilateral 8-mm conjunctival Müllerectomy. Left upper lid is undercorrected. (**d**) Final lid levels after undergoing revision of left upper lid with external levator advancement

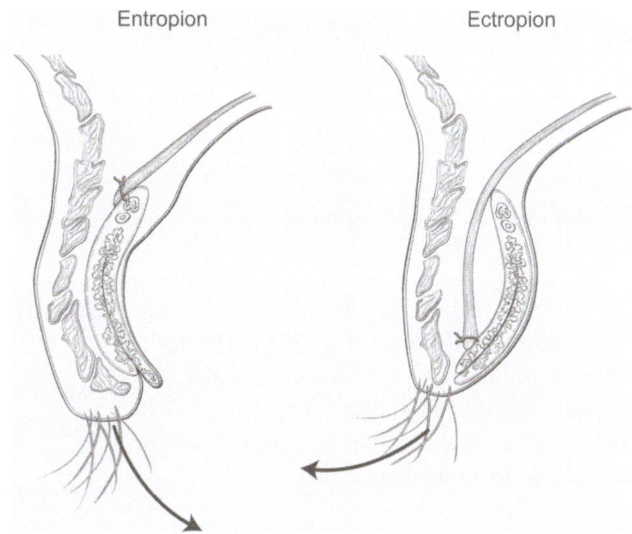

Fig. 30.4 Incorrectv ertical placement of suture can result in entropion or ectropion due to the upward pull of the levator

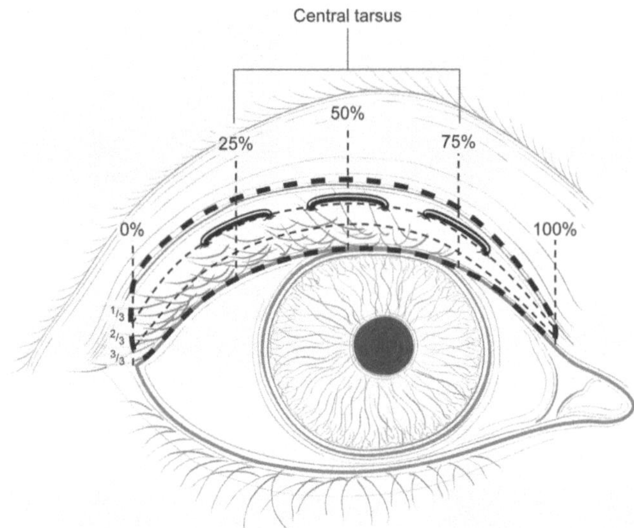

Fig. 30.5 Optimal placement of sutures is along the central 25–75% part of the tarsus horizontally and between the junction of the upper and middle thirds vertically

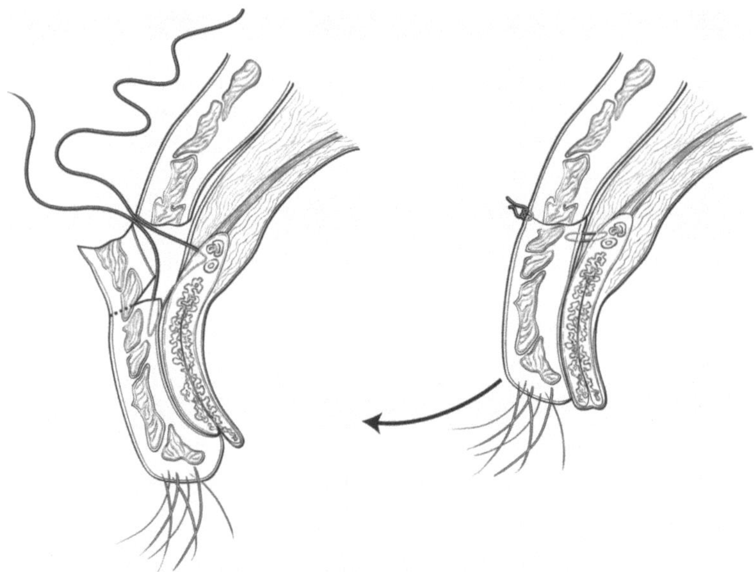

Fig.30.6 Anterior lamellar repositioning to evert upper lashes and correct upper lid entropion

vertical level on the tarsus. This creates excellent eversion of the lid margin (Fig. 30.6). This technique is useful during both levator resection and frontalis suspension surgery. Any excess skin above the lid crease can then be removed and the skin closed in a standard fashion.

Symblepharon

Excessive scarring in a posterior approach surgery can lead to cicatricial contractures creating excessive inward pull on the eyelid which in turn can also cause entropion. Treatment is aimed at releasing the scar, which allows the tissue to relax back to its normal configuration (Fig. 30.7a–c). In rare cases, if the symblepharon is severe enough to produce limitation of eye movement and/or binocular diplopia, placement of a mucous membrane or amniotic membrane graft may be necessary.

Ectropion

In general, ectropion occurs when there is excessive anterior and upward pull as opposed to posterior and inward tension on the eyelid. This can occur in several ways. In cases of a large levator resection, ectropion is usually due to the levator being sutured too far inferiorly on the tarsus. Likewise, in frontalis suspension, if the sling is attached too far inferiorly or if the sling is too superficial, the lid may elevate away from the globe when the brows are raised (Fig. 30.8a–c).

Finally, if excessive skin is removed along with any ptosis procedure, full thickness shortening of the eyelid will occur and ectropion can result, which is accentuated by the elevation of the brow. This may produce symptomatic lagophthalmos that is difficult to correct surgically without replacing skin via a graft or flap.

Treatment for ectropion involves adjustment of levator or sling attachments, such that the tarsal fixation point is more superior (further away from the lid margin). With frontalis suspension, passing the sling posterior to the orbital septum (while avoiding the arcus marginalis) prior to exiting near the brow should correct the

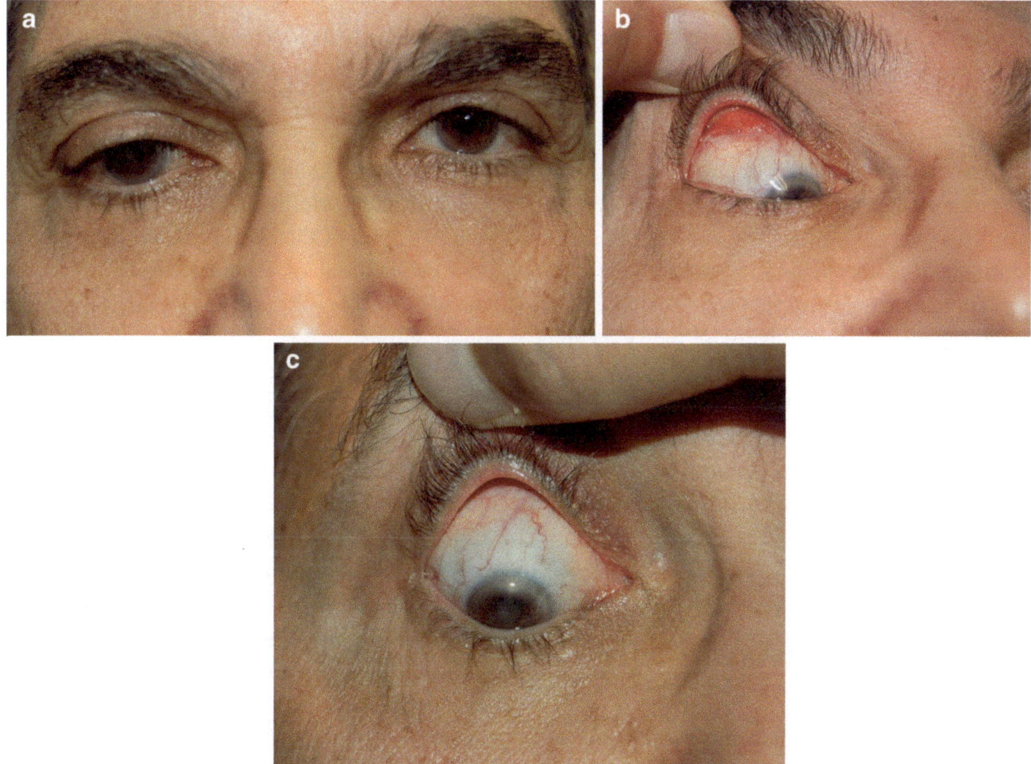

Fig. 30.7 (**a**) A 69-year-old male who underwent large Müller's muscle conjunctival resection (>10 mm) was referred for management of symptomatic entropion of the right upper eyelid. (**b**) On upper lid eversion, symblepharon noted, causing cicatricial entropion. (**c**) After release of symblepharon and placement of amniotic membrane graft to rebuild fornix. Note the deepening of fornix

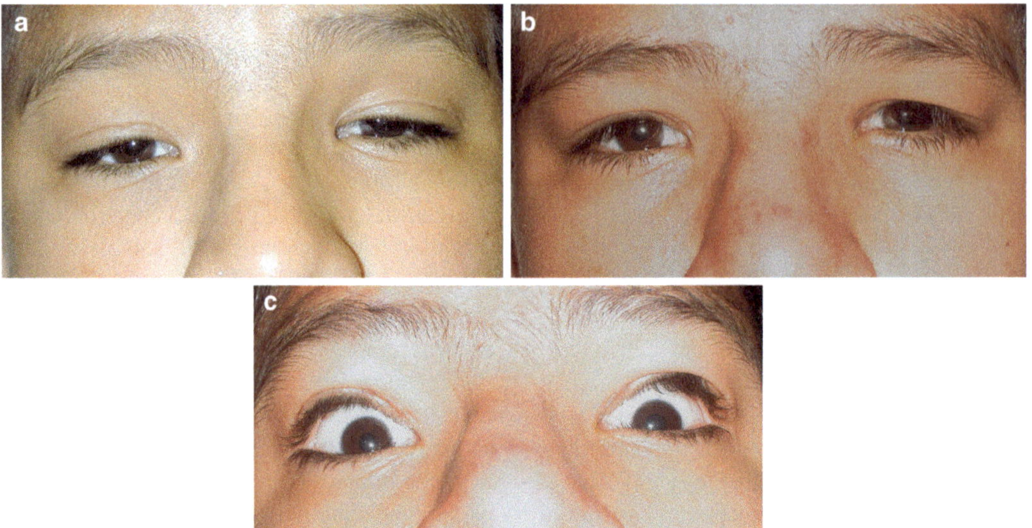

Fig. 30.8 (**a**) 12-year old male with poor function bilateral ptosis. (**b**) After bilateral upper lid frontalis suspension with autologous fascia lata. Note satisfactory lid position in primary position. (**c**) With maximal with frontalis elevation, upper lid ectropion occurs

ectropion. This provides a more favorable, posteriorly and superiorly directed vector force that lessens the tendency of the lid to pull away from the globe with eyebrow elevation. An excessively lax upper eyelid increases the chances of developing ectropion, and occasionally horizontal tightening of the eyelid is warranted.

If longstanding ectropion is present after frontalis suspension, an eyelid crease incision can be made, with release of the sling's tarsal attachments to allow the eyelid to "relax" downward. Although the tarsal attachments are lysed, the fibrous tracts that formed around the sling material (autologous or alloplastic) will continue to allow eyelid elevation with frontalis contraction.

ContourD eformity

Postoperative contour deformity is largely aesthetic in nature and rarely functionally significant. It can occur with any type of ptosis repair. In assessing the deformity, some time should be given for resolution of edema and inflammation before considering treatment, particularly if there is significant eyelid swelling. This must be weighed, however, against the fact that as the healing process progresses, dissection becomes more difficult, i.e., it is quicker and easier to do a brief touch-up, such as repositioning the tarsal sutures, during the first 2 weeks after surgery.

Contour deformities can manifest in several ways. Peaking of the eyelid nasally, centrally, or temporally, nasal or temporal drooping, and a flat eyelid contour are all types of contour abnormalities.

Contour deformities occur most commonly following levator surgery and frontalis suspension. Improper suture placement is usually the cause of the deformities (Fig. 30.9a, b). If the sutures are placed too far apart from each other on the tarsus, it can lead to an eyelid that has a flat contour without the natural curvature of the eyelid that has its highest point just nasal to the pupil [10]. On the other hand, if the sutures are placed close to each other, the pull vector will concentrate too much in the middle leading to unnatural peaking. Length of the suture pass in the central tarsal bite can also be a factor. A horizontally long tarsal bite can also cause flattening, while a short tarsal bite can cause peaking (Fig. 30.10). Contour abnormalities are more common in patients with very thin, floppy tarsal plates and also in vertically shortened tarsal

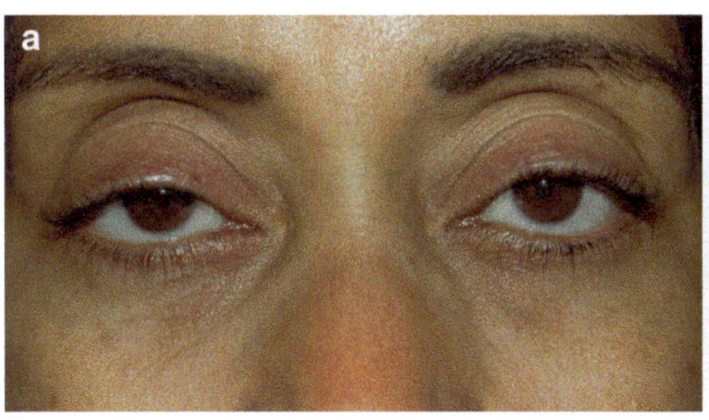

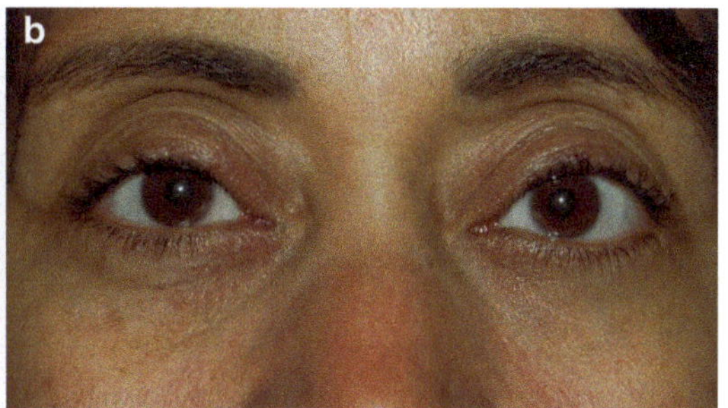

Fig. 30.9 (**a**) A 52-year-old female with bilateral acquired ptosis with good levator function. (**b**) Same patient after undergoing bilateral external levator advancement. Note satisfactory lid levels but lateral peaking in left upper lid due to temporal placement of centrals uture

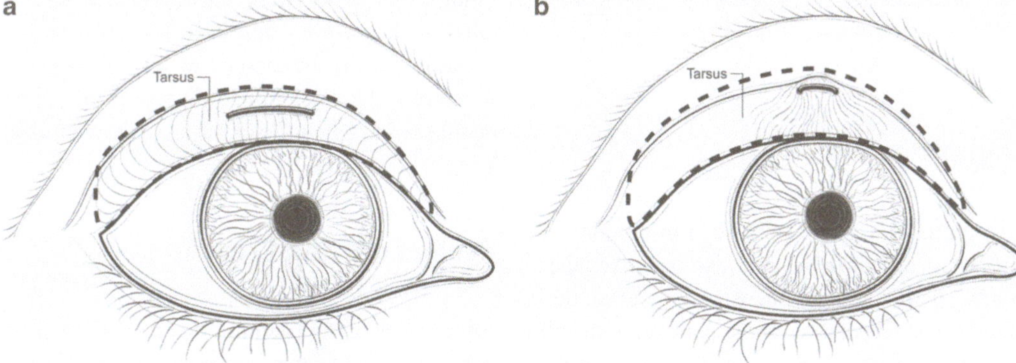

Fig. 30.10 (**a**) Flattening of the lid due to a long tarsal suture bite. (**b**) Peaking of the lid due to a short tarsal suture bite

plates from prior surgery, such as a Fasanella–Servat or Hughes procedure. In these cases, a temporal tightening, lateral canthopexy can help to achieve favorable eyelid margin contour. Nasal or temporal peaking can usually be corrected by shifting the tarsal bite in the opposite direction and possibly higher on the tarsal plate.

If the contour irregularity has not resolved after some time, then conservative management such as massage or stretching can be attempted. Definitive treatment, however, usually requires reoperation to release and place the sutures at the appropriate location. If the levator is well anchored on the tarsus, then the levator must be dissected, freed, and resutured.

For mild contour defects, anterior or posterior tarsectomy on the portion of the eyelid that appears flat can be a useful technique. This technique should be reserved for patients who have not undergone prior tarsal resection; otherwise, the patient may end up with deficient tarsus and is at risk for developing eyelid instability with any additional tarsal resection. For patients with a more severe contour deformity, opening of the wound and suture replacement is necessary. A central suture fixated from levator to the tarsus can be placed if the contour is too flat, and two sutures can be placed nasally and temporally if central peaking has occurred.

Patients undergoing the posterior lamellar approach can also develop abnormal eyelid contour. This complication usually occurs due to resection of tissue that is not centered over the pupil. This complication is best avoided by marking vertically, where the pupil is located with the upper eyelid everted prior to placing the resection clamp. This may also result from improper hemostat placement if one is using two curved hemostats instead of the modified Putterman clamp to perform a Fasanella–Servat procedure.

In frontalis suspension, contour deformity occurs if tarsal anchor points are poorly positioned on the eyelid. Due to the variety of suspension patterns and material used, there is no uniform method to correct contour abnormality. Nonetheless, the most efficacious way to correct contour abnormalities in patients who have undergone frontalis suspension is to open the wound, release and replace the sutures at different fixation points from the original placement, and move them either temporally or nasally. Broadening the fixation point with additional sutures, depending on the contour abnormality, may also be attempted.

Lagophthalmos

Lagophthalmos is typically seen in conjunction with overcorrection but can also occur independently, particularly if there is any orbicularis oculi muscle weakness. Most patients with mild overcorrection have complete or nearly complete eyelid closure. Lagophthalmos mostly occurs with large levator resections and frontalis suspension operations. It can also occur when the levator is inadvertently sutured to a structure that is not moving in synchrony with the eyelid, such as the orbital septum or the tendon of the superior oblique or superior rectus muscle. If this is suspected, releasing the suture to exclude the septum or tendon can resolve the lagophthalmos.

Lagophthalmos, particularly when mild, can be tolerated quite well in the presence of a good Bell's phenomenon, satisfactory tear production, and a healthy cornea. However, in patients with poor protective mechanisms (poor Bell's phenomenon or third nerve palsy) or preexisting corneal issues (due to chronic blepharitis, anterior basement membrane dystrophy, or neurotrophic keratitis, for example), lagophthalmos can be very detrimental to the ocular surface and can cause significant exposure keratopathy or corneal ulceration and perforation. If encountered early, observation is appropriate, with the use of ocular lubricants and taping of the eyelids closed during sleep, if necessary.

In cases of more severe lagophthalmos, an anterior or posterior approach levator recession is performed. If the amount of levator recession to correct the lagophthalmos passes the upper tarsal border, a hang-back suture can be utilized.

Eyelid Fold and Crease

Asymmetry of the eyelid fold and crease is probably the second most common complication of ptosis surgery, following over- or undercorrection. Creation of the eyelid crease is a crucial part of ptosis surgery. In the case of unilateral surgery, efforts should be directed at matching the opposite crease. In the case of levator advancement or resection, this can be accomplished by placing sutures to attach the levator edge to the skin or orbicularis muscle at the level of the proposed eyelid crease (Figs. 30.6 and 30.11a, b). The upper eyelid skin fold, which includes the skin and the orbicularis, drapes over the crease.

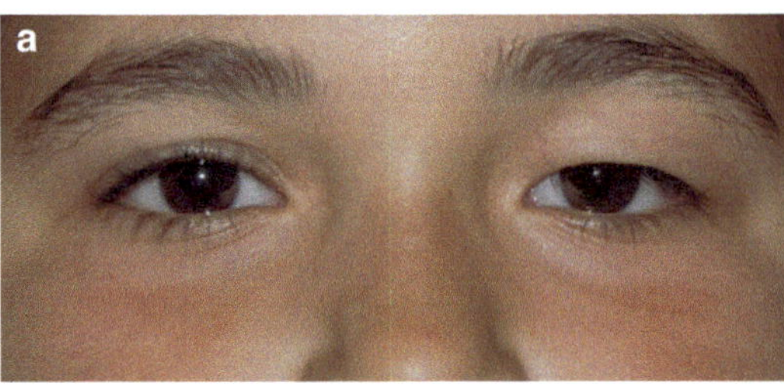

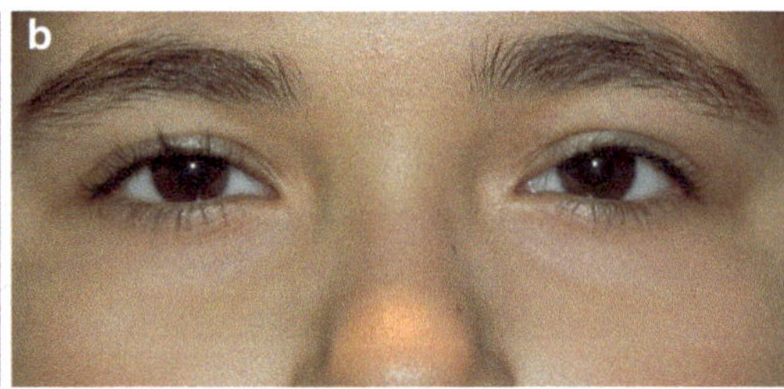

Fig. 30.11 (**a**) A 8-year-old female after levator resection for left upper lid congenital ptosis. Note subsequent entropion and poor crease formation. (**b**) Same patient after undergoing lid crease fixation and entropion repair witha nteriorl amellarr epositioning

Most congenitally ptotic eyelids have some degree of skin excess as the chronically droopy eyelid stretches the skin. We typically include a small amount (1–2 mm) of skin excision as part of our standard levator repair in children.

Symmetry between the two eyelid creases is very important cosmetically, and it is important to make the new lid crease and fold in harmony with the ethnic background of the individual. For example, in Asian patients, levator surgery will likely result in the formation of a crease, which may or may not be the patient's wish. This should be disclosed to the patient, but if the eyelid crease incision is kept low (5–6 mm above the lash line), the results can be very natural. One can try to avoid the creation of an inadvertently higher eyelid crease by limiting or foregoing resection of preaponeurotic fat. If the patient wishes to avoid the crease altogether, a posterior conjunctival approach is the more logical choice to correct mild ptosis. For unilateral levator surgery in an Asian patient, elevating or creating a low-lying crease on the opposite side is an excellent option for likely asymmetry that is due to the creation of a surgical crease on the operated side [11, 12].

In general, it is much easier to raise an eyelid crease than to lower one. If the surgical eyelid crease has been formed too low, then the desired place for the crease should be marked and incised. From this point, the skin and the orbicularis are undermined inferiorly down to the location of the old crease. The skin and orbicularis are then pulled up to the point of incision and sutured through the levator aponeurosis. A small amount of redundant skin can be excised before skin closure. The downside is that the lower incision scar may be visible below the new, higher eyelid crease.

If the crease has been formed too high, depending on the degree of asymmetry, several techniques can be applied. For more mild cases, soft tissue fillers or free fat injected above the crease deep to the eyelid fold provides an excellent way to enhance volume to allow the skin fold to rest lower, obscuring the elevated crease. For more severe cases with adequate skin, the new crease is marked below the elevated crease, and the intervening skin segment is excised. The orbital septum is then opened, and preaponeurotic fat is advanced and sutured to the superior tarsal border. This fat creates a barrier to prevent the levator from readhering to the upper skin edge. Skin closure is then performed.

ConjunctivalPr olapse

The superior fornix is held by the suspensory ligament, which may be inadvertently severed during larger levator resections [13]. This can lead to prolapse of the conjunctiva. Excess edema and/or a hematoma can also cause conjunctival prolapse. The superior fornix should be checked at the end of ptosis repair to look for prolapse. If present, horizontal mattress sutures can be placed through the fornix to attach the conjunctiva to the undersurface of the levator muscle intraoperatively (Fig. 30.12). If the conjunctival prolapse occurs postoperatively, conservative management with observation or repositioning of the conjunctiva with muscle hooks can be attempted under topical anesthesia in the office. If resolution does not occur with conservative measures, surgical repair is likely necessary. One option is to excise the prolapsed tissue with direct closure. The other is to place full-thickness horizontal mattress sutures from conjunctiva and exiting on the skin surface to recreate the fornix.

Hemorrhage/Hematoma

Hematomas can cause several complications including suture release and conjunctival prolapse. The most feared complication of retrobulbar hemorrhage is rare but has been described in the literature [14]. Use of anticoagulants and uncontrolled hypertension increases the risk of vision-threatening hemorrhage, and discussion should be held with the patient and his/her internist regarding the pros and cons of stopping blood thinners before surgery.

Preseptal hemorrhages are more common and can typically be observed. Bleeding and an ensuing hematoma can occur if there is trauma to the

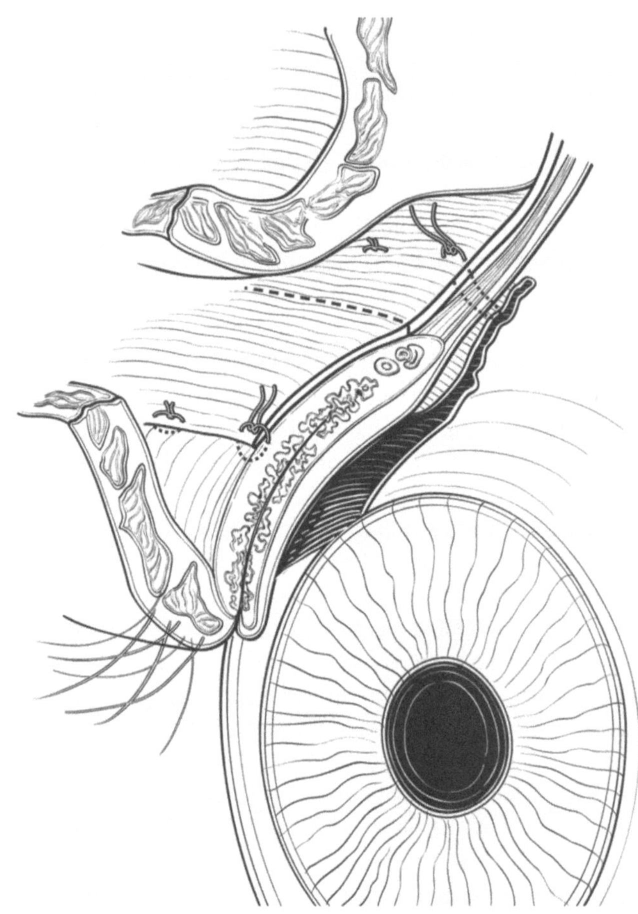

Fig.30.12 Diagram of conjunctivalprola pser epair

eyelid postoperatively. Children are especially at risk for postoperative bleeding since they are more prone to falling or running into objects or rubbing the operative eye. Patients should be advised to avoid sleeping face down for at least 1 week after surgery, as it can increase pressure and possibly cause direct trauma to the surgical site.

Infection

Risk of infection after eyelid surgery is low given the rich blood supply of the face. Although the risk is small, an infection can have devastating consequences if it migrates postseptally into the orbit. At the very least, it causes discomfort, swelling, and delayed healing. The septum may have been intentionally or inadvertently violated surgically and provide a path for spread of infection. Certain patients, such as diabetics, smokers, and those on chronic immunosuppressive medications, are at greater risk of infection and require closer monitoring and patient education regarding wound care. Community-acquired methicillin-resistant *Staphylococcus aureus* (MRSA) has become increasingly prevalent in recent years, likely exacerbated by the excessive use of antibiotics. Any site of possible infection postoperatively should be monitored very closely for the onset of cellulitis or an abscess. The wound may need to be incised and drained, with cultures sent for identification and sensitivities. The patient should be started on broad-spectrum oral antibiotics. Several oral agents have been reported to be effective against MRSA. These include trimethoprim/sulfamethoxazole, clindamycin, rifampin, and doxycycline [15]. If the clinical signs do not improve, or if there are signs of orbital involvement, the patient should be hospitalized and started on intravenous vancomycin. Currently, there are no recommendations regarding preoperative antibiotics for patients with history or colonization of MRSA, nor is there a recommendation for usage of routine prophylactic systemic antibiotics in the garden-variety, sterile ptosis procedure.

CornealA brasion/Ulceration/ Perforation

When performing levator advancement or resection, partial-thickness tarsal sutures should be used at all times to prevent suture perforation through to the conjunctival surface. Inadvertent full-thickness sutures that are exposed through the conjunctiva can cause corneal abrasion or ulceration. It is a prudent practice to evert the upper eyelid after placement of the tarsal sutures to be certain that no sutures are exposed on the inside of the upper eyelid. Avoidance of exposed sutures can be more challenging in those patients with very thin tarsal plates. In addition, we advocate the use of intraoperative corneal protectors to prevent accidental corneal puncture during tarsal suture placement.

Conclusion

Although ptosis repair may seem straightforward, all surgeons are likely to encounter complications due to the structural complexity, nuances, and intricacies of ptosis surgery. In addition to being well versed in each technique of ptosis repair, a thorough understanding of potential complications, focusing on prevention and management, is essential for every ptosis surgeon.

References

1. Cetinkaya A, Brannan PA. Ptosis repair options and algorithm. Curr Opin Ophthalmol. 2008;9(5):428–34.
2. Spahiu K, Spahiu L, Dida E. Choice of surgical procedure for ptosis correction. Med Arh. 2008;62(5–6):283–4.
3. Ahmad SM, Della Rocca RC. Blepharoptosis: evaluation, techniques, and complications. Facial Plast Surg.2007; 23(3):203–15.
4. Whitehouse GM, Grigg JR, Martin FJ. Congenital ptosis: results of surgical management. Aust N Z J Ophthalmol.1995; 23(4):309–14.
5. Cates CA, Tyers AG. Outcomes of anterior levator resection in congenital blepharoptosis. Eye. 2001;15 (Pt 6):770–3.
6. Dortzbach RK, Kronish JW. Early revision in the office for adults after unsatisfactory blepharoptosis correction. Am J Ophthalmol. 1993;115(1):68–75.
7. Lee MJ, Oh JY, Choung HK, Kim NJ, Sung MS, Khwarg SI. Frontalis sling operation using silicone rod compared with preserved fascia lata for congenital ptosis a three-year follow-up study. Ophthalmology. 2009;116(1):123–9.
8. Ben Simon GJ, Macedo AA, Schwarcz RM, Wang DY, McCann JD, Goldberg RA. Frontalis suspension for upper eyelid ptosis: evaluation of different surgical designs and suture material. Am J Ophthalmol. 2005;140(5):877–85.
9. Pang NK, Newsom RW, Oestreicher JH, Chung HT, Harvey JT. Fasanella–Servat procedure: indications, efficacy, and complications. Can J Ophthalmol. 2008;43(1):84–8.
10. Kakizaki H, Zako M, Ide A, Mito H, Nakano T, Iwaki M. Causes of undercorrection of medial palpebral fissures in blepharoptosis surgery. Ophthal Plast Reconstr Surg. 2004;20(3):198–201.
11. Park DH, Kim CW, Shim JS. Strategies for simultaneous double eyelid blepharoplasty in Asian patients with congenital blepharoptosis. Aesthetic Plast Surg. 2008;32(1):66–71.
12. Kikkawa DO, Kim JW. Asian blepharoplasty. Int Ophthalmol Clin. 1997;37(3):193–204.
13. Wolfley DE. Preventing conjunctival prolapse and tarsal eversion following large excisions of levator muscle and aponeurosis for correction of congenital ptosis. Ophthalmic Surg. 1987;18(7):491–4.
14. Hass AN, Penne RB, Stefanyszyn MA, Flanagan JC. Incidence of post blepharoplasty orbital hemorrhage and associated visual loss. Ophthal Plast Reconstr Surg.2004; 20(6):426–32.
15. Gorwitz RJ, Jernigan DB, Powers JH, Jernigan JA, and Participants in the Centers for Disease Control and Prevention-Convened Experts. Strategies and clinical management of MRSA in the community. Summary of an Experts' Meeting Convened by the Centers for Disease Control and Prevention. March 2006.

Chapter31
Commentary: Perspective of a Risk Manager: 12St epso faSuc cessfulSur gicalEnc ounter

John Shore

Abstract Patient satisfaction is dependent on more than just a favorable anatomic result. Good communication with the patient during the entire process is essential, making certain that you have the opportunity to hear and address the patient's concerns and to be sure that the patient and you are "on the same page." This chapter provides invaluable advice regarding how to optimize the surgeon-patient relationship and increase the chances of a happy patient postoperatively.

Surgeons recognize results of ptosis surgery as being unpredictable and therefore a source of patient dissatisfaction. Many ophthalmologists, as well as other surgeons with the knowledge and technical skill to perform ptosis surgery, avoid it because they do not like to deal with unpredictable results and unhappy patients. Yet those who perform ptosis repair on a routine basis proclaim that ptosis correction yields great patient satisfaction. How is it that some patients who have a marginal result are happy and others who may have achieved a very reasonable result are so unhappy? The answer is that successful ptosis surgeons manage patient expectations and guide their patients through the surgical experience with compassion and understanding. They anticipate and manage problems as the problems arise and help patients control their frustration and remain patient as they treat such things as asymmetry, abnormal contour, under- and overcorrections, lagophthalmos, discomfort, and dry eye, to name a few. They explain to patients the unpredictable nature of ptosis surgery. They intervene at appropriate intervals and choose appropriate adjustments to enhance results when needed. They very carefully inform their patients that results cannot be promised and that even in the best hands, the desired outcome cannot be achieved every time.

Ptosis surgery humbles the surgeon. I have been performing ptosis surgery for 31 years and may have done as many as 10,000 ptosis operations during that time. I do not believe that I am any better at achieving anatomic success today than I was 5 years after completing fellowship training. I think I have happier ptosis patients now than earlier in my career – not because I am better at technical execution or because I quit tackling difficult cases. I believe it is because I am better at matching patients to procedures and managing patient expectations than in the past. Experience has given me a better feel for the problems encountered during and after ptosis surgery. Over time, one learns how to anticipate and identify problems more quickly and develop better judgment concerning the appropriate time to adjust the eyelid position and contour or intervene in other ways to enhance results. Also, I am better at communicating to patients what to expect when things are not working out, as I now have a better feel for what the final result will be than I did years ago. Patients want to know their surgeon has seen and can manage complications and unsatisfactory results that occur with ptosis correction. Reasonable patients hope for, but do not expect, perfect results. They

J.Shore (✉)
TexasO culoplasticC onsultants, Austin, TX, USA
e-mail:j shore@tocaustin.com;j shore@austin.rr.com

A.J. Cohen and D.A. Weinberg (eds.), *Evaluation and Management of Blepharoptosis*,
DOI 10.1007/978-0-387-92855-5_31, © Springer Science+Business Media, LLC 2011

give their surgeon vast leeway in managing suboptimal results as long as they are confident that their surgeon will bring his or her skill, knowledge, and experience to bear to overcome obstacles and achieve the best result possible for them. They want their surgeon to stand with them during this time, explain what is going on, and keep them abreast of plans to solve the problem.

I have asked myself many times why it took me so long to realize that technical execution and anatomic alignment are not the most important criteria on which to judge results. Patient satisfaction is elusive and unpredictable. I have pondered how I could have acquired insight earlier in my career into the nuances of the patient–physician relationship that lead to a happy postoperative ptosis patient. I now realize that setting and managing patient expectations is as important, or perhaps more important, than technical execution in obtaining "happy patient status." I have gained an appreciation for how important listening is to managing patient expectations. When communication fails, patients do not feel "connected" to their surgeon. They are less forgiving and more apt to express displeasure with suboptimal results than patients who "like" their surgeon. These patients are far less likely to lose confidence and criticize their surgeon when problems occur. An average or even a mediocre surgeon may have a thriving and growing practice if he is good at communication and building patient rapport. Likewise, the technically skilled, uncommunicative surgeon may be frustrated because patients go elsewhere for care. Having studied medical-legal cases for many years, I am familiar with how important communication skills, compassion, and conveyance of a concerned and caring attitude are to avoiding malpractice suits, complaints to medical boards, and word-of-mouth discontent in the community where one practices.

How do surgeons acquire communication and patient management skills so important to building a successful practice? During residency and fellowship, the surgeon acquires the technical expertise to perform surgery. Surgeons must meet specific technical performance standards before they can graduate. They are tested on their knowledge and judgment throughout training and during board certification examinations that follow. There are no standards to meet regarding the acquisition of communication and listening skills, however, and certification boards do not test this skill. Performance varies widely, as one might expect. For a few physicians, the ability to communicate and convey compassion is innate. Others acquire these skills over many years. Some never get there. They may be outstanding technicians, but they never acquire the ability to communicate with patients in a meaningful way. In short, they struggle to build patient rapport, and they do not manage unhappy patients very well. Managing the unhappy patient is perhaps the single most important part of building a successful ptosis, or, for that matter, a successful ophthalmic plastic surgical practice. It is a skill that can be acquired if one has the insight to recognize how important it is. For most, it is an acquired skill and one that can be learned. This chapter is written with the hope that it will help surgeons acquire these skills early in their career.

Twelve Steps to a Successful Surgical Encounter

Consider for a moment a surgical encounter beginning with a patient arriving at the office with ptosis. The surgical experience takes place over the course of 2–4 months with three or four office visits, one or more surgical procedures and ends with (hopefully) a happy patient, one who is satisfied with his or her final result. There are twelve steps involved in a successful surgical encounter. Each step is important because it provides the physician an opportunity to communicate and connect with the patient. If a surgeon sets up his or her practice in such a way that staff is going to be the primary interface with the patient in the office, these steps are even more important as opportunity for direct and personal communication between patient and surgeon is limited.

1. Establish a diagnosis: The diagnosis of ptosis is not a difficult one to make and takes little time. The office evaluation is short, and the

decision tree is easily mastered. Rarely is diagnostic testing necessary. Documenting the visual field and taking photos for insurance purposes are quickly performed. Since the evaluation is straightforward in many cases, it is easy for a physician to divert his attention to other patients and leave the evaluation of the ptosis patient to trained staff. If the patient's expectations are met, this can work. However, if the surgeon does not invest quality time in direct face-to-face discussion with the patient, he misses an important opportunity to connect with the patient. This in turn sets the stage for patient dissatisfaction if the outcome is suboptimal. In addition, there are nuances in evaluating the ptosis patient that may be overlooked by staff. Only the surgeon has the knowledge and experience to observe, sort out, and work these nuances into a good surgical plan. The patient's initial office visit is the first opportunity one has to communicate with the patient. Taking the patient's history personally provides sufficient time to interact with the patient and family. The surgeon who takes the time to interview and thoroughly examine the patient gains valuable insight into the patient's personality, emotional state, visual difficulties, and suitability for surgery. Admittedly, it takes a substantial investment of physician time to do this. Some feel taking the history personally is not efficient use of a physician's time as much of the information can be gathered by a technician or nurse. Conversely, the time invested up front leads to a favorable patient–physician relationship and serves the surgeon well whether the outcome is good or bad. If the office policy is to delegate the intake history and initial examination to technicians, the surgeon still must find time for a direct discussion with the patient regarding the chief complaint, physical findings, and plans for surgery. It is possible, and a huge mistake in my opinion, to delegate too much to staff in this area. The opportunity to gain the patient's confidence may be lost if the surgeon does not take the time to sit and talk to the patient and the family for a sufficient length of time at the initial visit. In addition, the personal time invested will result in higher surgical conversion rates. Too many times one hears statements such as these from patients dissatisfied with the care they get in another office: "I never got a chance to get my questions answered," "He never explained the operation to me," "He was in and out of the office in under 3 min", "Why didn't he tell me that?" "I was never told that could happen;" "I tried to tell him but he did not listen;" "He never explained what went wrong". It is human nature to fill a void with suppositions when answers and explanations are not forthcoming. Thus, the physician who leads the discussion, listens, anticipates the patient's concerns, and answers all questions will fare well in practice. The stage is set at the initial office visit. It should be noted the quotes above are presented purposefully in the masculine gender because it is well known that, in general, female physicians listen and communicate more effectively than their male colleagues.

2. Analyze the anatomic, medical, psychological, and social factors that affect the surgical decisions and outcome: All operations are (or should be) anatomically based. Every surgeon recognizes truth in that statement. When planning surgery, physicians have choices to make. Often, the patient's anatomy and physiology, i.e., levator function, drives the surgeon to select one procedure over another. For instance, in recurrent ptosis in an Asian configuration eyelid, one might decide to perform posterior surgery to avoid altering the eyelid crease rather than a repeat anterior approach where the eyelid crease may be more difficult to control. After considering anatomic variables, the surgeon must consider comorbidities that may affect the outcome of surgery. For instance, if a patient has a mechanical heart valve and must remain anticoagulated during and after surgery, one might choose an operation known to have a lower risk for bleeding complications over an alternative procedure that carries with it an increased risk for bleeding. Likewise, if a patient has severe rheumatoid arthritis, keratitis sicca, and compromised ocular host defense coupled with

severe ptosis and poor levator function, the surgeon may alter his preference for a fascia lata sling and opt for a silicone sling instead. The assessment of anatomic and medical variables is intuitive to surgeons but, if not considered, can lead to avoidable complications.

What is often overlooked in surgical planning is the need to assess psychological and social factors that affect outcomes. A good example is the management of a patient with severe unilateral congenital ptosis with absent or very poor levator function. The conventional teaching is to disable the levator on the unaffected side (first operation) followed by a bilateral frontalis sling as a staged procedure (second operation). This operation is rarely performed today. Parents simply will not accept it. When managing moderate Marcus Gunn Jaw winking ptosis, surgeons may compromise and accept moderate jaw winking with better correction of ptosis than absence of jaw winking with a sling and two operations to extirpate the levator and substitute the frontalis muscle to provide the lifting power for the eyelids. Both operations are anatomically based, but the decision is made by the patient or parents following very specific discussion between the surgeon and patient or among surgeon, patient and family members. For patients to be happy with surgical results, they must be educated about the anatomy that governs what can be done at surgery, and their surgeon must take into account psychological and social concerns that affect patients' (parents') decisions. In a very complicated or high-risk case, or when dealing with a difficult patient, the surgeon must take time to review the risk factors in each category (anatomic, medical, psychological, social) individually and collectively. The surgeon then can select an appropriate procedure to solve the patient's problem while taking these risks into account.

3. Match the patient to the procedure (patient selection/procedure selection): More often than not there is more than one solution (procedure) available to achieve a given result. When either solution will work, the decision of which to use may boil down to surgeon preference, patient preference, or medical problems that shift the risk such that one procedure becomes the operation of choice. For instance, when confronted with the need to correct 2 mm of ptosis in a patient who has ocular cicatricial pemphigoid, most surgeons will avoid the internal approach for ptosis repair to avoid surgical manipulation of the conjunctiva. When making surgical decisions, one needs to assess all factors that may affect outcome and strive to match the patient to the operation. This is a very critical step in surgical planning. Take coloboma repair in a newborn. Everyone recognizes the need to avoid amblyogenic eyelid sharing procedures in these cases. The objective is to find alternative means to achieve corneal coverage without occluding the visual axis. Sometimes, this is not possible. In such a case, the only option may be to accept the risk of amblyopia and do one's best to manage it. The parents must be informed so they will understand and accept the consequences of that decision. For patients with severe disease and complex anatomic, medical, psychological, or social problems (as presented in paragraph 3), surgeons may find it helpful to prepare a list of options and consider each when planning surgery. It may help them focus on how they are going to establish and achieve the result they hope to obtain (Table 31.1). Each of the surgical options will have advantages and disadvantages to consider, as choices are weighed.
4. Establish and communicate the goals of surgery (informed consent process): Once the surgeon has selected his preferred procedure, he must explain the operation to the patient in terms the patient can understand (planned procedure). At the same time, the surgeon must (1) explain why he is making that specific recommendation and what he expects to accomplish (goals of surgery), (2) other options (both surgical and nonsurgical) available to solve the patient's problem (alternatives), (3) give his best estimate concerning the anticipated results (expected results), (4) explain potential pitfalls and problems that may occur with the options he presents (possible complications), (5) and what is likely to happen if the patient elects not to have any treatment (informed refusal).

Table31. 1 Options for complex ptosis repair, Sally Sue 2-26-10

Surgicalne ed
Ptosis correction to achieve functional vision
Better ocular surface protection
Anatomicproble ms
Prior upper eyelid surgery to repair complex eyelid laceration
Lagophthalmos and incomplete closure due to shortage of skin
Weakened orbicularis function, posttraumatic. Good frontalis function
Prior corneal ulcer in eye for planned ptosis correction
Blind in nonsurgical eye, therefore dependent on the planned surgical eye for vision
Socialproble ms
Livesa lone
Transportationprob lems
Financialha rdship
Psychologicalproble ms
Unreliable for follow-up appointments
Lack of understanding due to prior brain injury
Surgicaloptions
Nos urgery
Levator shortening surgery combined with lower eyelid recession (graft) to maintain size of the palpebral aperture while elevating the upper eyelid
Levator shortening surgery combined with lateral tarsorrhaphy
Staged surgery including release of upper eyelid with skin graft followed by silicone frontalis suspension at a later date
Posterior upper eyelid lengthening with tarsoconjunctival graft from the opposite upper eyelid combines with laterally based skin muscle flap to add vertical length of the upper eyelid followed by staged elevation of the eyelid by frontalis silicone suspension

This information is often summarized in the informed consent document that the patient should be asked to sign after the discussion. Procedure specific consents are available from several sources including the Ophthalmic Mutual Insuance Company (OMIC0 and can be found at www.omic.com. The informed consent document needs to be signed prior to surgery. The mere signing does not guarantee that a court (jury) will hold that informed consent has taken place. In fact, in complicated cases, or when there is a language barrier, a court may decide that informed consent was not given despite the presence of a signed document. For this reason, I find it helpful to enter into the medical record-specific language confirming that I have completed the informed consent process and that in my opinion the patient comprehends and consents to the planned procedure (Table 31.2). It is important to include as part of that statement case-specific concerns, plans, and discussions that have taken place. Most importantly, this process should take place any day other than the day of surgery. This document along with the written informed consent document signed in the physician's office and signed by the patient provides strong evidence that the informed consent discussion took place and the patient agreed to the planned procedure on a day other than the day of surgery. The facility consent, often signed in the hospital or ambulatory surgical facility, is a separate consent that covers the facility and should not be used as a substitute for the informed consent document signed in the physician's office. There are rare exceptions where state law (Texas for example) governs the informed consent documentation.

There is a second advantage to this process. The statement can be used by the surgeon to review his concerns about the case, his surgical plan, and goals of surgery and confirm his preop discussion with the patient immediately before entering the operating room or when the patient is being marked in the holding area. As previously mentioned, the informed consent discussion and formal execution of the office informed consent document should take place prior to the day of surgery. Since many patients do not go to the hospital or surgical facility until the day of surgery, the facility informed consent document may not be signed until the day of surgery. Reliance upon a consent document signed on the day of surgery and in the facility where surgery is to take place and immediately prior to surgery as the sole means of documenting the informed consent discussion is suboptimal at best. The handwritten document or dictated note, as set forth in Table 31.2, establishes that the informed consent discussion took place well before the day of surgery and that the patient was not "coerced" or "enticed" to give his or her consent on the day of surgery.

5. Clarify patient expectations immediately prior to surgery (confirm the surgeon's and patient's expectations match): Once the discussion in paragraph 4 is complete, it is wise to have a brief discussion on the day of surgery whereby the most important goals of surgery are reviewed and reinforced and last minute questions answered. At this time, it is also important to once again go over what the patient (and family) will see and experience immediately following surgery. This is the ideal time to reiterate what the surgery is intended to accomplish, remind the patient what is *not* going to be accomplished, and confirm the agreed surgical plan. One should be positive and supportive. While it is OK to remind the patient of concerns you have and the problems you expect to encounter, now is the time to reassure the patient that you are prepared to meet the surgical challenges ahead. Patients should enter the OR confident, calm, and trusting the surgeon. Involved discussions of complications and alternatives at this stage may cause the patient or family to call into question the surgeon's planning

Table31 .2 Consentf ors urgery

(Patient unique information, e.g., dictated at the preop visit). Sally Sue is a 35-year-old woman who presents for complex ptosis repair following delayed repair of trauma. She has had two previous attempts at ptosis repair and is left with residual ptosis encroaching up on the visual axis (MRD 1 = +1 mm). The levator function is graded as poor (6–7 mm). She has compromised eye protection manifest by diminished corneal sensation and decreased tear production. In addition she 3 mm of lagophthalmos on gentle eyelid closure due to posttraumatic and postsurgical scars in the anterior and midlamella of the affected upper eyelid. There is shortage of skin as well. She is blind in the opposite eye and needs improvement in the eyelid position in order for her function in her daily life. She is very aware of the risks of ptosis correction in this case
This is the first stage of a planned staged reconstruction. The goals for this surgery are to release the scar in the upper eyelid through an upper eyelid crease incision. A posterior lamellar vertical eyelid procedure will be accomplished utilizing a graft of tarsus and conjunctiva from the contralateral upper eyelid. A musculocutaneous, laterally based flap from the temporal region will be used for mid- and anterior lamellar augmentation. A lateral suture tarsorrhaphy will be placed to stabilize the wound during the initial stages of wound healing; however, the visual axis will not be occluded. Second stage eyelid elevation is planned using a frontalis silicone sling if possible. The patient is aware this may not be possible due to corneal exposure problems and that she will be left with an eyelid that rests lower than at present
(Information common to each consent, e.g., in a macro). The patient has been informed of the diagnosis, proposed treatment, feasible alternatives, the likelihood of success, and the prognosis with and without surgery. I have discussed the planned surgical procedure with the patient in terms that can be understood. The patient is aware of the goals of surgery, alternatives including operative and nonoperative options, the expected results and possible complications. I have explained specific risks including, but not limited to, postoperative infection, hemorrhage, loss of vision (blindness), and failure to achieve the intended goals of surgery. The possibility of further surgery being required has been discussed with the patient in detail. The patient is aware that results cannot be promised and the revision or adjustments and even further surgery may be necessary. The patient expresses understanding of these risks and with no further questions has decided to proceed with the proposed surgery. The patient has given me written and verbal permission to proceed. I have obtained informed consent. I have also answered all questions to the best of my ability and to the satisfaction of the patient

and preparedness. The surgeon will instill confidence if, by his demeanor and verbal communication, he lets the patient and family know that he is prepared to follow the surgical plan as outlined and manage any problems that may present in the OR. If there are particular concerns that have been previously discussed yet need to be reinforced, they can be revisited briefly at this time. One should not undermine the patient's confidence with negative comments, however. A typical discussion might go something like this, "You may recall that we discussed the fact your ptosis is due to prior trauma and that the existing scar tissue will make surgery more difficult. My biggest concern is not whether I can find the muscle inside the eyelid but whether or not I can use it effectively to lift the eyelid. If so, we are all set. If it is involved in the scar and cannot be used, remember we have a backup plan. That plan includes the use of a small silicone sling device that will allow you to use your forehead muscle to lift the eyelid." By reading the previously prepared consent document (Table 31.2) just before greeting the patient in the preop area, the surgeon is reminded of points that require emphasis. One should strive to keep such discussions brief and use them only in difficult cases. In the routine situation, cautionary comments are not necessary. Instead, one should remain positive and emphasize what needs to be done after surgery depending on the case (e.g. ice, inactivity, use of ointment, elevation of the head, no nose blowing, etc.). The goal of this discussion is to keep the patient and family focused on the essential elements of surgery and recovery that are important to the success of the operation.

6. Surgical planning: Planning the actual procedure is something that does not involve communication with the patient or family. Surgical planning is the identification and selection of the specific elements of surgery that will be used to obtain the desired results. Surgical planning in complex cases begins long before the surgeon arrives in the OR and may include such things as selection of implants, methods for obtaining clear margins in tumor cases, determining surgical incisions (length, configuration, how they are made, e.g., laser, scalpel, etc.), instruments and supplies necessary for the conduct of the operation, whether an assistant or another specialist is needed, type of anesthesia, etc. The most important element of surgical planning is identification of the specific surgical steps and their sequence in the conduct of the operation. If alternative steps may be necessary (intraoperative change in surgical steps), these are planned as well. For instance, plans on how one is going to handle enucleation for melanoma if extrascleral extension is unexpectedly found should be made before the surgeon enters the OR. Surgical planning begins before the day of surgery and is continuously updated during the case. The surgical plan is modified and refined as the case progresses just as a pilot modifies his approach to landing as the weather or wind changes during the course of a flight. The basic plan must be in place before surgery begins. Small problems that could have been anticipated have a way of becoming large problems during surgery particularly when the surgeon has not planned alternative solutions. In the cockpit, a pilot uses a checklist to complete his flight safely. Likewise, surgeons should have a road map to follow in complex cases. It may help to put the surgical plan (checklist) in writing and post it next to the patient's picture to insure all elementsa rea ccomplished(T able 31.3).
7. Technical execution: When asked, many surgeons will state that technical execution is the most important determinant of a successful surgical outcome. I disagree. Average surgeons will achieve acceptable results in all but the most difficult cases if they follow the twelve steps discussed in this chapter. The most technically astute surgeon may well falter if he relies too heavily on his technical ability and ignores one or more of the other eleven elements. It is true that technical expertise is an important determinant of surgical outcome (making the correct incision, staying in the correct plane of dissection,

Table31 .3 Surgical plan for Mary Jane 2-26-10

Endo forehead lift
3.0 mm endotines
Move tines medial to pick up central brow
Lift right brow 3–4 mm more than left
Internal ptosis repair by CCMR, bilateral
10 mm right
9 mm left
External upper blepharoplasty, bilateral
Following CCMR ptosis repair
Limited subbrow fat resection
Minimal central fat removal
Eliminate double crease left upper eyelid
Lower blepharoplasty, bilateral
Percutaneous with horizontal lower tightening
Rotate lower puncta right only, with 2-snip punctoplasty
TCA peel lower eyelids and cheeks
Juvederm to nasolabial folds, bilateral

designing flaps, establishing the correct amount of wound tension, suture, and implant placement). However, nature is kind to surgeons. Time is the surgeon's friend. The ability of the body to heal over time corrects for average or even suboptimal technical execution of a surgical procedure by the surgeon. It will not make up for poor communication or lack of patient rapport.

8. Observe initial results, anticipate patient concerns, and inform the patient what to expect at every stage of normal healing: Patients want to know how their surgeon feels about their operation. They look for nonverbal clues and listen for the confidence (or lack of it) in the surgeon's voice as he reports on the results of the operation. They look for a confirmation of success by comparing what the surgeon has previously told them to expect with what they hear and see at the end of the case. They factor in feedback from family and friends which explains why it is important to keep the family informed at every step of the surgical encounter.

Patients are not sure what they will see when they look in the mirror the first time following surgery, especially if they have never had surgery before. The surgeon can ease anxiety (thereby lessening pain as anxiety exacerbates pain), reduce phone calls to the office, and alleviate needless worry for the patient and family by reinforcing to patients what to expect during the postoperative period. As the time of surgery approaches, patients and families forget, ignore, or lose focus about what they have been told to expect following surgery. They direct their attention to the actual procedure and especially anesthesia. As soon as they know that they or their family member is safe, they redirect their attention to pain control, wound healing, and avoidance of infection. They want to know what they can do to care for the wound, avoid disrupting the wound, and improve the chance for successful healing and a good scar. Comments that explain what to expect in the first hours and days following surgery make for a smooth and uneventful early postop course. Instructions should be given verbally and in writing. Instructions from the nursing staff should not contradict those given by the surgeon. Surgeons who rely solely on the nursing staff to give instructions are missing an opportunity to connect with patients. Invariably, the instructions will not be taken as seriously as when the surgeon stresses the importance of following the instructions given by the nursing staff and provided to them in writing at discharge. The written instructions and the oral instruction given by the nurse must be in sync and reinforce the physician's instructions. Thus, training staff on what to say and providing them with written instructions to use is a very important part of the team approach to postsurgical care. The surgeon will have happier and better informed patients if he takes just a few moments to stress to the patient and family the importance of following the postoperative instructions. If problems are anticipated due to medical, social, psychological situations, or the inability of the patient and/or family to comprehend and follow instructions, it is important to address them. All questions need to be answered before the patient is discharged, no matter how many times asked or how trivial. At each visit following surgery, the surgeon should reinforce expectations, comment on the progress (or lack of it) since the last visit, and give some indication of the expected final outcome. If this does not happen, patients and families will fill in the gaps with erroneous assumptions that only increase anxiety or/or lead to improper activity or faulty wound care. One should be mindful that it is impossible to convince a patient that there is no problem when it is obvious that there is a problem (eyelid is closed when it should be open, eyelid will not close, contour is way off, etc.). The better strategy is to acknowledge that you see what it is that concerns the patient, that you also are concerned, and that you will be monitoring the problem closely to determine what action is needed, if any. If no intervention is necessary, at least the patent and family will sense you are concerned and are more likely to follow your instructions and accept your reassurance things are going well. If you are unsure of what is going on, and cannot identify a cause for what the patient is seeing and experiencing, it is best to admit it. Then, follow with possible explanations (excessive swelling, allergic reaction, splinting due to pain, altered wound healing, smoldering or early infection, etc.). Up to a point, patients will accept reasonable explanations and will look for guidance from the surgeon regarding unusual or unexpected early results. Once a true problem is identified, it is best to confront it and address it as soon as it is discovered. If a patient feels the surgeon is withholding information, bluffing, not being truthful, or making excuses that do not add up, they will look elsewhere for answers, try self-remedies, and discuss it with family members, friends, nurses, or other doctors. Obviously, this is not helpful and can lead to patient complaints and eventually legal action. During the postoperative period, the surgeon should listen to his patient, be attentive to the concerns expressed by his patient, and not fail to address those concerns. The physician should not allow a patient to leave the office after any visit with unanswered questions.

9. Identify outcome (good or bad) and disappointing results early on: Let the patient know how they are doing. If a patient is doing well, they will usually recognize it. Offer congratulations and give them credit for their cooperation and contribution towards a successful result. What about the patient who is not doing well? During surgery or immediately following oculoplastic surgery, the surgeon has a pretty good idea of what the outcome will be. In ptosis correction this is not always the case. However, within a week, the surgeon has a very good idea of how things will turn out. The earlier the surgeon identifies a problem and deals with it, the better. Addressing a problem does not necessarily mean bringing questionable results to the attention of the patient and family right away, but it does mean that cautious optimism or pessimism is in order when talking to the patient and family. If the surgeon identifies a problem at surgery that may affect results, it is a good idea to bring the problem or finding to the attention of the spouse or family as early as the postrecovery meeting. By informing the spouse or family, the surgeon gains their support and understanding that will ease the patient's anxiety when the complication is disclosed to the patient at a later time. The surgeon will have to decide on the time and place for this discussion to take place. For patients remaining in the hospital overnight, opportunities exist on the afternoon or evening following surgery (patient must be alert), the following morning, or later during the hospital stay. In the ambulatory setting, the surgeon may counsel the patient at the time of ASC discharge or bring the patient back the following day for an earlier-than-normal postoperative visit. The 1-week visit for suture removal is another time when minor problems can be revealed. If the discussion is going to be delayed, it is critical that the spouse or family be fully informed, as the patient will turn to them for answers in the absence of input from the surgeon. This must not occur. There may be legitimate reasons to delay telling the patient (unstable psychological state, obtundation, etc.); however, the surgeon should not give the patient the opportunity to fill the void created by his failure to inform and educate the patient with erroneous conclusions given by an uninformed

family member. If information is to be withheld from the patient for a short period of time, there must be a good reason, and it is essential the family be informed, brought into the discussion, and agree with the decision. They in turn will be more likely to reinforce the surgeon's decision. A good general rule is to identify and address all problems with the patient and family early, honestly, and with compassion. Working to keep the family informed and involved, and bringing problems to their attention, gives them confidence the surgeon has a grasp on the problem and is capable of finding a solution. Patients and families trust their surgeon. They do not expect perfection. They do understand that problems can happen. They do not know what to expect when problems arise. They want to know their surgeon has identified the problem, has a solution in mind, and is using his experience, knowledge, and good judgment to resolve the problem. They expect honesty and openness. When they see that, they will give the surgeon great leeway in getting the problem resolved. The ability of one surgeon to guide the family and patient through disappointing results separates the physician who is loved and respected by his patients from the surgeon who is looked down upon by his patients. As problems are identified, not only is it important to discuss how the problem might affect outcome but also what can be done to enhance the result or solve the problem. It is also wise to let the family know the time period until improvement is expected. Once the time frame has been set, it should not be changed without further explanation. In other words, the family must be in the loop at all times.

10. Actively manage complications: Every surgeon has complications. Some manage complications better than others. Some do not manage them well at all and are frustrated to learn patients have left their practice to seek care elsewhere. Having a patient leave the practice and go elsewhere for care is the worst possible outcome, particularly if the surgeon is unaware the patient is seeing someone else. It is far better to direct an unhappy patient to another provider and coordinate the referral than to have a patient lose confidence and leave on his own accord. Worse yet is the patient who leaves the practice without notice at the urging of his spouse or family. Patients can sense immediately when a surgeon is in over his head and will observe how the surgeon addresses his inability to manage the complication. If the surgeon is unsure what to do, he should not be shy. Instead he should admit it and get help. Patients appreciate frankness and the effort a surgeon makes to get them in the hands of someone who can solve the problem (another specialty, a more experienced surgeon, or one who is well known for managing a specific yet unusual complication).

The more typical situation is one in which the surgeon handles his own complication. In this case, the surgeon needs to manage the patient's care actively and not delegate it to others. Personal phone calls, personal attention during office visits, blocked private time reserved for the patient at the end of the day, and uninterrupted patient visits are important strategies. In this way, the surgeon can maintain personal contact with the patient and direct his full attention to the patient and the problem. The mistakes made far too often are these: remaining aloof, not returning phone calls promptly, ducking questions, and cutting visits short, leaving the family or spouse out of the conversation, and interruptions during counseling sessions. The surgeon must invest personal time as he addresses the patient's and family's concerns. He must do it privately without making the patient wait in public, or in a busy waiting room where embarrassing encounters may occur. At times, it may be necessary to offer touch-up or follow-up surgery at no or minimal cost. It may also be important to assign a senior or experienced staff to personally coordinate office appointments and schedule tests or surgery. Certainly, it is no time to pursue collection activity, allow office staff members to hassle the patient over small financial matters, late or missed appointments, or last-minute requests for appointment changes. Whether or not to have a technician or staff member in the room during the office visit is a decision that must be made on an individual basis. One should be careful about having private one-on-one discussions with a member of the opposite sex and never after hours. In most cases, when the complication is severe, or the family is confrontational, it is best if a family member and an experienced staff member are present in the room.

11. Assess outcome openly and honestly: Patients do not expect perfection. They like to hear that they are doing well. They also appreciate an honest assessment when their results are mediocre. They want to know when they have achieved their final result, good or bad. It is not good for an enthusiastic staff member to exuberantly proclaim how good a patient looks when it obviously he does not. Staff should only make positive comments when it is obvious the outcome is good.

One cannot put off the final outcome discussion forever. Patients do have unrealistic expectations regarding the time necessary for complete wound healing, however. Therefore, the surgeon must provide consistent, realistic, and honest assessments of the patient's postoperative progress. Photos are a powerful tool that the surgeon can use to review results and guide future intervention. Often patients will point out imperfections of concern to them. The discussion is over when the surgeon can show the "blemish" was present on the preoperative photograph and is unrelated to the surgery. If the "blemish" is due to surgery, an honest assessment of the blemish or imperfection and an explanation as to what is going on, coupled with an offer to correct the problem (if indicated) will usually satisfy the patient. Similarly, when an early postop ptosis patient inquires about her observation that the eyelid position is lower than anticipated; one can use serial photos to document and show improvement (or lack of it) as swelling resolves. If a patient is unhappy with the result, the surgeon must not blow the person off. Instead he must listen, commiserate, and provide solutions that will satisfy the patient (up to a point).

Some patients will not be satisfied no matter how hard the surgeon tries to make the patient happy. If an impasse is reached, it is clear that the patient is unhappy, and in all attempts to convince the patient that the result is reasonable and within normal limits, the surgeon must accept the situation, avoid further confrontation, and seek an alternative resolution. A good option is to consult a colleague or refer the patient to another physician for care. In doing so, it is important the patient feels the referral is someone who is independent and will give an honest opinion based on his or her assessment and not on a bias introduced by the referring surgeon. The referral may need to be to someone outside the practice but not always. The decision has to be individualized and with input from the patient and family. Another option is to offer referrals to several physicians and let the patient decide whom he wants to see. In any event, the handoff is important. The patient's wishes must be respected, but important information also needs to get into the hands of the physician to whom the patient is referred.

12. Revisit patient expectations: At some point before releasing the patient from care, it helps to revisit the goals of surgery in the context of the original problem and the final outcome. If the goals were achieved, remind the patient and family at the final office visit and send a follow-up letter and photos to the referring doctor and the patient. This cements the patient/physician relationship and drives referralstothe pra ctice.

The comments on managing surgical encounters as presented above are not specific to ptosis surgery or to surgeons who perform oculoplastic surgery. They apply to all surgery and surgeons. These steps will not always improve results, but they provide a process leading to patient satisfaction with the surgeon and the result much of the time. It also provides a mechanism for dealing with unhappy patients or unexpected results. If followed, these steps will reduce stress associated with any surgical encounter and lead to happy patients most of the time. Happy patients are less unlikely to seek legal remedy or file a medical board complaint when the outcome is less than anticipated.

Chapter32
Conclusion

Adam J. Cohen and David A. Weinberg

Abstract Ptosis is a very common eyelid disorder, and yet may be quite challenging both diagnostically and therapeutically. Due to a certain degree of inherent unpredictability regarding eyelid position, ptosis surgery requires surgical revision more often than many other periocular procedures. Often such touch-ups may be done in the office within one to two weeks after surgery. There has been some evolution in ptosis surgical techniques over the years, while major advances in ptosis management have taken place in the area of molecularge neticdia gnosis.

Ptosis, a widely prevalent eyelid disorder, presents a number of challenges to the clinician, both diagnostically and therapeutically. Ptosis correction, which epitomizes the art and science of surgery, can humble even the most experienced and capable surgeon. Not all factors are under the surgeon's control, such as the severity of postoperative eyelid edema. Despite careful preoperative planning and meticulous surgical technique, ptosis surgery is more often met with a suboptimal result than other commonly performed eyelid procedures, such as entropion and ectropion repair. An unfavorable outcome may necessitate a surgical revision. If a patient is forewarned of the possible need for reoperation, that may assuage any potential anger or frustration on the part of the patient should a suboptimal surgical result be encountered.

Ptosis surgery is a slowly evolving field, without the major "high tech" instrumentation breakthroughs seen in keratorefractive surgery or radical changes in therapeutic approach, as with the management of age-related macular degeneration. Nevertheless, there have been advances in biomaterials, such as sutures and frontalis sling materials, and in newer techniques and procedural modifications that have been described. Surgical procedures will continue to evolve, and perhaps a local anesthetic that provides complete sensory anesthesia but no motor paralysis will be developed, making levator resection surgery in adults easier and more comfortable for patients. Better bioadhesives may expedite wound closure. One area that has seen exponential growth in recent years is molecular genetics, which has greatly facilitated diagnosis. This has bearing on a wide range of heritable disorders, such as the myogenic ptoses, congenital ptosis in general, and familial ptosis. Laboratory studies with genetic analysis have now generally supplanted the need for tissue biopsy. Gene therapy carries the hope of potentially obviating the need for ptosis surgery in patients with certain genetic disorders some day in the future. That being said, since ptosis is the final common pathway for so many disparate pathologic conditions, ptosis surgery will likely remain a common procedure in our surgical repertoire for the foreseeable future.

D.A.W einberg (✉)
ConcordEye C are, Concord, NH
and
Department of Ophthalmology, Dartmouth Medical School, Hanover, NH, USA
e-mail:da weinberg@hotmail.com

A.J. Cohen and D.A. Weinberg (eds.), *Evaluation and Management of Blepharoptosis*,
DOI 10.1007/978-0-387-92855-5_32, © Springer Science+Business Media, LLC 2011

Index

A.J. Cohen and D.A. Weinberg (eds.), *Evaluation and Management of Blepharoptosis*,
DOI 10.1007/978-0-387-92855-5, © Springer Science+Business Media, LLC 2011

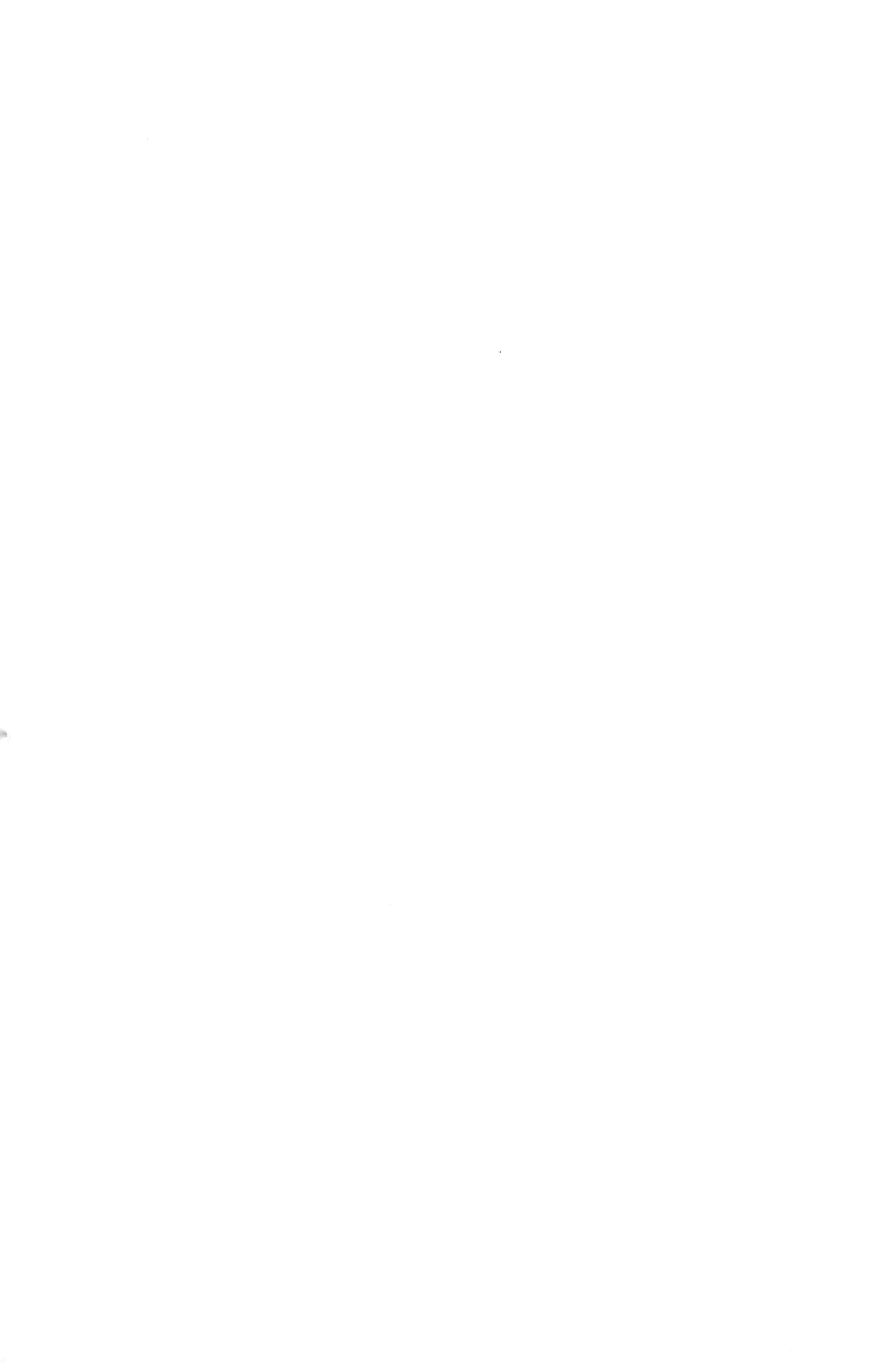

MIX
Papier aus verantwortungsvollen Quellen
Paper from responsible sources
FSC® C105338

If you have any concerns about our products, you can contact us on
ProductSafety@springernature.com

In case Publisher is established outside the EU, the EU authorized representative is:
Springer Nature Customer Service Center GmbH
Europaplatz 3, 69115 Heidelberg, Germany

Printed by Libri Plureos GmbH
in Hamburg, Germany